DATE DUE			
M.H.C. LIBRARY DEC 2 78			
M.H.C. LIBRARY MAR 10 79			
U.S. Library APR 25 '85			
DEC 3 '85 Library			
U.C. DEC 02 '89			
OCT 0 8 1998			
NOV 2 8 2007			
GAYLORD			PRINTED IN U.S.A.

THE DYING PATIENT

The Dying Patient

EDITED BY

Orville G. Brim, Jr.
Howard E. Freeman
Sol Levine

AND

Norman A. Scotch

WITH THE EDITORIAL CONSULTATION OF

Greer Williams

RUSSELL SAGE FOUNDATION
NEW YORK

PUBLICATIONS OF RUSSELL SAGE FOUNDATION

Russell Sage Foundation was established in 1907 by Mrs. Russell Sage for the improvement of social and living conditions in the United States. In carrying out its purpose the Foundation conducts research under the direction of members of the staff or in close collaboration with other institutions, and supports programs designed to improve the utilization of social science knowledge. As an integral part of its operations, the Foundation from time to time publishes books or pamphlets resulting from these activities. Publication under the imprint of the Foundation does not necessarily imply agreement by the Foundation, its Trustees, or its staff with the interpretations or conclusions of the authors.

©1970 RUSSELL SAGE FOUNDATION

Standard Book Number: 87154–155–6

"A Flat One" from *After Experience* by W. D. Snodgrass. © 1960 by W. D. Snodgrass. Reprinted by permission of Harper & Row, Publishers.

Library of Congress Catalog Card Number: 77–104181
Printed in the United States of America

CONTRIBUTORS

RICHARD M. BAILEY, Associate Professor of Health Economics, School of Public Health, University of California, Berkeley.

ORVILLE G. BRIM, JR., President, Russell Sage Foundation.

DIANA CRANE, Associate Professor, Department of Behavioral Sciences and Department of Social Relations, Johns Hopkins University.

HOWARD E. FREEMAN, Morse Professor of Urban Studies, Brandeis University, and Sociologist, Russell Sage Foundation.

BARNEY G. GLASER, Associate Research Sociologist, University of California, San Francisco.

ROBERT J. GLASER, Vice President for Medical Affairs, Dean of the School of Medicine and Professor of Medicine, Stanford University.

RICHARD A. KALISH, Associate Professor, School of Public Health, Division of Behavioral Sciences, University of California, Los Angeles.

ANDIE L. KNUTSON, Professor of Behavioral Sciences, School of Public Health, and Research Behavioral Scientist, Institute of Human Development, University of California, Berkeley.

LOUIS LASAGNA, Associate Professor of Medicine and of Pharmacology and Experimental Therapeutics, School of Medicine, Johns Hopkins University.

MONROE LERNER, Professor, Department of Medical Care and Hospitals and Department of Behavioral Sciences, School of Hygiene and Public Health, Johns Hopkins University.

SOL LEVINE, Professor and Chairman, Department of Behavioral Sciences, School of Hygiene and Public Health, and Director of Center for Urban Affairs, Johns Hopkins University.

BAYLESS MANNING, Dean and Professor of Law, School of Law, Stanford University.
ROBERT S. MORISON, Chairman, Division of Biological Sciences, Cornell University.
OSLER L. PETERSON, Professor of Preventive Medicine, Harvard Medical School.
DAVID L. RABIN, Associate Professor, Departments of Medical Care and Hospitals and Behavioral Science, School of Hygiene and Public Health, Johns Hopkins University.
LAUREL H. RABIN, Freelance Editor and Writer.
JOHN W. RILEY, JR., Vice President–Corporate Relations, The Equitable Life Assurance Society of the United States.
ELISABETH K. ROSS, Assistant Professor of Psychiatry, University of Chicago, La Labida Children's Hospital and Research Center.
NORMAN A. SCOTCH, Professor of Social Anthropology, Departments of Behavioral Science and Social Relations, School of Hygiene and Public Health, Johns Hopkins University.
ANSELM L. STRAUSS, Professor of Sociology and Chairman, Graduate Sociology Program, University of California, San Francisco Medical Center.
DAVID SUDNOW, Assistant Professor of Sociology, University of California, Irvine.
GREER WILLIAMS, Assistant Professor of Preventive Medicine (Communications), Tufts University School of Medicine.

CONTENTS

CONTRIBUTORS v

PREFACE
 Robert S. Morison ix

INTRODUCTION New Dimensions of Dying
 *Howard E. Freeman, Orville G. Brim, Jr.,
 and Greer Williams* xiii

PART ONE THE SOCIAL CONTEXT OF DYING

1. When, Why, and Where People Die
 Monroe Lerner 5
2. What People Think About Death
 John W. Riley, Jr. 30
3. Cultural Beliefs on Life and Death
 Andie L. Knutson 42

PART TWO HOW DOCTORS, NURSES, AND HOSPITALS COPE WITH DEATH

4. The Prognosis of Death
 Louis Lasagna 67
5. Physicians' Behavior Toward the Dying Patient
 Louis Lasagna 83
6. Innovations and Heroic Acts in Prolonging Life
 Robert J. Glaser 102
7. Patterns of Dying
 Anselm L. Strauss and Barney G. Glaser 129
8. The Dying Patient's Point of View
 Elisabeth K. Ross 156

9. Consequences of Death for Physicians, Nurses, and Hospitals
   David L. Rabin with Laurel H. Rabin   171
10. Dying in a Public Hospital
    David Sudnow   191

PART THREE   TERMINATION OF LIFE—SOCIAL, ETHICAL, LEGAL, AND ECONOMIC QUESTIONS

11. Dying as an Emerging Social Problem
    Sol Levine and Norman A. Scotch   211
12. Control of Medical Conduct
    Osler L. Peterson   225
13. Legal and Policy Issues in the Allocation of Death
    Bayless Manning   253
14. Economic and Social Costs of Death
    Richard M. Bailey   275

CONCLUSION   Dying and Its Dilemmas as a Field of Research
Diana Crane   303

Death and Dying, a Briefly Annotated Bibliography
Richard A. Kalish   327

INDEX   381

PREFACE

Nothing happens by itself any more, and there are no acts of God. Man is to blame for almost everything.

How far will man accept the new responsibilities thrust upon him by his own ingenuity? This book is about a particularly personal and compelling set of such responsibilities. It explores the medical, social, economic, and ethical issues raised by man's increasing control over death and dying. In doing so, it incidentally reveals how the pursuit of a "value-free" science and technology brings us to a whole new range of value-loaded questions. It also provides us with another equally interesting paradox: the same science that has knocked many of the supports from the ethical structures of the past now demands a more thorough ethical understanding than could ever have been conceived of when the world operated according to God's will.

One reaction to these new burdens is to be found in what Paul Goodman has defined as the New Reformation. It may indeed be prophetic in its "drastic comment on the dehumanization and fragmentation of modern times" but it has not yet convinced Mr. Goodman, much less the rest of us, that its vision of the "warmth of assembled animal bodies" provides a faith that will save us from our own contrivances. Not only do "today's young" repudiate the science and technology they blame for our predicament, they "do not even remember their own history." Disinclined to serious study of society, and hostile to the very idea of wise and effective action, they are caught, as Mr. Goodman sees it, "in the religious dilemma of Faith vs. Works."

To continue the metaphor, we may perhaps look upon this collection of essays as among the first steps in a counterreformation. Most of the physicians and social scientists who have contributed are, in Mr. Goodman's possibly pejorative terms, monks of the university if not mandarins of the establishment. Though clearly uneasy about supporting themselves by continued sale of the old indulgences, they are far from abandoning reason and works altogether. Instead they summon the courage to mold these timeworn but still reliable instruments into a new dispensation. They would be the first to point out that they have only suggested how a small part of the blueprint ought to look; but at least they have made a beginning.

The book deals principally with two somewhat different aspects of the dying patient. The first includes the large range of professional analyses and decisions, as well as the intensely personal feelings, involved in determining how and when an individual's death should occur. The second concerns the process of dying: what actually goes on now and what might be done to make the process somewhat less graceless and more acceptable not only to the dying patient but also to those who love and attend him.

The complexities and dilemmas inherent in both situations are thoroughly explored; it would be both premature and presumptuous to suggest anything more definitive at this time. What has been accomplished gives confidence that the continued examination of the uncomfortable truths of our position will enable us to handle our new responsibilities for death as well as can reasonably be expected.

In several places the authors hint at, but scarcely develop, the impact of changing attitudes to death on man's continuing search for a sensible philosophy of life. It is pointed out that until very recently death struck almost at random, not only on the just and the unjust but also at infants and young adults, as well as on those who managed to survive to old age. More often than not its coming seemed both senseless and tragic, and most men lived under a constant shadow of fear for themselves and their children. As a consequence, many men spent much of their time trying to understand, explain, and render acceptable the fact that many lives came to "an untimely end." The formal religions in all cultures provide the most obvious examples, but much of secular art also devoted itself to justifying the ways of God to man.

It remains to be seen what happens to a society in which the great majority of deaths occur after the normal span is completed, and earlier deaths are regarded largely as examples of human error rather than divine will. Death is now more often than not accepted or even welcomed as an appropriate end to a life in which former joys are turning into present sorrows and previous achievements have given place to frustrations.

There seems to be some evidence that the reduction in anxiety about death is accompanied by increasing uncertainty about the meaning of life. Skepticism about the gods and speculations regarding the absurdities of life are maladies of the affluent. As long as the dominating human activity is the struggle for existence it scarcely seems sensible to develop elaborate questions about the value of life. Under such circumstances it is obvious that if death is bad, life must be good. As acquaintance with death recedes, doubts about life arise. Unable to resolve these doubts some men may actually invent artificial ways of looking death in the face so as to make life more real. Interviews with bullfighters and Grand Prix drivers suggest that death in the afternoon makes life sweeter in the evening. One might even seek an explanation for civilized man's peculiar propensity for making war on his fellows in the need to find something in life worth dying for.

However one may feel about speculations of this kind, it is clear that death is an important aspect of life and that we must still try to understand it as well as we can. The present volume gives tangible proof that death is a researchable phenomenon. As such it opens the door to the possibility that further research will enable us to die more reasonably. With this possibility before us we might even learn to live more reasonable lives.

ROBERT S. MORISON

INTRODUCTION

New Dimensions of Dying

Howard E. Freeman, Orville G. Brim, Jr., and Greer Williams

THE DEATH of an individual is about as significant to the survival of the community as the death of a cell is to the future of a complex biological organism. It happens all the time; the individual is dead but life continues in kind. The notion is well captured in the monarchic cliché: "The king is dead, long live the king."

At the same time, the human mystique requires that we treat the death of every individual as a universal tragedy, a loss to all as well as to him. "Any man's death diminishes me," John Donne said. Such a view appears to be not only a logical extension of a democratic philosophy of individual freedom and responsibility, but also an apparent consequence of the intellectual and emotional uniqueness of human experience. To the extent that we fail to appreciate the singular value of human life, so the humanist argument goes, we reduce our humanness by that much. The case can be restated, of course, in terms of *love,* love of self and love of others.

The Dilemma of Mortality

We have reiterated the old dilemma of individual versus social good, nothing more. The supreme irony in human life is that, whereas we can reason that the renewability of life—the facts of birth, of the young replacing the old, of metabolism, of the constructive *and* destructive processes of energy exchange—practically dictates the inevitability of death for any given unit, we find it emotionally difficult to admit the mortality of life in the individual case. Herein we may perceive a rationalization for a traditional belief in immortality. To release ourselves from the dilemma of personal death versus social survival, we have only to convince ourselves that no one really dies.

It is the intention of the editors and authors of *The Dying Patient* to address themselves to new dimensions of this ancient dilemma, not with any immediate hope of resolving it, but with the definite desire to describe what seems to be, in certain aspects, a new phenomenon involving a shift of attitudes and expectations about life and death—particularly about the quality of life in the period preceding death—as seen from the standpoint of the individual and society. The new dimensions involve the impact of science, technology, economics, and communications. We hope not only to illuminate what is happening but also to identify some of the problems and issues, and to define the outstanding questions that may be answered through social research.

To provide the reader with a frame of reference—one might even call it a plot line—we must indulge in a few historical generalities at this point. Some, of course, may regard our generalizations about attitudes and trends as suspect, since any effort to generalize engenders staggering problems of variation and complexity in people, their character, and custom, as well as in place and time. We are well aware that institutions for dealing with the dying person and, after death, his body, are not uniform among societies; indeed, they vary widely within the American, or Western-style, community.

Some persons, for example, die in complete isolation from medical attention; some are attended, but inadequately; others have the benefit of what has aptly been called "medicated survival," involving the employment of virtually every technique and therapeutic intervention known to practitioners in highly sophisticated medical complexes. In addition, the cause of death, the duration of illness, the individual's age, his social, economic, or ethnic background, his good or bad fortune in where he lives and in whose hands his fate is placed, and indeed the community's respect or lack of respect for him, all may determine whether his life is to be prolonged and for how long.

Such variables have been at work throughout history, yet we do feel justified in speculating that a change in outlook has occurred in the last hundred years. That long ago, when annual death rates, particularly among children, were at least twice as high as they are now, even more fortunately situated families were compelled to live amid the dying and sometimes to care for them personally. For many, death was a household event, not only involving the loss of the elderly but also of young children and young parents. A comparative few reached maturity without witnessing the passing of a loved one or friend, often of several such persons.

Confrontation and Evasion of Death

In those times, as we now may reconstruct the life style, there was no turning away, no escaping from association with the Grim Visitor. At any rate, such rejection was not socially respectable. The survivor was obliged to stand by or lend a hand during the terminal illness of a family member or neighbor, and to feel the presence of death in the house. The only possible way of softening the emotional impact, of circumventing tragic reality, it seemed, was to define death as a beginning, not an end. Every well-established family had its death-bed scenes and, often enough, the off-stage drama of the absent kin racing against time, not in any hope of forestalling death but just to be present and be able to say farewell, and so to join with the clan in common alarm and then grief. In the social circumstances we describe, an individual's death was treated as a Great Event as well as a loss. A person about to meet his Maker deserved attention.

All this investment of interest and feeling in the *rite de passage* has not disappeared, as anyone can see from the impressive hearse-and-ten-Cadillac funerals as they roll by, headlights on. Yet, as we look around us and examine the facts, death has not continued to be a central feature in the lives of many people. Even in our well-organized, well-exploited anxiety about heart disease, cancer, and stroke, our concern is not in a mastery of the event but in simply avoiding death from these major causes. For instance, it does not seem that we are much inclined to obey Freud's injunction, "To endure life, prepare for death." Rather, many of us appear to gaze upon death with a frozen stare, as if it were not there, or as if we were looking through a pane of glass at something of which we were not a part.

As some of the authors in this book suggest, death in the twentieth century has replaced sex as the socially taboo topic. In this view, it has become the fashion in youth-idolizing America to focus attention on living, on a longer life, on a better life, on "living it up." People turn their backs on death as much as possible, symbolically taking out and renewing all the life insurance they can get. They cannot help but note that others die, a reason perhaps for turning the music up, but on the whole there now seems to be a tendency in American society to regard death as a technical error, to write off the dying as if they were a business loss.

A reawakened interest in death and dying appears to be developing, however, as if we now have found time (or reason?) to examine a subject that we had felt justified in putting aside during a period of rapid scientific progress and social change. The decision to write and publish this book is but one evidence of this interest. More can be found in the annotated bibliography at the end.

A New Social Phenomenon?

How can we be sure that we are describing a social phenomenon, an actual trend in modern society? We cannot, in the present state of knowledge. The lines of information, of fact and interpretation, weave in and out, do not quite cover the holes in the fabric, and sometimes are frightfully snarled. What, to shift the metaphor, can a goldfish tell us about life in a goldfish bowl?

But there are some things we know on evidence.

American death rates for more than fifty years followed a sweeping downward curve, a trend that continued until 1954. During a half-century normal life expectancy increased from 40 to 70 years. By far the greatest gain, as already suggested, was among children. Nowadays, children do not frequently die; they get sick and suffer injuries, but they usually recover. More than nine out of ten born alive will still be alive at age 40. Finally, whereas half the population used to die before the age of 40, half now live beyond the age of 70.

These days, statistics show that the opportunity to die or to witness death among one's peers has greatly diminished, and does not become statistically overwhelming until old age. Except for the news media—they never cease to remind us—dying remains only a small cloud on the horizon during the young and middle years *for people as a whole.*

We have another piece of evidence that is not quite as solid but is impressive and permits us to presume a good deal. We know that "in the old days" sick persons did not go to the hospital as much as they do today. Indeed, from the information handed down, it appears that it was mainly the poor who died in institutions, if they lived to reach one. Physicians delivered medical care, such as it was and as much as there was, mainly in the home.

Current information, on the other hand, indicates that the majority of deaths now occur in hospitals, nursing homes, or similar institutions, and that this number is growing. Unmistakably, the more common scene of "natural death" has shifted, and is continuing to shift, from the home to the institution, just as the more common age of death has shifted from the younger to the older age groups.

"Well and good," the scientist or technologist might say, "this is progress." The effects of this shift, the special concern of the social sciences, are more difficult to measure. Certain corollaries of the trend are hard to dispute, however. Apparently it has become the fashion among American families to delegate the care of their dying relatives to someone else, who functions as a third-party agent or stand-in.

We can easily discern who this someone else is, collectively. It is often a community hospital, small or large, that must organize itself bureaucratically in order to handle hundreds and thousands of patients as they come and go; this operation must be carried out rather commonly in the face of certain shortages of staff and financial resources, meaning priorities of need and attention have to be established. It may be a chronic disease hospital or a mental hospital. Or the place of assignment for dying may be a nursing home; increasingly this is so. This institution, while quite unlike any home the patient has known, may meet every sensible test of considerate care, professionally administered; or it may be a grossly inadequate facility, perhaps with a primarily proprietary and profit-taking motive.

Low Quality in Care of the Dying

Apparently the terminal patient is progressively losing the privilege of dying in old, familiar surroundings, with his family around him, with himself as a center of interest and therefore, in an important human sense, in control of his environment, master of his fate. Still, we may ask, since the American home is no longer competent to this responsibility, and because of the advancement of scientific and technical competence and the need for special equipment, is it not better to find a good hospital or a good extended-care facility and put the sick person in competent hands, trained and experienced in such matters?

Theoretically this alternative appears reasoned and sound. Yet the specific point made by some of our authors on the basis of close scrutiny of health professionals and their institutions is that, outside of any fortunate native endowments of personality that they may have, the professionals are quite unprepared to cope with the needs of the dying patient. For example, few physicians and nurses receive any training qualifying them to deal with the approach of death; indeed, their training emphasizes healing and prolongation of life almost to the exclusion of how to provide care once death is inevitable.

Wholly consistent with their own technical objectives and the death-avoidance attitudes of the society they serve, health professionals commonly avoid discussions of impending death with the patient or his relatives; when their efforts to forestall the dying process fail, or when any effort is useless, they customarily lose interest and withdraw from the scene. In effect, death offends their profession!

The patient is left to face the end alone in many instances, depending on circumstance, as still another species of alienated individual in a society increasingly scolded for its gaps in the communication of the meaningful and relevant, its gaps in social transactions, its gaps in interpersonal relationships. We have heard so much about the depersonalization, or dehumanization, of medical care as it has become technology-based and more specialized, that the extension of the phenomenon to the dying patient should come as no surprise, even though it may shock the humanist.

There are some ironic features of incidental interest, one concerning the hospital and the other the physician. The traditional hospital was a place where the sick poor, deserving of charity, were sent to die. It evolved in our time into the modern hospital where people of any class went to recover, hopefully. The hospital is again being identified as the place where people, now of any class, go to die (as well as to recover). What effect, if any, this new view may have on the future of hospitals is uncertain. Because of their marked tendencies toward overutilization and high expense and the concurrent failure to meet the need for primary care in the community, however, there is presently some agitation among health care leaders to keep patients out of hospitals. There are signs that many technically and scientifically well-trained physicians themselves are not content to let the human, the comforting, the reassuring side of the doctor-patient relationship go by default; some of them, along with some community health leaders, are trying to keep alive and revitalize the spirit that the old family doctor was supposed to have and that, in its absence, we are supposed to miss.

There is, as we suggested, some evidence of a new willingness to face the individual and social issues of death and dying. It is not possible to measure the increase in interest quantitatively, but it is fair to say that we are in a period where the prolongation and termination of life is receiving unusual attention from a good many people—medical educators, scientists, practitioners, social scientists, legal scholars, students of ethics, the mass media, policy makers, and the informed public.

Some of the interest naturally stems from the fact that dying is a matter on everybody's agenda. The fact presses harder when we pass middle age and find ourselves in a no-win foot race against time. The question then turns, in some minds, to whether it is the idea of decline and discomfort—the period of dying—or the end result of death that we fear and hate the more. Whatever, the normal human ego is such that it finds it difficult to visualize a world in which it does not exist.

Part of the interest also arises from the unsolved and unresolved moral and human issues that confront both individuals charged with deciding the course of care for seriously and terminally ill patients and those engaged in the development of social policies on health at a local and national level.

The casualties of the Vietnam War have provided a special area of preoccupation, not so much because they include American boys, because American boys "have given their lives for their country" many times before. Rather, popular concern with their deaths arises from the fact that minorities, including youth, have had the courage to confront national policy makers and say that these youths are not giving their lives in defense of their country but essentially in defense of a mistaken policy. In this instance, the protest against death, visited upon bombed civilians as well as our soldiers, has had major political manifestations.

Of course, part of the recent interest in death and dying reflects simply the fact that the behavior of the community and its health professionals, and the organizational and operational mechanisms they have developed to deal with the terminally ill, are the legitimate concerns of the social sciences. Attitudes toward the dying reflect many of the problems of social deviance and disorganization that pervade our society.

Much of the interest, and certainly a leading journalistic topic, arose from the further development of radical surgical procedures, especially in the transplantation of the human heart. Other forms of organ transplantion, such as the older and more successful kidney transplant, have lacked the dramatic appeal of replacement of a heart, preceded, of course, by death of the donor. (A Belgian patient broke all records by surviving the more delicate transplantation of a lung for ten months.)

Crucial Issues and Need for Decisions

These surgical innovations and heroic acts, the subject of Chapter 6, have presented the practitioner in his relationship with the individual patient and the health care system vis-à-vis the community, as well as government itself, with the need for a number of critical decisions leading to the reformulation and refinement of legal norms and social policies. When is someone "dead," so his organs may be removed for transplants? Should a "technically dead" man be flown halfway across the country so his organs can be delivered in living condition to waiting patients who need them? Should, or does, the clinical judgment of the transplant surgeon lie outside the law, or is it superior to administrative regulation? What length of time constitutes a "useful" or "worthwhile" prolongation of life in a person receiving a transplanted organ? How does one justify the large expenditure of public funds to save a single life in the face of the unmet needs of unhealthy thousands? Who should be selected and who should be rejected for costly periodic treatment with the limited number of lifesaving artificial kidneys? These are only a few of the questions now being discussed not only within the medical profession, which carries the primary responsibility, but also by the press, by lawyers, by legislators, and by economists.

Part of current concern about the quality of medical care available to people of all classes might be interpreted as a backlash in the perennial promise by some health leaders of mass life-saving as justification for Federal support of biomedical research. Beyond question, the application of research results related to the major causes of death have prolonged many individual lives but, overall, the mortality trends in heart disease and cancer have been upward, and the gains made have not been reflected in increased average life expectancy. Knowledge of these diseases is still not sufficiently advanced to bring them under general control, and what is known suggests that the only hope for substantial reductions of incidence, disability, and mortality lie not in medical care but in changes in such individual responsibilities as one's habits of eating, exercising, and smoking.

Also essential to our understanding is a subject that has received relatively little attention; it has been conveniently labeled "the mythology of American medicine"; René Dubos called it *The Mirage of Health*. Vocal elements of the American public and medical profession, it has been observed, share the conviction that the historic decline in death rates was primarily the result of medical science; this is in part true, but illusion enters in when, as commonly happens, this is interpreted as meaning "medical care" or "the private practice of medicine." Epidemiologists for the most part do not see health progress in this way. The role of medical care, they conclude, has been secondary to improvement of living conditions, including sufficient food, housing, sanitation, and the elements that go into a safe, clean, home environment, including the educational opportunities and purchasing power that make it possible. The greatest gains have been made, and are still being made, in the prevention of infectious diseases through sanitation, control of insect vectors, and immunization. Except for the antibiotics in the control of pneumonia and other bacterial infections, plus certain types of emergency surgery that are truly life-saving, there is nothing in therapeutics to compare with public health approaches to disease prevention.

The Unfulfilled Promises of Public Health Policy

Ironically, typical private practitioners, while perhaps too busy openly to disavow the heroic role bestowed upon them, do not see themselves—when their opinion is invited—as primarily engaged in saving lives. Rather, they are engaged in taking care of the sick within the limits of their time and competence, part of their responsibility being to relieve anxiety in the needlessly alarmed and other concerns being to reduce discomfort, distress, and disability. With the exception of a few specialties like brain, heart, cancer, or traumatic surgery, death is an adversary rarely encountered in medical practice.

It is certainly true that public campaigns against infectious diseases —smallpox, tuberculosis, typhoid fever, venereal disease, diphtheria, malaria, and so on—have been sold to the public on the basis that they would prevent sickness and death. It is also true, but generally overlooked, that the application of the same kind of appeal in the chronic degenerative diseases, mainly diseases of late life, has led to distortion and misrepresentation. Neither the target populations, the nature of the disease, nor the methods of attack generally have been comparable. As a consequence of misguided strategy and the limitations of science, as well as deficiencies of manpower and system, those who have made government health policy have left the public with a collection of unfulfilled promises (e.g., to save us from "dread diseases").

It is for the complex of reasons set forth that some sectors of medicine, both clinical and preventive, both private and public, have become concerned with the nontechnical, the human, and social aspects of medical care, including, of course, the economic reality that little or no adequate medical care is available to those who cannot afford it.

It is difficult to establish how widely such concerns are felt throughout the medical profession, whether in clinical medicine of the private-practice or academic group type. There is ample recent basis for assuming that organized medicine in its leadership expresses less public than it does political and professional interest.

In addition to the resistance within medicine to the equitable provision of services, health care leaders have charged that an insufficient concern has been shown in improving the quality of care available. The medical educator and medical scientist come as much under criticism as the average practitioner in this regard.

The target area of constructive criticism reveals itself most sharply in problems in the care of the mortally ill: Physicians emerge from their long years of specialized training without a systematic consideration of how to relate to the dying or their relatives; badly run, poorly staffed, and inadequately planned medical facilities result in increased discomfort and even technically incompetent care for dying patients. The lack of a realistic program for developing personnel and facilities to care for the terminally ill has resulted in a lack of continuity of care and a disorganized system of facilities characterized at its worst by some nursing homes that are hardly more than dying bins.

The Unsettled Question of Terminating Life

Concern with the social consequences of life and death reflect, and are reflected in, shifts that have occurred in more general social values. Concern with medical care and particularly with prolongation of life is associated with a long-term trend toward increased humanitarianism in Western society; suffering is no longer regarded as having special value in character-building or spiritual purification. The quality of dying, like the quality of life, is being scrutinized. A related, but perhaps more recent, trend is an increased belief in the feasibility and propriety of human intervention at both the beginning and end of life. A majority of the population no longer accepts either birth or death fatalistically; contraception and abortion are more acceptable; the community's evaluation of suicide and "mercy killings" may be somewhat more liberal. All of this seems to be associated with a decline of belief in an afterlife.

Such value changes have had their effect on the conduct of the physician and on social policy regarding the producing, prolonging, and terminating of life. There is considerable evidence that doctors do terminate lives in certain situations. Some have been criticized for failing to do so. The long-time argument against euthanasia seems to be essentially twofold. First, there is the question whether people could enjoy the therapeutic benefit of faith in their physician if they knew his commitment to keeping them alive was not an absolute one. Opposed to this view would be patients in pain who beg the doctor to end their lives. A second argument against legalizing euthanasia is the difficulty of regulating decisions to terminate a patient's life. This position implicitly assumes that such decisions do not occur. Since they are occurring, is not some sort of public regulation desirable?

Dying as a Field of Inquiry

Finally, the social sciences have changed; the field of medicine has become an important research area for sociologists, psychologists, and anthropologists. Most recently, social scientists have reawakened to the important interface between social and biological behavior. Moreover, the appropriateness of being critical of existing patterns of organization, of social inequities, and of the existing norms and values of community life has increased. It is just as fair to question what happens to dying patients and to examine the conduct of those responsible for their care as it is to inquire into other disturbances of social life and social order, such as crime and violence.

Although a reasonably strong case can be made for an increased interest in the dying and in the social consequences of their medical care—one of the strongest reasons is that those involved professionally have not shown much interest—there is but limited systematic social research on the prolongation and termination of life, minimal agreement on the resolution of the moral and social dilemmas that dying provokes, less than full consideration of the legal and economic ramifications of the current state of affairs, and a lack of systematic programs of research and scholarship to remedy the limitations in knowledge and its dissemination.

An attempt to unravel the reasons for past attitudes toward death and medical conduct would be instructive, but a more constructive alternative, in our opinion, is to make known existing works and hopefully to codify and integrate them. The desired consequence of such an effort is not only to stimulate additional professional and public interest but to promote increased research and scholarly inquiry as well. Hence, this book. We feel this work should be interesting not only to physicians and nurses—whatever the problems of the dying patient, they have to deal with them every time a patient becomes terminally ill—but also to political leaders and social critics concerned with what is and what ought to be, including the wise allocation of economic and manpower resources.

It had been our intention to include in this introduction brief remarks on each of the fourteen chapters as our authors—physicians, sociologists, lawyers, economists—have tackled them. We have decided, however, to refrain from such a pedestrian exercise. Rather, we have attempted in spirit, if not in a complete summary, to capture the content of the book, and in so doing have leaned heavily on the contributions of each author.

The breadth, depth, and variety of viewpoints the contributors have brought to the subject of the dying patient is clear from the book's contents page. It begins with three chapters describing the social context of dying—when, where, and why people die, what they think about death, and the cultural background of their attitudes.

The book moves into the heart of the matter in seven chapters on how doctors, nurses, and their institutions cope with terminal illness—on the prognosis of death, the physician's behavior toward the dying patient, the impact of mortality on the health professions and their institutions, patterns of dying, how terminally ill patients themselves react, and the dismal "social death" role played by many patients dying in a public hospital.

The book closes with four chapters examining the social, ethical, legal, and economic questions arising from the prolongation and termination of life—dying as an emerging social problem, control of medical conduct, legal and policy issues in the allocation of death, and the economic and social costs of death. Finally, a concluding chapter deals with the research questions arising from dying and its dilemmas.

The editors would like to call the reader's attention to the fact that, although this is a book of primary interest to health professionals and social scientists, we have gone to some length to free it of terminological and semantic sins against literary nature. Doubtless, some readers variously will point out that we (1) have not wholly succeeded, and (2) have been too simplistic. Nevertheless, it is our hope that the work will be of interest to many general readers. In a period of social activism, we believe it will be.

THE DYING PATIENT

PART ONE

The Social Context of Dying

1

When, Why, and Where People Die

Monroe Lerner

Perhaps one of man's greatest achievements in his endless quest to extend the limits of his control over nature has been his success in increasing the average duration of his lifetime. This success has been particularly substantial in the modern era, beginning with the mid-seventeenth century, and during the second third of the twentieth century it extended even to the far corners of the globe. During this period, and possibly for the first time in human history, the lifetimes of a substantial proportion of the world's population have been extended well beyond even the economically productive years, so that most people can now reasonably expect to survive at least into their retirement period.

The ability to do this has always been highly valued, at least as an ideal, and perhaps especially in those societies able at best to struggle along only at the subsistence margin and with almost no economic surplus to support life during the barren years. But even in other circumstances, more than one conception of the "good society" has had a component notion that survival beyond the productive years could be within the realm of possibility for all. Nevertheless, only in the technologically advanced Western nations of today does the *average* duration of life reach, and even in some instances exceed, the famous Biblical standard of threescore and ten. If the average duration of life—life expectancy, to use the technical term of statisticians and actuaries—is conceived of as an important indicator of man's control over nature and at the same time also as a crucial element in the moral evaluation of society, then surely man's difficult journey down the long paths of history may be described as social progress rather than merely as evolution.

In any case, whether progress or evolution, man certainly has extended his average lifetime. This chapter first traces that process, as much as it is possible to do so from the inadequate historical data, and only in the most general terms, from prehistory down to the present situation in the United States. Life expectancy, however, is in one sense simply a refined measure of mortality, and for some purposes it is more useful to deal with mortality rates rather than with life expectancy. Mortality, then, becomes the focus of the remainder of the present discussion.

Later, mortality trends in the United States are traced from 1900 to the present, for the total population and separately by age and sex. Young people—infants, children, and young adults—and females at all ages have clearly been the chief beneficiaries of this process, although other segments of the population have also gained substantially. The major communicable diseases—tuberculosis, influenza and pneumonia, gastritis and duodenitis, the communicable diseases of childhood, and so on—have declined as leading causes of death, to be replaced by the "degenerative" diseases, that is, diseases associated with the aging process—heart disease, cancer, and stroke—and by accidental injury.

Populations may be perceived not only as consisting of sex and age groups, but also as individuals and families ranged along a multidimensional, socioeconomic continuum. The problem then becomes: How do people at various points or in various sections of this continuum fare with regard to mortality risk or, in a more literal meaning of the term than was intended by the German sociologist Max Weber who coined it, what are their life-chances?

Perhaps the most meaningful way of dealing with this question, if the objective is to identify large groups or strata in the population who actually do experience gross or at least identifiable differences in mortality risk, is to assume the existence of three major socioeconomic strata in this country, each characterized by a distinctive and unique life-style—the white-collar middle class, the blue-collar working class, and the poverty population. Various structural factors in the life-styles of these populations are conducive to different outcomes in

When, Why, and Where People Die [7

mortality risk. In general, the poverty population experiences relatively high mortality rates at the younger ages and from the communicable diseases, while the white-collar middle class, especially its male members, experiences relatively high mortality rates at mid-life and in the older ages, from the "degenerative" diseases. The blue-collar working class, to the extent that it avoids both types of disabilities, appears for the moment at least to be experiencing the lowest mortality rates among the three strata.

Finally, the place where death occurs—that is, in an institution, at home, or elsewhere—has long been a neglected area of mortality statistics. From national data presented later in this chapter, it seems clear that the proportion of all deaths in this country occurring in institutions has been rising steadily, at least for the last two decades and probably for much longer than that. It may now be as high as, or higher than, two-thirds of all deaths. Almost 50 per cent of all deaths occurring outside an institution in 1958 were due to heart disease, and especially to the major component of this cause-of-death category, arteriosclerotic heart disease, including coronary disease, which accounted for 37 per cent of the total. Cancer, stroke, and accidents comprised the remaining major components of the total, accounting for another 30 per cent of the out-of-institution deaths.

History and the Duration of Human Life

Scholars can only estimate, in the absence of direct data, what the average duration of life must have been during prehistory. Such estimates have been made, however, and they appear to be roughly consistent with the fragmentary data available from the few surviving contemporary primitive groups, in Africa and elsewhere, whose conditions of life resemble those of our remote ancestors at least in some of their major relevant aspects. Prehistoric man lived, according to these estimates, on the average about 18 years (Dublin, 1951:386–405); life during prehistory was, in the Hobbesian sense, indeed nasty, short, and brutish. Violence was the usual cause of death, at least judging from the many skulls found with marks of blows, and man's major preoccupation was clearly with satisfying his elemental need for survival in the face of a hostile environment including wild beasts and other men perhaps just as wild. Survivorship in those days was very seldom beyond the age of 40. Persons who reached their mid-20s and more rarely their early 30s were *ipso facto* considered to have demonstrated their wisdom and were, as a result, often treated as sages.

With the rise of the early civilizations and the consequent improvements in living conditions, longevity must surely have risen, reaching perhaps 20 years in ancient Greece and perhaps 22 in ancient Rome. Life expectancy is estimated to have been about 33 years in England during the Middle Ages, about 35 in the Massachusetts Bay Colony of North America, about 41 in England and Wales during the nineteenth century, and 47.3 in the death-registration states of the United States in 1900.* Thus a definite upward progression in life expectancy has been evident in the Western world throughout its history, and this progression is, furthermore, one in which the pace has clearly accelerated with the passage of time.

The upward progression has continued during the twentieth century and, at least in the United States, its rate of increase has accelerated even further. Thus, life expectancy continued to rise in this country after 1900, even if somewhat erratically; by 1915 it had reached a temporary peak at 54.5 years. The 1918 influenza epidemic caused a sharp drop in life expectancy, to just below 40 years, a level probably typical of "normal" conditions in the United States during the first half of the nineteenth century (Lerner and Anderson, 1963:317–326). But thereafter the upward trend in life expectancy resumed and, between 1937 and 1945 and following the development of the sulfa drugs and the introduction of penicillin during World War II, its increase was extraordinarily rapid. From 1946 to 1954, however, although life ex-

* All life expectancy and mortality figures presented in this chapter pertaining to the U.S. in 1900 or subsequent years, unless otherwise specified, are based on various published reports of the National Vital Statistics Division of the National Center for Health Statistics (formerly the National Office of Vital Statistics), U.S. Public Health Service. The reports themselves are not specifically cited here, but the source for each figure is available upon request. Rates for years prior to 1933 are based on the "death-registration states" only. In 1900 this group consisted of ten states, primarily in the northeastern part of the country, and the District of Columbia. However, the number of states included in this registration area gradually increased over the years, and by 1933 all states in the continental U.S. were part of it. For comparison purposes, figures for the death-registration states are customarily considered as satisfactorily representing the experience of the entire country, and this practice is followed in the present discussion.

pectancy in this country continued upward, the *rate* of increase tapered off. And from 1954, when life expectancy was 69.6 years, to 1967* when it had reached only to 70.2, the gain was at a snail's pace compared to what it had been during the earlier period.

In broader perspective, that is, during the first two-thirds of the twentieth century that we have now experienced, life expectancy rose by almost twenty-three years, an average annual gain of about one-third of a year. This is a breathtaking pace compared to any period of human history prior to this century, and it clearly could not be sustained over a long period of time without enormous social disruption. In line with this, however, life expectancy in the country may now have reached a plateau at, or just above, 70 years.

Where does the United States stand in life expectancy compared with other nations, and what can we anticipate as the reasonable upper limit, or goal, that this country *should* be able to attain in the present state of the arts? Although international comparisons of this type appear to be a hazardous undertaking, in large part because of the substantial obstacles to comparability, a number of other nations clearly have higher life expectancies than we do, and at least in some instances the differences are fairly substantial. Even cursory observation of a recent international compendium of demographic statistics (United Nations, 1967:562–583) reveals, for example, that in Australia, Denmark, The Netherlands, New Zealand, Norway, and Sweden life expectancy may be as much as two to three years higher than the comparable figure in the United States. Countries such as Belgium, France, East Germany, the Federal Republic of Germany, Switzerland, England and Wales, and many others, also exceed us in life expectancy, but not by so wide a margin. Surely this country should at least be able to reach the level of those listed above, if not to exceed them. It is possible that these countries may be nearing an upper limit, however, one that may persist unless some major medical breakthrough occurs. Returning to our own country, future projections of life expectancy and mortality made prior to 1954 now appear to have been much too conservative (Dorn, 1952); on the other hand,

* All 1966 and 1967 figures shown in this chapter are provisional. Based on past experience, however, the provisional rates are likely to be identical, or nearly so, to the final rates.

those made subsequent to 1954 were clearly too optimistic. Tarver (1959), for example, projected a life expectancy of about 73.5 years in 1970, but it now appears that we may be a long time in reaching this goal.

Life expectancy by definition is equivalent to the average duration of life. But how are the numbers obtained for this measure? Starting with a hypothetical cohort of one hundred thousand persons at birth, the mortality rates by age and by sex of a given population in a given year are applied to this cohort as it ages and moves through its life cycle, reducing it in number until no survivors of the original cohort remain (Spiegelman, 1968:293). The number of years lived by the *average* person in this cohort is termed the given population's life expectancy. Clearly then, the life-expectancy figure thus obtained is simply the inverse of mortality experience; it depends entirely upon age-and-sex-specific mortality rates. Employment of the measure "life expectancy" as an indicator of the mortality experience of a population is useful for comparison purposes both currently and across time. This is especially true because this measure eliminates the disturbing influence on the mortality rate of variation in the age-and-sex composition of populations. It is precisely because of this characteristic that life expectancy was used in the preceding discussion to make comparisons across the long span of history. For discussion of the immediate past and current situations, however, it is perhaps best to shift the locus of the discussion from life expectancy to mortality.

Mortality in the United States, 1900 to 1967: Trends and Differentials, Overall and by Age and Sex

Paralleling inversely the increase in life expectancy from 1900 to the present, the mortality rate (deaths per 1,000 population) of the United States population has declined sharply during this century. Thus in 1900 the mortality rate was 17.2 per 1,000 population, but by 1954 it had dropped to 9.2 per 1,000, the lowest ever recorded in the United States. Since that time it has fluctuated between 9.3 and 9.6, and in 1967 the rate was 9.4, representing a decline of about 45 per cent since 1900. These figures understate the extent of the "true" decline, however, primarily because the age composition of the United

When, Why, and Where People Die [11

States population has changed drastically since 1900. This change has generally been in the direction of increasing the high-mortality-risk age segments of the population as a proportion of the total and at the expense of the low. With age composition held constant, that is, using the 1940 age composition of the United States population as a standard, the hypothetical "age-adjusted" death rate in this country declined between 1900 and 1967 from 17.8 to 7.2 per 1,000, a drop of about 60 per cent.

Age and Sex The pattern of mortality rates by age in this country during 1900 was generally similar to that prevailing today (see Table 1).

TABLE 1
Mortality Rates per 1,000 Population by Age and Sex, United States, 1900 and 1966

AGE (IN YEARS)	1900			1966		
	BOTH SEXES	MALES	FEMALES	BOTH SEXES	MALES	FEMALES
All ages	17.2	17.9	16.5	9.5	11.0	8.1
Under 1	162.4	179.1	145.4	23.1	25.7	20.4
1–4	19.8	20.5	19.1	1.0	1.0	0.9
5–14	3.9	3.8	3.9	0.4	0.5	0.4
15–24	5.9	5.9	5.8	1.2	1.7	0.6
25–34	8.2	8.2	8.2	1.5	2.0	1.0
35–44	10.2	10.7	9.8	3.1	3.9	2.3
45–54	15.0	15.7	14.2	7.3	9.7	5.1
55–64	27.2	28.7	25.8	17.2	23.6	11.2
65–74	56.4	59.3	53.6	38.8	52.0	28.1
75–84	123.3	128.3	118.8	81.6	98.5	69.5
85 and over	260.9	268.8	255.2	202.0	213.6	194.9

Thus in 1900 the mortality rate was high during infancy, 162.4 per 1,000, in comparison to the rates at other ages; it dropped to the lowest point for the entire life cycle, 3.9, at ages 5–14; but thereafter it rose steadily with increasing age until at ages 85 and over the mortality rate was 260.9 per 1,000 population. In 1966 the comparable rate was only 23.1 per 1,000 during infancy; the low point was 0.4 at ages 5–14; and again the rates rose steadily with increasing age, to 202 per 1,000 at ages 85 and over. Between 1900 and 1966 the largest *relative* declines in the mortality rates took place at the younger ages, especially during infancy and childhood. Although the declines at the older ages are less impressive percentages, they are, nevertheless, very substantial in absolute numbers. For example, at ages 85 and over the mortality rate dropped by about 59 deaths per 1,000 population, that is, from 261 to 202 per 1,000.

Although the mortality rates for both males and females in the United States population declined substantially since 1900, the *rate* of decline was much sharper for females. Thus the mortality rate for females dropped from 16.5 in 1900 to 8.1 in 1966, a decline of 51 per cent. For males the corresponding drop was from 17.9 to 11.0, or by 39 per cent. The male death rate has been significantly higher than the female death rate in this country throughout the twentieth century, but the relative excess of male over female rates has increased over the years, from 8.5 per cent in 1900 to 36 per cent in 1966. When these rates are age-adjusted to a standard population, the excess of male over female rates in 1966 is considerably larger, about 70 per cent.

In 1900, the relative excess of male over female mortality rates by age was largest during infancy, at 23 per cent. At ages 5–14, the mortality rates for males were actually slightly lower than the comparable rates for females; at ages 15–34, rates were about the same for each sex; and in each of the age groups at 35 and over, the mortality rates for males exceeded the comparable rates for females only by a relatively slight amount, that is, by from 5 to 11 per cent. By 1966, however, although the mortality rates at each age were lower for each sex than the comparable rates in 1900, the decline in almost all cases was larger for females. As a result, the percentage excess of male mortality rates over female rates was larger in most age groups during 1966 than it had been during 1900. It was largest (an excess of almost 200 per cent in 1966), at ages 15–24.

Mortality in the United States, 1900 to 1967: Trends and Differentials by Cause of Death

One of the most significant changes in the mortality experience of this country since 1900 has been the decline in the major communica-

When, Why, and Where People Die [13

ble diseases as leading causes of death* and the consequent increase *in relative importance* of the so-called chronic degenerative diseases, that is, diseases occurring mainly later in life and generally thought to be associated in some way with the aging process. Accidents, especially motor vehicle accidents, have also risen in relative importance as causes of death during this period, but mortality during infancy and maternal mortality, that is, mortality associated with childbearing, have declined sharply.

The Communicable Diseases The leading cause of death** in 1900 was the category: "influenza and pneumonia, except pneumonia of the newborn." This major communicable disease category was listed as the cause of 202.2 deaths per 100,000 population in 1900 (see Table 2), and it accounted for 11.8 per cent of all deaths in that year. By 1966, however, the mortality rate for this category was down to 32.8, it ranked fifth among the leading causes of death, and it now accounted for only 3.4 per cent of all deaths during the year.

Tuberculosis (all forms) and the gastritis grouping,† second and third leading causes of death, respectively, in 1900, were both reduced so significantly and to such low rates during the course of this

---

* Cause of death in U.S. mortality statistics is currently determined in accordance with World Health Organization Regulations, which specify that member nations classify causes of death according to the International Statistical Classification of Diseases, Injuries and Causes of Death, 1955. Besides specifying the classification, World Health Organization Regulations outline the form of medical certification and the coding procedures to be used. In general, when more than one cause of death is reported, the cause designated by the certifying physician as the underlying cause of death is the cause tabulated (cf. World Health Organization, 1957).

** The method of ranking causes of death used here follows the procedure recommended by the *Public Health Conference on Records and Statistics* at its 1951 meeting. Only those causes specified in the "List of 60 Selected Causes of Death" were included in the ranking, and the following categories specified in that list were omitted: the two group titles, "major cardiovascular-renal diseases" and "diseases of the cardiovascular system"; the single title, "symptoms, senility, and ill-defined conditions"; the residual titles, "other infective and parasitic diseases," "other bronchopulmonic diseases," "other diseases of the circulatory system," and "all other diseases"; and all subtitles represented within a broader title. Causes of death are ranked on the basis of rates unadjusted for age or to a specific Revision of the International List of Diseases and Causes of Death, and the above discussion is based on these "crude" rates. But the *titles* used, and the 1966 rates, are those of the Seventh Revision.

† The full title of this cause-of-death grouping, in the nomenclature of the Seventh Revision of the International List of Diseases and Causes of Death, is: gastritis, duodenitis, enteritis, and colitis, except diarrhea of the newborn.

TABLE 2
The Ten Leading Causes of Death, by Rank, United States, 1900 and 1966

1900

RANK	CAUSE OF DEATH	DEATHS PER 100,000 POPULATION	PER CENT OF ALL DEATHS
	All causes	1,719.1	100.0
1	Influenza and pneumonia	202.2	11.8
2	Tuberculosis (all forms)	194.4	11.3
3	Gastritis, duodenitis, enteritis, etc.	142.7	8.3
4	Diseases of the heart	137.4	8.0
5	Vascular lesions affecting the central nervous system	106.9	6.2
6	Chronic nephritis	81.0	4.7
7	All accidents	72.3	4.2
8	Malignant neoplasms (cancer)	64.0	3.7
9	Certain diseases of early infancy	62.6	3.6
10	Diphtheria	40.3	2.3

1966

	All causes	954.2	100.0
1	Diseases of the heart	375.1	39.3
2	Malignant neoplasms (cancer)	154.8	16.2
3	Vascular lesions affecting the central nervous system	104.6	11.0
4	All accidents	57.3	6.0
5	Influenza and pneumonia	32.8	3.4
6	Certain diseases of early infancy	26.1	2.7
7	General arteriosclerosis	19.5	2.0
8	Diabetes mellitus	18.1	1.9
9	Cirrhosis of the liver	13.5	1.4
10	Suicide	10.3	1.1

century that neither category was listed among the ten leading causes of death in 1966. Tuberculosis had caused 194.4 deaths per 100,000 in 1900, or 11.3 per cent of all deaths, while the gastritis grouping, with 142.7 deaths per 100,000, had accounted for 8.3 per cent of the total. By 1966 the comparable rates for these two categories were 3.9 and 3.3, respectively, with each accounting for substantially less than one-half of 1 per cent of all deaths in that year. The percentage declines for each from 1900 to 1966 were by 98 per cent.

Diphtheria had been listed as tenth leading cause of death in 1900, with 40.3 deaths per 100,000 population. In 1966 this condition accounted for only forty deaths all told in this country, that is, considering the entire United States population as at risk, so that the death rate was about one death per five million persons. Other major communicable diseases with impressive declines in mortality were some of the other communicable diseases of childhood, such as whooping cough, measles, scarlet fever, and streptococcal sore throat, and syphilis, typhoid and paratyphoid fevers, rheumatic fever, and typhus.

Hillery *et al.* (1968), comparing recent mortality data from forty-one countries, have shown that the communicable diseases ("infectious diseases" in their terminology) as causes of death decline significantly as a proportion of all deaths in each country as these countries move "up" in the demographic transition, that is, as their birth and death rates decline, and as they concomitantly become at least presumably more "advanced" technologically and socially. Thus, in the "transitional" countries (low death rates but high birth rates), communicable diseases account for about one-third of all deaths on the average, while in the demographically "mature" countries (both death rates and birth rates low), the comparable proportion is about one in twelve of all deaths. This finding is generally in conformity with past experience in this country and elsewhere.

The Degenerative Diseases "Diseases of the heart" ranked fourth among the leading causes of death in this country during 1900; this category caused 137.4 deaths per 100,000 and accounted for 8.0 per cent of all deaths. By 1966, however, it had risen so far in importance that it had become the leading cause of death, far outranking all others. Its mortality rate had risen to 375.1 deaths per 100,000 population, and it accounted for nearly 40 per cent of all deaths in that year. Between 1900 and 1966 the unadjusted death rate from this disease rose by 173 per cent; the rise was much less if the age-adjusted rates for these two years are compared, but even this rise was very substantial.

The pattern of increase for malignant neoplasms (cancer) as a cause of death was generally quite similar. This disease ranked eighth among the leading causes of death in 1900. It accounted for 64 deaths per 100,000 population and less than 4 per cent of all deaths. By 1966, however, its rank among the leading causes had risen to second, its rate per 100,000 to 154.8, and its proportion of the total of all deaths exceeded 16 per cent. Vascular lesions of the central nervous system, although remaining relatively stable in number of deaths per 100,000 (106.9 in 1900 and 104.6 in 1966), nevertheless rose in rank (fifth to third) and as a proportion of all deaths (6 to 11 per cent).

How can we account for the increases, in both absolute and relative terms, in these "degenerative" diseases as causes of death? As the classification implies, these are diseases occurring later in life and closely associated with the aging process. Whereas formerly people died on the average much earlier in life, victims primarily of the communicable diseases, they survive today to a much later age, only to succumb in due time to the degenerative conditions. Hillery and his associates (1968) in their interesting study have generalized this trend also. Thus in their demographically transitional countries (low death rates but high birth rates) the degenerative diseases account for less than one-third of all deaths, whereas in their demographically mature countries (both death rates and birth rates low) these diseases account for just under two-thirds of the total. The net overall gain has clearly been an extension of life by many years.

Mortality and Socioeconomic Status

There appears to be a good deal of confusion in this country today, and perhaps especially among social scientists, demographers, and health statisticians, as to the precise nature of the relationship between mortality and socioeconomic status. This confusion has existed, and perhaps will continue to exist for some time, despite the fact that quite a few studies in the past, and a number of ongoing studies, have attempted to clarify the relationship. Part of this confusion may be occasioned by what is perhaps the changing nature of that relationship, a change which in turn may have been brought about by the tremendous improvements in medical technology and therapies during the past century and by the increasing general affluence of the American population. But part of it results also from the lack of a generally accepted method for the construction of an overall index of socioeconomic status (Lerner, 1968).

In turn, the failure of social scientists to develop a generally accepted method for the construction of an overall index reflects their lack of general agreement on the number or composition of social classes or social strata in the United States, especially when this entire culturally diverse country is considered as the unit of analysis. Different numbers of classes or strata have been identified, depending on definitions and operational purposes, but none of these is a real entity. Various measures of socioeconomic status have been related to mortality, and the results of one very large study along these lines are now beginning to appear (Kitagawa, 1968). Nevertheless, the overall pattern continues to remain quite unclear at this writing.

For present purposes—to relate socioeconomic status to mortality—it appears that the most meaningful division of the United States population from a conceptual, rather than an operational, standpoint is into three socioeconomic strata. These strata are set apart from one another, in the most general terms, by a distinctive and unique life-style, even though the boundaries between these strata are not sharp, and there may be a considerable movement of individuals and families among them. The life-styles of these strata, in turn, are dependent upon or associated with income, wealth, occupation and occupational prestige, dwelling, ethnic origin, educational attainment, and many other factors, all of which, in some as yet unspecified way, add up to the total. The life-styles, in turn, are directly relevant to the health level, and more specifically the mortality experience of each stratum. The structural factors in each of the three major life-styles through which the relationship to mortality operates include at least these four: the level of living (food, housing, transportation, or other factors); degree of access to medical care within the private medical care system; occupation of the family head (sedentary or involving physical activity); and the nature of the social milieu for that stratum (that is, its degree of economic or social security).

The highest stratum consists of those who are usually designated as the middle-and upper-class white-collar business executives at all levels and professionals, and all those who are above this category. It even includes the highest echelons of skilled blue-collar workers (tool-and-die makers), foremen, supervisors, or the like. Although the range of variation *within* this stratum is great, the group as a whole shares the essential elements of a "middle-class" way of life, that is, residence in "better" neighborhoods and suburbs, general affluence, and so on.

This group will subsequently be designated in the present discussion as the middle class.

The second stratum consists of this country's blue-collar working class—mainly the semi-skilled and unskilled workers in the mass-production and service industries, but also small farmers and possibly even farm laborers, and lower level white-collar workers. These people are also relatively affluent, but not to the same extent as the middle class. Again, although the range of variation *within* this stratum is great, they also share a unique style of life distinctively different from that of the higher stratum. This group will subsequently be designated in the present discussion as the working class.

The lowest of the three strata includes those who are generally designated as the poverty population. By definition, these people generally do not share in the affluence characteristic of this country. It consists of the poor in large-city ghettos and the rural poor (residents of Appalachia or the Deep South, as well as others); the Negro, Puerto Rican, Mexican, and French-Canadian populations, and the other relatively poor ethnic minorities in this country; Indians on reservations; the aged; migratory laborers; and the dependent poor.

Although, as stated above, this mode of classification of socioeconomic status appears to be the most meaningful from a conceptual standpoint in terms of relating it to mortality, it clearly lacks merit from the operational point of view. This is because there would appear to be no ready way of segregating these groups from one another in the available national statistical data, relating either to population data or health statistics, and especially to study their respective mortality experiences. Nevertheless, here and there some attempts have been made; and some studies, mostly local and regional in character and particularly of the poverty population, have been carried out (cf. Chicago Board of Health, 1965; and Lerner, 1968). What follows, therefore, is to be understood as more of an overall gross impression and prediction, rather than anything else, and one based on a general familiarity with the literature of what would be found if the data were available in the form required by the present framework.

The poverty populations generally are likely to have the highest death rates of the three strata on an overall basis, but especially from the communicable diseases. This has been true historically between rich and poor nations in the modern era and still represents the situation in the world today at various levels of wealth and technological advancement (Pond, 1961; Anderson and Rosen, 1960). Within this country, a considerable amount of evidence exists to show that mortality rates among the poverty population are likely to be highest during infancy, childhood, and the younger adult ages. The communicable diseases of childhood, gastrointestinal diseases, and influenza and pneumonia are still a relatively serious health problem among this population, even where public health facilities and services are relatively adequate, as, for example, in the slums of large cities in this country today. What this population lacks most, perhaps, is adequate access to personal health services within the private medical care system. Although these services are to some degree available under other auspices (Strauss, 1967), they may be relatively ineffective and not oriented to the life-style of their recipients, while the cultural impediments to their use appear to be substantial.

In contrast, the white-collar middle class does enjoy relatively adequate access to personal health services under the private medical care system, and their mortality rates during infancy, childhood, and even young adulthood are substantially lower than that of the poverty population. This is especially true for mortality from the communicable diseases, but appears to extend almost to the entire spectrum of causes of death. The higher levels of living enjoyed by this stratum in general buttress its advantage during the younger years. During mid-life and especially during the later years, however, its mortality rates appear to become substantially higher than those of the rest of the population, primarily for the "degenerative" diseases, especially heart disease, cancer, and stroke.

One possible hypothesis that has been offered in explanation of this phenomenon merits comment here. It may be that, because of improved survival by members of this stratum at the younger ages, many persons are carried into mid-life with a lower "general resistance" factor than that which characterizes persons in the poverty stratum, and that these individuals are perhaps therefore more vulnerable to the diseases and hazards most prevalent at mid-life and beyond. At the moment, at least, there seems to be no possible way of testing this hypothesis.

Another hypothesis is that this excess mortality at mid-life is a concomitant of the general affluence characterizing the life-styles of the middle class and of their sedentary occupations (executive and white-collar). Both of these, in turn, may result in obesity, excessive strains and tensions, excessive cigarette smoking, and perhaps ultimately premature death. Men aged 45–64 (mid-life), especially white men, appear to be particularly vulnerable to coronary artery disease and respiratory cancer. Middle-class women, on the other hand, appear to be less affected by these affluence-related forms of ill health than middle-class men, perhaps because of innate resistance, social pressures to avoid obesity, cigarette smoking without inhalation, and generally less stressful lives, or perhaps some combination of these factors. In any case, women in this stratum appear to have the best of all possible worlds, that is, they have none of the health disabilities associated with the sedentary occupations characteristic of their spouses while at the same time enjoying adequate medical care.

The blue-collar working class appears to have the best overall mortality record. This group appears to have relatively low mortality during the younger ages and from the communicable diseases, especially because they do have access to good medical care in the private medical care system. At mid-life, moreover, they appear to suffer from relatively few of the disabilities associated with middle-class affluence.

Where Death Occurs

Where people die—in a hospital or other institution, at home, or in a public place—has been a relatively neglected aspect of mortality statistics in this country during the past few years. Although this information is contained on each death certificate and relatively little additional effort or expense would be required to code and tabulate it, this has not been done, perhaps because it has not been at all clear that the returns would be commensurate to the additional expense. As a result, the last national tabulation of these data based on the regular vital statistics data-collection system relates to 1958, and these data were far from complete; many of the cross-tabulations that could have been made were not, in fact, carried out. Some of the states and

When, Why, and Where People Die [21

cities here and there have published tabulations since that time, however.

Recently, some new interest has been expressed in this question among public health circles, possibly stimulated by the coming into being of Regional Medical Programs throughout the country. These in turn were set up under the Heart Disease, Cancer, and Stroke Amendments of 1965 (P.L. 89-239), which provided for the establishment of regional cooperative arrangements for improvement of the quality of medical care through research and training, including continuing education, among medical schools, research institutions, and hospitals, and in related demonstrations of patient care. The new legislation was aimed generally at improving the health, manpower, and facilities available, but one specific purpose was to make new medical knowledge available, as rapidly as possible, for the treatment of patients (Yordy and Fullarton, 1965). The assumption in public health circles was that the place of occurrence of some deaths, and the circumstances, may have been related to an inability to obtain proper medical care either at the moment of death or immediately preceding it, as in cases of sudden death, or at some point during the illness or condition leading to death in other cases. The extent to which this assumption is true is, of course, difficult to test given the present paucity of relevant data.

In 1958, according to the most recent *national* data available (see Table 3), 60.9 per cent of all deaths in this country occurred in institutions, that is, in hospitals, convalescent and nursing homes, and in hospital departments of institutions or in other domiciliary institutions. This figure represented a considerable rise over the comparable 49.5 per cent recorded in 1949, the most recent preceding year for which a national tabulation was made. On the basis of these data it appeared that the proportion was rising by an average of better than 1 per cent annually.

National data to test whether the trend continued beyond that year are unavailable, but state and local data appear to indicate that this, in fact, may have been the case. In New York City, for example, the proportion of deaths occurring in institutions rose steadily, with only one very slight fluctuation, from 65.9 per cent in 1955 to 73.1 per cent

TABLE 3
Number and Per Cent of Deaths Occurring in Institutions by Type of Service of Institution, United States, 1949 and 1958

TYPE OF SERVICE OF INSTITUTION	1958 NUMBER	1958 PER CENT	1949 NUMBER	1949 PER CENT
Total deaths	1,647,886	100.0	1,443,607	100.0
Not in institution	644,548	39.1	728,797	50.5
In institution	1,003,338	60.9	714,810	49.5
Type of service of institution				
General hospital	784,360	47.6	569,867	39.5
Maternity hospital	1,862	0.1	2,249	0.2
Tuberculosis hospital	9,097	0.6	13,627	0.9
Chronic disease, convalescent and other special hospitals	24,180	1.5	12,402	0.9
Nervous and mental hospitals	57,675	3.5	45,637	3.2
Convalescent and nursing homes, homes for the aged, etc.	98,444	6.0	22,783	1.6
Hospital department of institutions, and other domiciliary institutions	3,646	0.2	41,841	2.9
Type of service not specified	24,074	1.5	6,404	0.4

in 1967 (see Table 4). These same data indicate that the proportion of deaths occurring at home dropped commensurately during these years, from 31.4 per cent to 24.2 per cent. The proportion of deaths occurring elsewhere, primarily in public places, remained relatively constant. Data from the Maryland State Department of Health also indicate a substantial upward progression in the proportion of all deaths occurring in institutions, from 64.4 per cent in 1957 to 71.8 per cent in 1966 (Maryland State Department of Health, 1967).

Most of the deaths occurring in "institutions," as the data of Table 3 indicate, occurred in hospitals, the vast majority of which were general hospitals. Nervous and mental hospitals during each of the two years to which the table relates, however, accounted for somewhat more than 3 per cent of all deaths. The proportion occurring in convalescent and nursing homes, homes for the aged, and similar estab-

When, Why, and Where People Die [23

TABLE 4
Number and Per Cent of Deaths by Place of Death,
New York City, 1955–1967

	NUMBER OF DEATHS				PERCENTAGE			
	TOTAL	IN INSTI- TUTION	AT HOME	OTHER	TOTAL	IN INSTI- TUTION	AT HOME	OTHER
1955	81,612	53,746	25,598	2,268	100.0	65.9	31.4	2.8
1956	81,118	54,716	24,193	2,209	100.0	67.5	29.8	2.7
1957	84,141	57,141	24,609	2,391	100.0	67.9	29.2	2.8
1958	84,586	57,946	24,230	2,410	100.0	68.5	28.6	2.8
1959	85,352	58,859	24,127	2,366	100.0	69.0	28.3	2.8
1960	86,252	59,413	24,341	2,498	100.0	68.9	28.2	2.9
1961	86,855	60,061	24,524	2,270	100.0	69.2	28.2	2.6
1962	87,089	60,409	24,315	2,365	100.0	69.4	27.9	2.7
1963	88,621	61,588	24,677	2,356	100.0	69.5	27.8	2.7
1964	88,026	62,391	23,602	2,033	100.0	70.9	26.8	2.3
1965	87,395	62,308	22,879	2,208	100.0	71.3	26.2	2.5
1966	88,418	63,599	22,576	2,243	100.0	71.9	25.5	2.5
1967	87,610	64,083	21,222	2,305	100.0	73.1	24.2	2.6

Source of basic data: Personal communication from Mr. Louis Weiner, New York City Department of Health.

lishments increased substantially between 1949 and 1958, from 1.6 per cent to 6.0 per cent.*

Table 5 shows the per cent of deaths, by color, that occurred in institutions in 1949 and 1958, for the entire country and for each geographic division. In both years the proportion of deaths occurring in institutions was substantially lower for the nonwhite population than for the white when the country as a whole is considered as the unit. However, for the New England, Middle Atlantic, and East North Central states in both years and the West North Central states in 1949 the reverse pattern was true, that is, the proportion of deaths occurring in institutions was higher for the nonwhite population than for the white. In general, the proportions in both years for the East South

* However, there is some lack of comparability between these two figures, and this increase, although undoubtedly substantial, may not be quite as large as these figures indicate.

Central, West South Central, and South Atlantic states, and especially for their nonwhite populations, were very low in comparison to the rest of the country. In Mississippi, even as late as 1958, only 31.0 per cent of the nonwhite deaths occurred in institutions. (These data are not shown in Table 5.)

By cause of death, as Table 6 indicates, the most important cate-

TABLE 5

Per Cent of Deaths Occurring in Institutions by Color and Geographic Division, United States, 1949 and 1958

	1958			1949		
GEOGRAPHIC DIVISION	TOTAL	WHITE	NON-WHITE	TOTAL	WHITE	NON-WHITE
United States	60.9	61.9	53.2	49.5	50.4	43.2
New England	64.2	64.0	72.4	52.2	52.0	67.1
Middle Atlantic	62.8	62.3	68.9	53.2	52.2	69.0
East North Central	63.6	63.2	67.9	51.5	50.9	59.7
West North Central	63.8	63.9	61.5	50.7	50.6	54.4
South Atlantic	55.8	58.6	48.4	42.5	45.3	36.3
East South Central	47.6	51.8	37.3	34.6	37.8	27.6
West South Central	54.9	57.7	44.2	42.8	45.3	34.3
Mountain	63.5	63.4	64.1	55.2	54.9	61.0
Pacific	66.5	66.3	68.8	58.5	58.1	65.5

TABLE 6

Total Deaths and Per Cent Occurring in Institutions by Cause, for Selected Causes of Death, United States, 1958

CAUSE OF DEATH	TOTAL DEATHS, NUMBER	PER CENT IN INSTITUTIONS
Tuberculosis, all forms	12,361	80.0
Syphilis and its sequelae	3,469	71.7
Dysentery, all forms	407	62.4
Scarlet fever and streptococcal sore throat	139	57.6
Whooping cough	177	60.5
Meningococcal infections	746	87.9
Acute poliomyelitis	255	91.8
Measles	552	63.8

TABLE 6 (cont.)

CAUSE OF DEATH	TOTAL DEATHS, NUMBER	PER CENT IN INSTITUTIONS
Malignant neoplasms, including neoplasms of lymphatic and hematopoietic tissues	254,426	67.7
Benign neoplasms	4,961	82.5
Asthma	5,035	55.4
Diabetes mellitus	27,501	68.6
Anemias	3,195	72.4
Meningitis, except meningococcal and tuberculous	2,247	91.8
Vascular lesions affecting central nervous system	190,758	65.8
Diseases of heart	637,246	50.4
Arteriosclerotic heart disease, including coronary disease	461,373	48.5
Other hypertensive disease	13,798	68.5
General arteriosclerosis	34,483	61.8
Other diseases of circulatory system	17,204	79.5
Chronic and unspecified nephritis, etc.	13,827	67.6
Influenza and pneumonia	57,439	68.6
Influenza	4,442	43.1
Pneumonia, except pneumonia of newborn	52,997	70.7
Bronchitis	3,973	61.7
Ulcer of stomach and duodenum	10,801	88.2
Appendicitis	1,845	94.5
Hernia and intestinal obstruction	8,853	90.5
Gastritis, duodenitis, enteritis, etc.	7,838	78.7
Cirrhosis of liver	18,638	79.3
Cholelithiasis, cholecystitis, and cholangitis	4,720	90.0
Acute nephritis, and nephritis with edema, etc.	2,203	76.0
Infections of kidney	6,889	85.5
Hyperplasia of prostate	4,627	81.1
Deliveries and complications of pregnancy, childbirth, and the puerperium	1,581	85.5
Congenital malformations	21,411	86.5
Certain diseases of early infancy	68,960	94.5
Symptoms, senility, and ill-defined conditions	19,729	25.2
Accidents	90,604	47.6
Motor vehicle accidents	36,981	44.0
Other accidents	53,623	50.0
Suicide	18,519	18.5
Homicide	7,815	34.1

gories in which the proportion of deaths occurring in institutions was relatively small were the external causes of death (accidents, suicide, and homicide), diseases of the heart, influenza, and the catchall category, "symptoms, senility, and ill-defined conditions." Less than one-half of all deaths following accidents occurred in the hospital, and the comparable figure was only 44 per cent for motor vehicle deaths. Only about one-half of all deaths from diseases of the heart occurred in an institution, and somewhat less than that figure for arteriosclerotic heart disease, including coronary disease. In the case of each of these conditions, as well as for suicide and homicide, it seems likely that the short time-interval between onset of the condition and death is probably a major reason for the relatively small proportions occurring in hospitals. Finally, only about one-fourth of all deaths for which a cause could not clearly be delineated (deaths attributed to symptoms, senility, and ill-defined conditions) occurred in hospitals.

Considering the almost 645,000 deaths that occurred outside an institution in 1958, almost one-half (49 per cent) were accounted for by diseases of the heart (see Table 7). (Within this category, arteriosclerotic heart disease, including coronary disease, accounted for about 37 per cent of the total.) The next three most important causes of death in accounting for all deaths outside of institutions were malignant neoplasms, 13.1 per cent; vascular lesions, 10.1 per cent; and accidents, 7.4 per cent. These first four categories combined accounted for about 80 per cent of all deaths occurring outside institutions, but other causes of death—for example, influenza and pneumonia, suicide, general arteriosclerosis, and so on—were also important in the total.

Conclusions and Implications

It would appear, at least from the point of view and focus of the preceding discussion, that the implicit goal of the health establishment in this country, to "assure for everyone the highest degree of health attainable in the present state of the arts" has been far from realized. For example, with regard to mortality and its derivative, life expectancy, other nations have clearly outdistanced us, and by a substantial margin. It is true that most of these countries are smaller and more homogeneous, and the environmental hazards plaguing them may not

TABLE 7
Deaths Occurring Outside Institutions by Cause, for Selected Causes of Death, United States, 1958

CAUSE OF DEATH	NUMBER	PER CENT
All Causes	644,548	100.0
1. Diseases of the heart	316,074	49.0
Arteriosclerotic heart disease, including coronary disease	237,607	36.9
2. Malignant neoplasms, including neoplasms of the lymphatic and hematopoietic tissues	84,724	13.1
3. Vascular lesions affecting the central nervous system	65,239	10.1
4. Accidents, all forms	47,476	7.4
Motor-vehicle accidents	20,709	3.2
Other	26,767	4.2
5. Influenza and pneumonia	18,036	2.8
Pneumonia	15,528	2.4
Influenza	2,508	0.4
6. Suicide	15,093	2.3
7. General arteriosclerosis	13,173	2.0
8. Diabetes mellitus	8,635	1.3
9. Homicide	5,150	0.7

be operative in the same manner and to the same degree as they are among us. Nevertheless, we do appear to have fallen short of what has been achieved elsewhere, and it is therefore appropriate to raise questions about the reasons for this apparent failure.

Three broad lines of inquiry have been suggested as possible approaches in this chapter, and a fourth influencing and possibly underlying the others will be mentioned. When one considers the entire spectrum of causes of death and their "places of occurrence," it is not unreasonable to assume *as a working hypothesis* that many deaths are occurring from causes—disease conditions—that are amenable, at least under optimum conditions in the present state of the arts, to medical management and control. Of course, the sex and age of the patient, the general state of health and degree of "resistance" of the organism, and many other factors should be considered in the evaluation of each case before any death is characterized as needless or preventable. Furthermore, it may be very difficult to refrain from setting up, as working standards, ideal conditions that are unattainable anywhere, given the realities and the imperatives of social organization, the relatively low priority of health in the hierarchy of human values and "needs," the "mass" nature of society, and the vagaries and irrational elements in what is colloquially described as "human nature." Nevertheless, the social and economic differentials in mortality discussed in this chapter would appear to argue that there is much room for improvement, that the low mortality rates now attained by some could be attained, theoretically at least, by all.

If this is true, and if our goal is indeed to assure the highest degree of health attainable *for everyone,* then we must ask ourselves whether the social organization for the provision of health services to the population in some degree shares responsibility for the discrepancy between goal and reality. If responsible inquiry is directed toward this problem, the unknowns in this vital area of public policy may be reduced, and we may begin to reexamine the place of health in our presently implicit hierarchy of values as opposed, for example, to education, other forms of welfare, space exploration, urban crowding, rural poverty, national security, and the myriad national concerns to which we allocate community resources. We may even be able to move toward calm and rational discussion of some alternative forms of social organization of the health care system, including their economic and perhaps social costs, hopefully with the result that we ultimately arrive at intelligent decisions.

REFERENCES

Anderson, Odin W., and George Rosen.
    1960   "An examination of the concept of preventive medicine." Health Information Foundation, Research Series No. 12. New York: Health Information Foundation.

Chicago Board of Health; Planning Staff of the Health Planning Project.
    1965   A Report on Health and Medical Care in Poverty Areas of Chicago and Proposals for Improvement. Processed.

Dorn, Harold F.
    1952   "Prospects of further decline in mortality rates." Human Biology 24, 4(December):235–261.

Dublin, Louis I., in collaboration with Mortimer Spiegelman.
    1951   The Facts of Life—From Birth to Death. New York: Macmillan.

Hillery, George A., Jr., et al.
1968 "Causes of death in the demographic transition." Paper presented at the Annual Meeting of the Population Association of America, Boston, Mass., April. Processed.

Kitagawa, Evelyn M.
1968 "Race differentials in mortality in the United States, 1960 (corrected and uncorrected)." Paper presented at the Annual Meeting of the Population Association of America, Boston, Mass., April. Processed.

Lerner, Monroe.
1968 "The level of physical health of the poverty population: a conceptual reappraisal of structural factors." Paper presented at Conference on New Dimensions in Health Measurements, sponsored by Washington Statistical Society and American Marketing Association, Washington, D.C., January 25. Processed.

Lerner, Monroe, and Odin W. Anderson.
1963 Health Progress in the United States: 1900–1960. Chicago: University of Chicago Press.

Maryland State Department of Health, Division of Biostatistics.
1967 Annual Vital Statistics Report: Maryland, 1966. Also, same annual reports for earlier years to 1957. Baltimore.

Pond, M. Allen.
1961 "Interrelationship of poverty and disease." Public Health Reports 76(November):967–974.

Spiegelman, Mortimer.
1968 "Life tables." Pp. 292–299 in International Encyclopedia of the Social Sciences. New York: Free Press.

Strauss, Anselm L.
1967 "Medical ghettoes: medical care must be reorganized to accept the life-styles of the poor." Trans-action 4(May):7–15 and 62.

Tarver, James D.
1959 "Projections of mortality in the United States to 1970." The Milbank Memorial Fund Quarterly 37, 2(April):132–143.

United Nations.
1967 Demographic Yearbook, 1966. New York.

World Health Organization.
1957 Manual of the International Statistical Classification of Diseases, Injuries, and Causes of Death: Based on the Recommendations of the Seventh Revision Conference, 1955. Vol. I. Geneva, Switzerland.

Yordy, K. D., and J. E. Fullarton.
1965 "The heart disease, cancer, and stroke amendments of 1965 (P.L. 89–239)." Reprint from Health, Education, and Welfare Indicators, November.

2

What People Think About Death

John W. Riley, Jr.

During the next twelve months, nearly two million Americans will die. Throughout the whole world, between fifty and sixty million will die. Considering a phenomenon of such wide and deep personal significance, knowledge of how contemporary man relates to death is meager indeed. It has been said that man is loath to consider this most basic uncertainty (Feifel, 1959). It has been widely assumed that he prefers to ignore death—to take an ostrichlike view. Without historical insight, many of us have made this "truth" part of our own lore, an incorporation of that ancient taboo which man seems to have placed on thoughts about death, in part to deny its existence. These and related assumptions are now being called into question.

Indeed there are indications that what has seemed to be a pervasive silence about death was nothing more than a public silence. Today, under the influence of technological, cultural, and social changes, even that public silence may be in the process of being broken—in much the same way that, not long ago, the public silence concerning sex was shattered. Thus, as our attention was directed to the social concerns inherent in "the pill," legalized abortion, and new patterns of sexual behavior, it is now being directed to problems concerned with man's relationship to death:

1. Dilemmas confronting the medical profession; for example, when should treatment be terminated?

2. Risk-taking decisions by those in seats of power that may cause mass death; for example, the use of nuclear weapons.
3. Risk-taking by individuals; for example, cigarette smoking or the nonuse of automobile safety belts.
4. The complex moral and social implications surrounding the scientific control of death; for example, the individual's "right" to a dignified death, the allocation of scarce life-saving materials—blood plasma, transplantable tissues (see Fulton, 1965).

Death and Society

Death is a personal event that no one ever has been able to describe for himself. On the other hand, in no known society is the individual left to face death completely uninitiated (cf. Riley, 1968a). He is provided with beliefs about "the dead," and he is offered a range of theories about his own probable fate after death. Furthermore, every society has prescribed ways of dealing with the problems of death—the disposal of the corpse, help for the bereaved, modes of replacement in strategic posts, allocation of the property of the deceased, and countless other arrangements.

As a rule, social institutions have evolved to facilitate life and to prevent death. Indeed, the demographic history of man shows that he has been more interested in death control than in birth control. Mortality rates have tended to decline faster than fertility rates. This is documented in an impressive literature; but the larger problems inherent in the relationships of society toward death have drawn much less attention. No general theory of death and society has yet appeared. There are signs, however, of a developing theoretical concern with such problems.

One example of this widening concern notes that both the threat of early death and the prospect of suffering as a concomitant of dying have been greatly reduced by medical advances. Premature death is now more often adventitious; physical suffering *in extremis* can often be avoided. The weakening of these two traditional anxieties, it is now being argued, is leading to new orientations toward death (cf. Parsons and Lidz, 1967).

Another line of theoretical concern has begun to probe the relationships between death and human society through the application of such social science concepts as political succession, kinship structure, and socialization. No serious attempt, however, has yet been made to develop a fully articulated sociological theory of death (Blauner, 1966).

Death and the Individual

Empirical studies of the individual's relationship to death have also been comparatively few and comparatively recent (Kalish, 1965). Attempts are now being made to study individual feelings and attitudes about the meaning of death, however. Using techniques ranging all the way from projective tests to survey research, social scientists are exploring the intricate and complex patterns of individual responses to death.

Reactions have been obtained from widely disparate segments of the population. One study suggests that the child's conception of death develops in stages; among very young children who have not yet developed a concept of causality, death is seen as reversible, not final. Studies of the other end of the age spectrum suggest that a secure environment and close kinship ties become important for the dying patient, that elderly patients have less anxiety about death if they live in familiar surroundings or with relatives (or even in homes for the aged) rather than alone. These and other indications of the need for social support raise a paradox for our society where there is a growing tendency to hospitalize and isolate people who are dying (see Glaser and Strauss, 1965; Sudnow, 1967).

Other characteristics of the individual (sex, religiosity, education, health) are also being evaluated as possibly affecting attitudes toward death (Feifel, 1959). One series of studies investigating possible connections between people's religion and their attitudes toward death, for example, has thus far produced inconclusive findings. Some of the studies find that fear of death increases with spiritual orientation, while others find no association at all between religious conviction and beliefs about death.

These examples of the growing literature on death and the indi-

What People Think About Death [33

vidual testify to the emergence of new questions for systematic research within a broader conceptual framework.

An Empirical Study

As part of a continuing program of basic social research, the Equitable Life Assurance Society of the United States has sponsored studies of various aspects of the meaning of time and death in contemporary American society (for example, Moore, 1963; Riley, 1968b).

The rest of this chapter will report the results of a survey of individual attitudes and orientations toward death. The field work for the study was conducted by the National Opinion Research Center at the University of Chicago. The sampling involved a standard multistage area probability design with quota sampling at the block level based on sex, age, race, and employment status. A total of 1,482 adults thus selected were interviewed.

One finding that emerged from this study points to the public's high regard for doctors as advisers or counselors in dealing with death. Thus, when people were asked with whom they would feel most comfortable in discussing problems associated with death, only clergymen were mentioned more frequently than doctors. (Life insurance agents and lawyers were mentioned about one-third as often as acceptable counselors on death.)

The survey was designed to provide answers to five sets of questions:

1. *What is the everyday significance of death?* How frequently do people think about death? At what stage in the life cycle does death become an important concern? Under what kinds of circumstances are people led to think about death?

2. *What is the image of death?* What kinds of images of death do people have? Do these images tend to involve only the self? Or others as well? Is the imagery morbid or reassuring?

3. *Do people make plans about death?* To what extent are people inclined to avoid the "problem" of death? To what extent are they motivated to make plans in anticipation of death? What kinds of plans do they make? What kinds of people make what kinds of plans?

4. *How do people differ in their attitudes toward death?* Are there

differences between young and old? Men and women? Well educated and the less educated? And so on.

5. *Is the taboo on talking about death changing?* What kinds of evidence, if any, indicate changes in the public's definition of death? Is concern with death increasing or declining? Are people more concerned with the personal problems of death? Or with the problems that death creates for survivors?

We shall consider briefly each of these questions.

The Everyday Significance of Death

Throughout our studies we have tried to learn something of the extent to which thoughts of death intrude upon the everyday lives of people. It is relatively infrequent. In contrast to three out of four Americans who say that they think often about current money problems or health, only one in three reports that he thinks as often about the uncertainty of life and death (see Table 1).

In contrast, a surprising result has to do, not so much with people's

TABLE 1
Frequency of Thoughts About Death and Other Problems

THE QUESTION: *"How often do you think about (a) your own or family's health? (b) your present financial situation or responsibilities? (c) the world situation and threat of war? (d) your future financial situation or responsibilities? (e) the uncertainty of your own life or the death of someone close to you? Do you think about this quite often, only occasionally, or hardly ever?"*

PROBLEM	OFTEN	OCCA-SIONALLY	HARDLY EVER OR NEVER
Your own or family's health	76	20	4
Your present financial situation or responsibilities	74	21	5
Your future financial situation or responsibilities	60	31	9
The world situation or threat of war	50	38	12
The uncertainty of your own life or the death of someone close to you	32	36	32

$(N = 1482)$

tendency to inhibit *thoughts* of death, as with their willingness to *talk* about them. Thus, in a preliminary study in which skilled field interviewers talked at length with a small sample of adults from all walks of life, only one interview in fifty had to be broken off because the subject proved too painful to endure, and this turned out to be a case of one who had experienced a sudden and grievous bereavement. The interviews lasted from two to three hours with people being encouraged to talk about death in all its aspects. Almost without exception, the interviewers reported that people, typically toward the end of the discussions, expressed feelings of relief, almost as though some load of unexpressed anxiety had been lifted from them.

A result consistent with this observation lies in a comparison of answers to two questions asked of the national sample: *"When do you imagine people think most about death—as young children, as teenagers, in their middle years, or in their later years?"* and *"How about yourself? When would you probably think most about death?"*

Although individuals report that they would be most likely to think about death at their own age, there is a strong tendency for them to believe that *others* think about death mainly in the later years. Thus people seem to be quite willing to admit that death is not a complete stranger to their thoughts.

Nor is this unrelated to answers to the following question: *"Under what circumstances are you most likely to think about death?"*

The interesting finding here is that thoughts of death tend to be triggered by external events. Few people report that they think frequently about death in connection with family plans, as a consequence of religious activity or belief, or as a threat to financial status. Rather, the overwhelming majority report that they are stimulated to think about death under three deeply personal circumstances: an accident or a "near-miss," a serious illness, or the death of someone significant to them.

In short, people typically tend to think about death as a consequence of death-related experiences that impinge directly upon them.

Images of Death

Turning next to images of death, the survey suggests that, while people may not preoccupy themselves with thoughts of death, they

TABLE 2
Images of Death

THE QUESTION: *"People's beliefs and attitudes toward death are, of course, quite varied. I'll read you a few statements, and you tell me whether you agree or disagree with each one."*

STATEMENT	PER CENT WHO AGREE
Death is like a long sleep	54
To die is to suffer	14
Death is not tragic for the person who dies, only for the survivors	82
Death always comes too soon	53
Death is sometimes a blessing	89
	($N = 1482$)

do nevertheless carry about with them various images of death. Table 2 shows the relative importance of images as reported by the sample.

For some, death epitomizes a release from activity—"Death is like a long sleep"—an image that is particularly common among the disadvantaged and less well-educated. For large majorities at all socioeconomic levels, however, death assumes quite a different image as an event to be reckoned with, a reality that must be explained, and, if possible, excused. Thus, nine out of ten adult Americans agree that "Death is sometimes a blessing," and almost the same proportion believe that "Death is not tragic for the person who dies, only for the survivors." Indeed, once encouraged to do so, most Americans are inclined to be quite expressive on the subject.

In reply to the question: *"What is it that first comes to your mind when you think of death?"* people are far more likely to express concern for others than they are for themselves. Thus, for every person who thinks morbidly of such things as "the cold ground," or "the horror of accident," there are eight who express worry about the future of their families or how their "loved ones" will "get along." This concern for others bears a strong relationship to socioeconomic status. The lower the status, the greater the concern for self; the higher the status, the greater the concern for others. It is almost as if they said, "If you have lived a good life, death poses no threat."

Two other images are of particular theoretical interest. Throughout most of human history the tragedy of death has been closely identified with the suffering that often accompanied dying and the anxiety of dying at an early age. During the past century, however, Americans have been moving away from a human condition in which these twin threats were grim but constant companions in everyday life—moving toward a mode of life in which both physical suffering and the incidence of early death have been reduced. (Witness the remarkable pharmacological developments in medicine and the striking changes in tables of life expectancy.)

The survey findings offer some insight into modern man's response to these threats. Relatively few Americans, nowadays, identify death with suffering, and this fact is related not only to medical advances but also to social change. For example, the higher the person's educational attainment, the less apt he is to make this connection. Thus, those with only a grade school education are more than three times as likely as those with a college education to believe that death and suffering go together. Furthermore, education makes a difference at every age level.

As for premature death, this image is held by little over one-half of all American adults. And, like suffering, this belief tends to be more typical of the poorly educated. Pessimistic thoughts of impending personal calamity seem to be characteristic of the poor and disadvantaged.

Do People Make Plans About Death?

Apart from questions having to do with the images of death and its significance, questions were asked concerning the steps people take in anticipation of death.

The issue was first posed in the abstract: *"Do you feel it's best to ignore the subject (of death) and not to try to make any kind of plans for when that time comes, or do you feel it's best to try to make some plans about death?"*

Our expectation, based upon hunches about the pervasiveness of the death taboo, had been that many people would admit to a reluctance to make plans. It was, consequently, of considerable interest, when over 80 per cent replied that they thought it was better to make some plans about death. And when people were encouraged in follow-up questions to talk about different ways in which to cope with the uncertainty of life, it turned out that:

1. One out of every four adults reported having made a will.
2. About the same proportion said that they had made some kind of funeral or cemetery arrangements.
3. Just about one-half said that they had made a point of talking about death with those closest to them.
4. And over 70 per cent reported that they had purchased some form of life insurance.

With the exception of the purchase of life insurance—the incidence of which has not changed markedly over recent decades—there are no very good trend data on the plans that people make in anticipation of death.

Individual Difference in Attitudes

We have alluded to differences in the beliefs and attitudes toward death according to individual characteristics. His age, sex, family status, and education all seem to be related to a person's view of death and to the approach he adopts in planning for it. Among these, education and age appear to affect his perceptions and attitudes most.

Within each age category, the higher the educational level, the less likely are people to feel threatened by death. Just as the poorly educated view death often as an almost welcome release from activity, they are also more likely than their educated counterparts to think often about the uncertainty of their own or another's life. They are somewhat more likely to think about death at their present age, suggestive perhaps of a more immediate concern with death. Nor is this educational difference restricted to thoughts about death; the less well-educated are also comparatively more preoccupied with matters of health and finances. Only on the topic of the world situation and the threat of war are the better-educated more likely to show concern. In thinking about death, the less well-educated tend to focus more on self, the better-educated being more concerned with others.

Contrary to popular speculation, a person's age seems less clearly related than his education to his view of death. Older people are a little more likely than younger to agree that "Death is like a long sleep," or that "Death is sometimes a blessing"; but there is little indication that such attitudes constitute a general set of views which change with age and which condone a passive acceptance of death. Although older people may think somewhat more often about the uncertainty of life, there is no consistent tendency for personal worries to increase with age.

If the better-educated are less prone toward passive acceptance than the less well-educated in their view of death, and less preoccupied with it, they are typically *more* active in the actions and plans they take in approaching death. As we have noted, larger proportions of them report having purchased life insurance, made a will, and talked about death with those closest to them. More of them disavow the idea that one should ignore death or avoid making plans. One finding was particularly striking: older Americans take a more active approach toward death than younger Americans on all such counts. Thus, by and large, the better-educated and the older persons are more likely to take positive action in regard to death.

Such tendencies in the data fit into our sociological understanding

TABLE 3*
Age and Images of Death

STATEMENT	PER CENT WHO AGREE WITH EACH STATEMENT:				
	AGE 30 AND UNDER	AGE 31–40	AGE 41–50	AGE 51–60	AGE 61+
Death is sometimes a blessing	88	88	86	92	91
Death is not tragic for the person who dies, only for the survivors	78	81	83	84	85
Death is like a long sleep	46	54	53	64	62
Death always comes too soon	51	45	65	60	51
To die is to suffer	13	10	13	18	18
Total respondents = 100%	(348)	(389)	(280)	(211)	(249)

* See M. W. Riley, A. Foner, and associates, *Aging and Society: An Inventory of Research Findings* (New York: Russell Sage Foundation, 1968), I, 330 ff., for a detailed analysis of these materials by age.

of the roles played by people occupying differing positions in society. Thus, perceptions of death and anxieties about it seem to fit the broad pattern of mental health, in which the better-educated are generally favored. The approach to death appears as just another element in the individual's approach to life in which the better-educated are in general active, the less well-educated, passive. At the same time, the findings raise further questions. How, for example, can we reconcile the finding of an active orientation among older people with prevailing views of the passivity of the aged? Is the prevailing view largely a distortion arising from the preponderance of poorly educated in the generations recently past? And, if so, does this mean that increasing education in the future will mark an increasingly active adaptation to death, a decrease in anxiety, and an increase in realistic planning for death?

Is the Taboo on Death Changing?

Two lines of research evidence support the notion that the meaning of death in contemporary America may be changing and that the taboo on the topic is being relaxed. In the first place, as this volume attests, there has been lively debate in the medical fraternity as to how to define death and how to deal with it. In both medical and theological circles, there is a growing concern with the individual's "right" to die with dignity. There is heightened interest among basic scientists in the possibility of manipulating the genetic code and in the questions that this would pose for "the politics of creation." There is increasing attention being paid to death in the arts and in the mass media. And social scientists are showing a new interest in the relationship of death to the social structure as well as in the problems of bereavement.

The second line of evidence emerges from the empirical research that has been reported in this chapter. To the extent that the elimination of suffering and prematurity may permit a less threatening view of death, we may be on the verge of developing new attitudes and beliefs. Two aspects of possible change seem clear: one, individual; the other, social or interpersonal. For the individual, these data strongly suggest that death is feared because it will cut short the achievement of goals upon which current self-esteem depends. In this view, death is not denied; rather, it is seen as a threat to the activity of life. The individual with such a view is expressing less a fear of death than he is of being "caught short." If death is not premature, it can be seen as an event characterized by personal fulfillment and individual dignity. In contrast, from the social point of view, the data emphasize not so much the threat that death poses for the individual and his own identity, as the problems that death will create for his survivors. And here the evidence of concern is clear. In contemporary American society, concern with death prompts people to think of others far more often than it provokes anxiety about self.

REFERENCES

Blauner, Robert.
    1966   "Death and social structure." Psychiatry 29:378–394.
Feifel, Herman (ed.).
    1959   The Meaning of Death. New York: McGraw-Hill.
Fulton, Robert L. (ed.).
    1965   Death and Identity. New York: Wiley.
Glaser, Barney, and Anselm Strauss.
    1965   Awareness of Dying: A Study of Social Interaction. Chicago: Aldine.
Kalish, Richard A.
    1965   "Death and bereavement: a bibliography." Journal of Human Relations 13:118–141.
Moore, Wilbert E.
    1963   Man, Time, and Society. New York: Wiley.
Parsons, Talcott, and Victor Lidz.
    1967   "Death in American society." Pp. 133–170 in Edwin S. Shneidman (ed.), Essays in Self-Destruction. New York: Science House.
Riley, John W., Jr.
    1968a   "Death and bereavement." International Encyclopedia of the Social Sciences. New York: Free Press.
    1968b   "Old age in American society: notes on health, retirement and the anticipation of death." The Journal of the American Society of Chartered Life Underwriters. 22:27–32.
Riley, Matilda White, Anne Foner, and associates.
    1968   Aging and Society. New York: Russell Sage.
Sudnow, David.
    1967   Passing On. Englewood Cliffs, N.J.: Prentice Hall.

3

Cultural Beliefs on Life and Death

*Andie L. Knutson**

IN DEATH MAN experiences the most awesome unknown. Since primitive times he has been at once frightened and challenged by death and has engaged in a continuous search to understand it and to find means of adapting to it or controlling it. Lacking any personal evidence as to what occurs in death, he has been limited to individual and group observations of what happens in others. His interpretations have been guided by his beliefs, ethical values, and attitudes; his hopes, wants, and desires; his fears, doubts, and uncertainties. From his personal and group projections of life after death have emerged the most imaginative contributions of humanity.

The very existence of death as an empirical unknown, urgent in its demands, has served to stimulate some of man's greatest creative efforts. The richness of our culture as expressed in philosophies, religions, literature, science, and the arts is in good part a product of projections of human experiences into descriptions, chartings, and interpretations of death. This creative effort has been focused on attempts to control life itself through construction of social rules designed to influence or control death and the events assumed to occur after death.

It would be negligent to discuss beliefs, ethical values, and attitudes related to death without noting that even in this modern scientific world our knowledge of death remains projective in its origins;

* This investigation was supported by Public Health Service Research Career Program Award (Number K3–MH–20976). Joe Ballonn served as research assistant on the analysis of personal research mentioned.

the extent to which those projections permeate our culture and the cultures of other societies appears to be limitless.

An End or a Beginning?

Many conceptual themes have emerged from these efforts to understand the meaning of death. In our society death is viewed as the end of life or as the beginning of eternal life; as the time that life's books are closed or the time that life's books are opened for eternal judgment; as the time all is past, or the time the past is evaluated; as an avenue of escape or the beginning of dreaded uncertainties; as a final separation or a lasting reunion; as the object of an instinctual wish, or as an object of instinctual terror (Feifel, 1959; Lester, 1967). Or death may be viewed as the ultimate harmony of man and nature or the defeat of man by nature and the failure of man in his attempts to challenge nature (Howard and Scott, 1965/66:162).

As these themes suggest, Western society tends to dichotomize life and death. The transition from life to death tends to be viewed as abrupt, final, and irreversible. How different this is from the early Greeks who reported the coming and going of the gods and the visits of the living to the land of the dead. How different from the Buddhist concept of life as continuous, with death viewed as the time the soul migrates from one form of life to another, perhaps one day to return in a new human birth. How different from the Shinto concept of death as joining one's ancestors, who retain a consultant role with the living. And how different from the gradual patterns of change that are observed in many patients during senescence.

The meaning of death is tied to the meaning of life, for without life there would be no death; without death, life would be continuous, with neither termination nor change into a new pattern of existence. Even those who believe in an afterlife or in the continuity of life in other forms through transmigration experience the shock of death and recognize death as a psychological fact, for death is an inevitable crisis for all human life. It is not only a crisis for the dying individual but also for those about him, the family, social group, and society. The shock experience of death is tied in part at least to the disorder of routine relationships as well as the destruction of intimate ties. All societies have developed ways of interpreting death for their members and rituals to assist in the neutralization of the occurring shock. We do not yet know which of the many philosophical and religious interpretations employed best prepares the dying man and his associates for approaching this unknown.

Criteria of Death

Definitions of death are of considerable significance for an understanding of attitudes about death, for once an individual has been defined as dead, by whatever definition employed, the attitudes toward the person may be expected to change. By formal and common law and by professional ethical standards, the treatment due living persons differs markedly from that accorded the dead.

In our society the criteria usually employed for judging the termination of vital functioning include the cessation of breathing, heartbeat, pulse, or other autonomic and voluntary responses; the onset of rigor mortis; or evidence of the beginning of decomposition. Since necrosis may occur in some vital organs prior to the satisfaction of even the earliest of such criteria, the use of these measures has been judged inadequate from the standpoint of transmission of certain vital organs. Brain death as a criterion is under test and may serve the purpose. There are still questions regarding its validity, however, since brain death may precede the cessation of breathing or heartbeat (Knutson, 1968a).

Other definitions of death are employed. Sudnow (1967:65) distinguishes between "clinical death," the appearance of death signs upon physical examination; "biological death," the cessation of cellular activity, and "social death," the point at which a hospital patient is accorded treatment essentially as a corpse, though still alive.

Kalish (1968) employs the term "psychological death" to define the status of a patient who ceases to be aware of his own existence and the term "anthropological death" to refer to one who, like a traitor, has been rejected and cut off from his community. The term "civil death" was formerly used in England as a legal expression for one who left the realm or was incarcerated and thus lost his civil rights.

The above definitions all emphasize the degree to which the individual concerned is treated by observers as human. They parallel definitions held regarding a new human life and qualities that make it human during the developmental stages (Knutson, 1967a and 1967b). Attitudes toward an individual may be expected to change as he becomes more or less human in the mind of the observer, whether this occurs in the beginning of life or during some later phase in life.

Social Research on Death

Death as an area of study by social scientists has only recently broken loose from its taboo status. Although the fear of death has been recognized as a researchable topic since 1896, relatively little study of this important issue has been conducted prior to the past two decades (Scott, 1896; Lester, 1967). In the absence of systematic research evidence gathered from dying individuals and persons involved in the death setting, we have been obliged to lean on the observations of philosophers, theologians, clinicians, poets, writers, and artists for an understanding and an interpretation of the universal experience of personal death.

Suicide, murder, and, to a lesser degree, capital punishment, war, disaster, and accidents as modes of death have received considerably more attention from social scientists than death under more natural circumstances (Lester, 1967; Williams, 1966). One can only conjecture the reasons for this disproportional attention given to nonnormative patterns of death. In part, it may reflect the greater freedom of sociological entree to data from statistical sources and the availability of statistical tools. In working with statistical data the researcher may be less dependent upon others and the beliefs, ethical values, and attitudes of others may govern his work less directly, even though they do influence the quality of his data and the support for his work. One must recognize, however, that the social scientist who works with statistical data is himself socially and psychologically removed from his content. The direct experience of death is kept at arm's length. This does not apply, of course, to the psychological autopsies of suicides and other depth studies of recent years (Shneidman, 1963:33).

Suicide and murder are taboo in Western society. Is it more ethical to give attention to these experiences than to more normal ones? Or do these more dramatic forms of death offer special challenges for the researcher and his sponsor? Does the fact that these deaths may be reduced provide a special incentive for the researcher?

Feifel, who deserves major credit for bringing to attention the importance of studying death, experienced many difficulties in gaining the support of administrators and physicians for his investigations. At first he was asked: "Isn't it cruel, sadistic, and traumatic to discuss death with seriously ill and terminally ill people?" (Feifel, 1963:9). This legitimate question was answered by evidence that interviews with terminal patients tended to be supportive rather than destructive. Patients thanked Feifel for the opportunity to examine their feelings about death; most expressed the desire to be informed about their condition; some said discussions helped them to adjust to the experience of death. He learned that "realization of possible death seems to give permission, even freedom, to some to be themselves rather than extensions or mirrors of other people's values" (Feifel, 1963:11).

The frustrating and irritating blocks placed in Feifel's way as he attempted to extend his research, together with the administrative vetoes received in various medical settings, led him to realize "that death is a dark symbol not to be stirred, even touched—an obscenity to be avoided."

Although publication of Feifel's collaborative work, *The Meaning of Death* (1959), was certainly an important stimulus to the study of death, Feifel was in some ways a product of the times. The development of training and research programs in the social sciences occurring since the mid-1950's helped to stimulate the investigation of hitherto prohibited areas of society. The increased support of social science research and training by foundations and universities, the growth in medical research and training supported by the National Institutes of Health, and in particular the training of social scientists and mental health specialists, have helped to give impetus to a concern for the emotional behavior of patients. The shift in the predominant pattern of morbidity and mortality from acute infections to chronic conditions with slow patterns of death, together with a growing sensitivity of our society to the process of aging, has brought into focus the importance of maintaining an awareness of the problems of the dying patient. Communicating about death has become significant for more professional people; the moral issues involved are being opened to critical review.

Younger as well as older scientists are giving attention to death and dying and the number of studies under way is increasing rapidly (Kalish and Kastenbaum, 1968). Yet the taboos remain strong emotional barriers to effective investigations; investigators often find their paths blocked and meet with frustration in the search for empirical evidence.

The Loss of Self-Control

In our society death is no longer a common experience for children and youth, except, perhaps, in rural areas or under conditions of poverty where crowding is excessive and hospital care is not available or is not perceived to be available. Deaths now usually occur in hospitals or other community facilities, in settings considerably removed from children or young adults.

Where people die tends to be determined by who has control over their lives at the time, unless death is sudden and unexpected. The person who maintains an awareness of his status and social control over his behavior may choose to die at home or in the hospital, as he sees fit. People who are unaware of impending death or too debilitated to make such decisions for themselves are likely to die in places determined by members of the family, friends, the physician, nurse, or other professionals involved (Glaser and Strauss, 1965:6).

Many people lose control over where they die because prior to death they give up the right to govern their own lives—or have it taken from them. For example, they may join the military forces, or a religious or other closed social group; they may become charges of the courts or of the police and lack freedom of movement. When moving into housing developments for senior citizens, nursing homes, or centers for the aged, they may arrange in advance for terminal care.

When death of an older, absent member of the family does occur, this death is not as realistic for the child or youngster as a death immediately present. It is likely that this older person is one with whom the child has had less association and identification. His death from senility or from a chronic condition occurs gradually and is accepted by degrees during a period of separation and disassociation. The shock of death may thus be softened for those at home.

Depersonalization of Death

While direct exposure of children and youth to death tends to be decreasing, death has been given considerable, usually very unrealistic, attention by television, radio, newspapers, magazines, movies, and comic books. Punishment, revenge, violence, and torture are often highlighted in westerns, mysteries, adventure stories, superspy escapades, and in war stories that dramatize thrills, glamor, and romance. The patterns of dying presented in such stories show little semblance to what occurs under normal conditions of life.

More recently, on-the-scene television has brought into the family realistic presentations of death as it occurs on the battlefield, during disaster, in fires and floods, or in accidents. Major news figures have met death before the television cameras. Yet, these are abnormal death scenes. We have yet to observe on television the slow, drawn-out suffering of a terminal patient, or the disintegration of the personality during senility. Thus, even today, with our added means of mass communication, society remains protected from direct association with one of its most common experiences.

In our society we appear to have developed a wide range of defenses to protect ourselves personally and as a group against injury from the loss of a valued life. The avoidance of the topic of death in conversation, discussion, and in research may itself serve as one of these defenses. The pattern of facilities developed for dealing with the sick and aged reinforces a person's gradual withdrawal or disengagement during the period of debilitation. In this way the socially traumatic experience associated with death may be avoided. Although extended care facilities were certainly not intended for this purpose, they nevertheless serve as one means by which society disassociates itself from the problems of death and dying.

One should note that this way of life is dramatically different from that which existed in both urban and rural life until a few decades ago. In earlier American society death tended to be a family affair; the dying person was the center of attention for the family in many groups. In interviews with persons regarding their early life and death experiences, a number expressed concern with the changes that have occurred. Some told of early experiences in which the family was not able to be in attendance with the dying person who was away in a hospital or rest home. Their parents felt guilty and expressed concern that they could not be present, attentive, and helpful to a dying relative some distance away.

The Professional Viewpoint

Medical and health professionals tend to come from middle-class American society. We do not know how their early life experiences differ from those of other members of the society, but data obtained from some health professionals suggest that their exposure to death prior to professional training was very limited indeed (Knutson, 1968b).

About half of 124 health professionals recalled seeing a dead body before entering high school and three-fourths prior to college or professional training. Thirty per cent reported being in a home when someone died and 15 per cent witnessed someone's death prior to entering college or professional training. Those who witnessed death were more likely to have done so outside the home, as in an accident, than in the home. Very few had been in the presence of a person during the last moments of a natural death.

With respect to these early exposures to death physicians and nurses do not appear to differ from their professional colleagues. Most of the physicians and nurses in one group of seventy-six professionals interviewed said that they first witnessed death during medical training; for a number of physicians, first exposure to a dead body was on the autopsy table in a medical school. For some who had never had an intimate friend or member of the family die, death seemed to be an impersonal experience.

When the subject of death was openly talked about at home, the focus tended to be on religion and particularly the rewards for morality and the punishments for ill behavior. In many families death remained a hush-hush experience; children were protected from it during the earlier years of life; in very few families was death discussed objectively without moral implications.

Subjects who had seen dead bodies during childhood or youth tended to have this experience at funerals or wakes, and there appears to be a tendency for those of more conservative and fundamentalist religious families to have had this experience earlier, some as early as five or six years of age. The recollection of subjects ranged from "Funerals and wakes were horrible experiences" to "I used to look forward to wakes. They were so much fun."

Protecting younger children from the experience of death is probably the modal pattern of our society. Yet, in some groups, special efforts are made to assure that children are fully exposed to the death experience, are brought to view and talk to the dying person shortly before death, or gather around at the time of expiration. We recognize the need of a dying individual and his family for support and consolation, and attempt to be with dying friends or relatives in distant hospitals or institutional settings at considerable personal cost.

Discrimination and Value Judgments

Throughout human history there has been a tendency to define and evaluate individuals differentially in terms of position, status, role, and other distinctive characteristics. Members of one's own group are defined in ways different from nonmembers; enemies and traitors may be viewed with contempt. Slaves and other persons of low caste or status have often been treated in a degrading manner; persons suffering from strange disorders or diseases that are not understood have been judged dangerous, unclean, or unworthy of respect. Harsh treatment has been accorded persons with behavior judged immoral—drunkenness, drug addiction, attempted suicide, crime, unwed motherhood, bastardy, and other deviants from the accepted values of the group.

People also differ in their judgments regarding the relative worth of human life according to such factors as the stage in development, years of maturity, patterns of decline during aging, socioeconomic status, ethnic group identification, social roles performed, statuses held, or others.

Health and medical professionals must make judgments that involve the relative worth of one life as compared with another. In war, civil defense, disaster, epidemics, and mass starvation, decisions of emergency treatment directly involve one life or group of lives as compared with another life or group of lives. Physicians also make decisions of this type on more individual bases. They may have to decide whether to save a mother or child in hazardous childbirth; when to employ heroic efforts to save or prolong the lives of critically ill patients, of premature babies, defectives, or terminal patients; when to use equipment or heroics to extend lives when facilities and staff are limited. Often, the individual most likely to profit or most worthy of service must be selected.

Sudnow (1967) and others report instances in which efforts to save lives appeared directly related to social status and moral characteristics as evidenced by intoxication, drug addiction, suicidal tendencies, or criminal attempts. The very elderly as compared with youth and children tend to be less likely to receive strenuous, heroic efforts on the part of the medical staff when they enter the hospital in critical condition. Those judged to be of improper moral character may be treated with disgust, and are less likely to receive the extra efforts necessary for the prolongation of life.

Choices involving human survival have far-reaching implications for society. A choice may have to be made between a major effort to save the life of one person in the community by means of clinical intervention and long-term therapeutic support, or saving the lives of a group of persons who are farther away physically and psychologically, but dying for lack of adequate food, water, or sanitation. In this situation, the high emotional appeal of the dying member of one's own group may lead to giving priority to one life over the lives of several who may be dying in a sociologically distant ghetto a mile away or dying from starvation three thousand miles away.

Who Shall Be Saved?

These decisions are most difficult for health professionals to make, or even to talk about. In one study, public health professionals were asked: "In case of an epidemic in your society, who should be taken care of first in the family, in the community, in society? If, in your community, a serious long-term state of starvation occurred, who should be given the last food available in the family, in the community, in society? In case of a disaster or major emergency in your community, who should be given priority in rescue-saving efforts?" Some professionals respond to these questions with emotion and attempt to avoid specific answers. They say they feel uncomfortable; all those needing help should be helped. The idea of saving some persons before others appears to be a disturbing issue that ought not even to be openly discussed. Our ethical values appear to make one feel guilty even to *say* that one person should be judged as more valuable than another (Knutson, 1968a).

Some respondents question the ability and the right of man to play God, and say, "It is the kind of decision God should make." These persons may urge the use of a purely random procedure of selection once potential candidates for service have been identified. The random procedure avoids the trauma involved in making explicit the decisions that must be made on matters of survival or death, but it implies the complete absence of any agreement in our society on the relative value of different human beings.

Yet members of the health professions *do* make—and *must* make—decisions on issues concerned with epidemics, starvation, and disaster. These decisions *do* involve choices about the relative worth of people. They are decisions directly concerning the nature of the composition of our future population. Is it better to make these decisions on the basis of a careful weighing of alternatives? Or in the excitement of an emergency and without preparation (Knutson, 1968c)?

The discomfort of health professionals with these social responsibilities for judging the worth of other persons is further revealed by their responses to the question: "Who has the right to make decisions regarding the continuing of or ending of a human life after it has grown up?" Alternatives employed to obtain judgments on this question were developed on the basis of responses obtained during an exploratory interview. Subjects were given an opportunity to rank their responses and 19 per cent gave more than one answer (Knutson, 1968a).

Only 11 per cent of the public health professionals believe the physician has the right to decide whether to continue or to end a mature human life; 19 per cent assign that right to spouse or other responsible survivors; and 22 per cent believe society through its leaders has that right. The great majority say that only the individual himself has that right (49 per cent), that only God has that right (30 per cent), or that no one has that right (29 per cent).

Responses suggest that the physician who acts on his own prerogative or even with the approval of responsible survivors in deciding whether to continue or to end a mature human life is acting counter to the ethical judgments of most of his professional colleagues. One must recognize that these health professionals are stating a general position that may be at variance with the positions they might take in a specific critical situation with unforeseen or unconsidered conditions and alternatives.

Do these responses reflect the tough- or tender-mindedness of respondents? Some may be indicating their judgments about who has a right to terminate a life; the responses of others may reflect what one ought to say about it.

These subjects were asked: "Often we must make judgments concerning the relative value of one human life as compared with another human life. In making such judgments of value, which one of the following criteria do you consider the most significant? Which one do you consider next most significant?" When first and second choices are combined, almost three-fourths of the respondents consider service to mankind or service to society as the significant criterion. Of lesser significance was service to one's family or intimate group (33 per cent), service to God (20 per cent), and the personal achievements of the individual (19 per cent). Less than 1 per cent of the respondents regarded either contributions to one's country, political ideology, or service to one's religion per se as being significant criteria for judging the relative value of a human life.

This finding is interesting in view of the range of variation of the sample in terms of age, sex, marital and parental status, education, profession, religion, and experience. It suggests that public health professionals are in considerable agreement on broad criteria to employ in judging the relative worth of one human life as compared with others.

One must recognize that a person who is somewhat obliged to rank alternatives from a preselected list is perhaps responding in terms of what he feels he "ought to say" with these alternatives before him. The response may have little bearing on how he would act or what action he would approve on his own volition in an undefined setting without preparation or alternatives in mind. In that undefined and possibly unexpected situation requiring immediate action, will he recognize that a decision involving a choice between human lives is present? Will he be aware that such a choice is being made either explicitly and openly or implicitly and without dialogue? Will he be sensitive to the full range of alternatives actually present or possible? Or will issues like these create such feelings of conflict, discomfort, and guilt that he will be immobilized and a choice of one person's life and another person's death will be made by default?

Research on attitudes toward dying persons is one area in which taboos have been particularly strong, as suggested earlier, since such research may be viewed as threatening by the subjects whose beliefs, ethical values, attitudes, and behaviors are being evaluated. The research is further complicated by the importance of taking into consideration a wide range of complex variables: the general characteristics and conditions of the society at the time of study, the specific situation in which the persons are dying, the characteristics of dying persons and those attending them, the type of illness or mode of death and its social meanings, the types of control over death that may be possible, and so on. Unique problems of sampling and measurement will need attention in order to achieve the results necessary for a better understanding of this significant issue.

Fear of Dying

Attitudes toward death as a relatively new acceptable area of research have yet to reach a level of quality or a productive peak. Lester (1967), in a review of the literature, draws special attention to the paucity of systematic conceptualization, systematic sampling, new methods, or the standardization of approaches used. Williams (1966) notes particularly a paucity of new ideas and of the full development through study of good ideas previously explored. Narrow approaches have tended to be the mode: "Psychoanalysts have worked like moles, hardly interested in what goes on above ground, and sociologists, surveying the earth with their measuring apparatus, have hardly noticed the tremors from below" (Williams, 1966:422). Improvements are noted in research currently in progress.

The major focus of research reviewed by Lester has been the fear of death. Although this involves fear of one's own death, fear of the death of others, and fear of the effects of death (Becker and Bruner,

1931:27; Lester, 1967), investigators have failed to distinguish between these alternatives.

Lacking also are measures of attitudes toward death as compared to other life experiences and orientations. Perhaps few people judge their own lives of greater value than some other life or lives, or of greater value than certain beliefs, values, and loyalties or opportunities for experience. One would guess that the fear of dying or death is not often uppermost in the minds of most people, and when it is, as Jung (1934) has noted, it is suggestive of mental illness. Our orientation tends to be defensive: We view death as something that happens to others and not something that inevitably will happen to ourselves.

Studies of the relationship of attitudes toward death to age, sex, residence, marital status, health, and activity yield conflicting evidence, perhaps reflecting the wide variety of subjects used and the lack of representative sampling. The better-designed studies suggest that in general demographic variables have little effect on the attitudes of mature persons regarding death. "It would seem that personality factors and life experiences are the important determinants of the fear of death" (Lester, 1967:31).

A somewhat similar state of ambiguity prevails with respect to such variables as anxiety, psychopathology, and religious orientation. The studies of religion, for example, yield conflicting evidence depending upon the instruments used and populations studied. Religious belief does not seem to "affect the intensity of the fear of death, but rather channels the fear onto the specific problems that each religion proposes" (Lester, 1967:33).

Little attention thus far has been given to one's own experiences with death as related to his attitude under conditions of physical illness, accidents, death of a family member, early exposure to death in childhood, nearness to a catastrophe, and roles that lead one into settings where death occurs. Nor has much attention been given to some of the consequences of religious orientations, particularly belief in a God, belief in an afterlife, the concept of and belief in a human soul, expectations regarding the manner of disposal of one's remains, and beliefs regarding the sanctity of the body after death.

As research progresses, one would expect consideration to be given to the attitudes toward types or modes of death other than suicide, murder, and capital punishment. How does one view death while suffering from starvation, or faced with disaster, accident, war, crime, defense, punishment, or experimentation? As one takes risks in behalf of his country, his religion, his ideals, his personal honor, or for the mere sport and thrill of the experience, does he think of death as the possible consequence and fear this consequence? Needed are studies of attitudes toward dying in different situations and under varying conditions of status, responsibility, role, and concern.

The roles and responsibilities of members of the health and medical professions lead them to a major exposure in areas concerning death. Their viewpoints, only recently coming under study, may be of high significance to society. Feifel (1963:15) has posed the hypothesis that certain physicians enter medicine "to govern their own above-average fears concerning death. A study I have just completed on the attitudes of forty physicians toward death indicates that, though physicians think *less* about death than do two control groups of patients and one of nonprofessionals, they are *more afraid* of death than any of the control groups." His limited study deals with the attitudes of physicians after their experiences with death, rather than at the time they choose their professions. The issue posed is interesting, but his hypothesis still lacks rigorous investigation.

The Dead Body

How are bodies treated after death? Who owns the body after death? Is the body sacred? Did the person have a soul and when does this soul leave the body? What happens to the soul? To what extent is the status and value of a person while living transmitted to his body when he dies? The beliefs, ethical values, and attitudes regarding dead bodies have been of high significance to development of science, medicine, and the arts, for, historically, opposition to autopsies, dissections, and other uses of the body has been associated with religious concerns.

Throughout history there have been periods when autopsies or dissections have been permitted, followed by periods in which religious opinion has held sway and all dissections have been discontinued. Dissections may have been conducted in Egypt as early as 4000 B.C.; a treatise on anatomic investigations was written about 1600 B.C.

Rabbis in Babylonia and the Greeks of the Alexandria School at the time of Aristotle are reported to have conducted dissections. Prior to this period dissections were reportedly carried out in China, but discontinued at the time of Confucius. In ancient India, dissections were apparently opposed on religious grounds (Jakobovits, 1959: Chap. 12; Saphir, 1938).

In each of the above situations in which dissections were permitted, actions were later taken to discontinue the practice on the basis of religious grounds. Offenses to the body are prohibited by the Talmud and by the Koran and there have been various Christian edicts against autopsies or dissections. Over time, adaptations have been made by all three groups to permit autopsies or dissections under certain circumstances. It is of interest that at times, for each of these groups, edicts have favored the dissection of members of other religions than their own. The Koran, for example, while explicitly prohibiting the opening of corpses in Turkish, Persian, or other Muslim universities, was amended to permit the dissection of Jewish and Christian bodies; rabbis ruled that the ban on dissections need not apply to bodies of non-Jews under certain circumstances; and at Padua students specifically requested Jewish bodies for dissections since the Jewish practice of early burial assured fresh bodies. Bodies of other nonstatus persons have been approved for dissections even when such practices were not permitted for members of one's own group. The early Jews, for example, permitted prostitutes' bodies to be boiled to facilitate the study of flesh and bones; Cleopatra gave bodies of her slaves to the king for study; in fourteenth-century France the study of anatomy was largely limited to the use of criminal bodies. In recent history, general practice has been to approve the use of unclaimed bodies for dissection (Jakobovits, 1959).

With the growth of medical schools and research centers has come an increasing demand for human bodies for teaching, demonstration, and research purposes. Through research many new uses for body parts have been developed and methods for preserving them in body banks for future use have proved effective (viz., blood, eye, bone, and kidney banks).

The right of possession for purposes of legal disposition of a body generally rests with the surviving spouse, children, or other next of kin. Consent of this person is legally required for autopsy, although the coroner or legal examiner may take legal custody under certain circumstances to perform an autopsy to determine the cause of death. The right to perform an autopsy, whether granted or legally required, does not include the right to retain body parts. A specific authorization from the deceased during his lifetime or from the survivor is required for this action.

One study suggests that health professionals vary considerably in the ethical positions they hold regarding autopsies; exploratory operations; the use of bodies for study, teaching, display, or scientific research; and the removal of body parts or blood for use by others. Many hold ethical positions at variance with current laws which require the consent of the individual or a survivor except for legally required autopsies (Knutson, 1968a).

From 8 to 29 per cent of the health professionals consider one or more of these practices to be almost always ethical. "Performing an autopsy" receives highest acceptance and "the removal of body parts for display in teaching" and "performing a scientific experiment on the body" receive lowest acceptance. They generally agree, however, that all these practices are judged usually ethical with the consent of the person himself and/or consent of a responsible survivor.

These health professionals do not agree on the philosophical and religious issue concerning the sanctity of the body after death. About 10 per cent believe the body belongs to God and is sacred; 43 per cent, that the body itself, while not sacred, should be respected; 28 per cent, that the body itself has no meaning or value but the person who once occupied it should be respected; and about 18 per cent hold the position that the body is "only dead flesh," but the person who occupied it should be respected.

Relatively little attention has been paid by social scientists to beliefs about the presence and nature of a human soul and its significance to the treatment of the body after death. According to the Talmud it is an offense to leave a body unburied overnight, but the soul does not leave the body until three days after death and during this time the soul may hover over the body before it departs. Muslims tend to have similar views. Catholic moralists, on the other hand, tend to hold that there is a latent period between death and the departure of the soul which may vary from one-half to one hour if the death is preceded by a long illness or from three to seven hours if death is sudden (Jakobovits, 1959).

Subjects in the present sample were found to vary considerably in their beliefs about the nature and presence of a human soul. Almost half the group believe that a human soul is God-given and/or immortal; about 17 per cent judge the soul to be a confusing term but are uncertain whether or not there is a soul; 28 per cent consider the soul a useful humanistic term for sensitivity and awareness, but not immortal; 7 per cent say there is no such thing as a soul.

As expected, the relationship between religious identification and beliefs regarding a human soul and the sanctity of the body tends to be direct when religious groups are ordered in categories ranging from Catholic and Fundamentalist at one extreme to Secularist at the other. The findings suggest that beliefs about the sanctity of the body and the presence of the soul tend to serve as intervening variables in the relationship between religion and ethical judgments about uses of the body.

Ethical judgments appear unrelated to age, sex, education, or professional specialty; physicians and nurses, representing 45 per cent of sample, do not differ in position from other professionals with respect to the primary findings. Religiously based beliefs about the human soul, the sanctity of deceased bodies, and the definition and value of a human life are found to be significantly associated with judgments about the ethics of autopsies, dissections, exploratory operations, and uses of bodies or body parts for study, teaching, display, or transplantation. Low correlations and wide individual variation indicate the presence of unidentified variables.

Historical records and observations in hospital and medical settings suggest that the ethics regarding treatment of the body tend to be related to the definitions and values assigned to the individual when alive. Bodies of persons of higher statuses—presidents, generals, cardinals—are treated with great respect. Bodies of hobos, derelicts, criminals, traitors, and members of enemy troops are treated with indifference or contempt. Health professionals who perceive the body as declining in value with the approach of death tend to place less value on dead bodies.

We have witnessed significant contrasts on television: Bodies of our dead leaders and heroes have been treated with honor, but little attention has been given to persons of less status who have died under similar circumstances. The bodies of our own soldiers are treated as sacred, whereas the bodies of our enemies are treated in profane ways.

The Communication Problem

The basic issue of communicating with the patient concerning his impending death would seem to be, as Aronson (1959:251) has put it, "How to help the patient to be an individual human being even though gravely ill and dying." Application of this principle requires a sensitivity to the specific needs of the patient and a tact in communicating that are beyond the capacity of many individuals.

Glaser and Strauss (1965:6) have posed the issue as follows:

> From one point of view the problem of awareness is a technical one: should the patient be told he is dying—and what is to be done if he knows, does not know, or only suspects? But the problem is also a moral one, involving professional ethics, social issues, and personal values. Is it really proper, some people have asked, to deny a dying person the opportunity to make his peace with his conscience and with his God, to settle his affairs and provide for the future of his family, and to control his style of dying, much as he controlled his style of living? Does anyone, the physician included, have the right to withhold such information?

Some preliminary studies suggest that, while most physicians do not favor telling their patients about impending death (Feifel, 1963; Emerson, 1963; Glaser and Strauss, 1965, 1968), most patients desire to be told frankly though gently about their condition at the time of dying. When they do receive such information, they usually demonstrate a high capacity for handling the communication either in an open manner or in defensive ways that protect them from trauma.

Even when patients are not directly informed that death is imminent, they do tend to acquire this knowledge by themselves or with the indirect aid of others. They observe change in behavior of the staff, other patients, and visitors; they note changes in the type of treatment they receive as the physician changes from restorative to palliative methods. At times they demonstrate a psychological awareness of death on the basis of the information they have thus acquired.

The problem is complicated by the fact that the physician, nurses, and other staff members may themselves avoid direct discussion of the impending death. Even the language employed may be such as to avoid the terms "death" and "dying"; substitute terms include "growing weak," "sinking," "may not be with us long," or "passing on."

Emerson (1963:330–331) suggests:

> Humor provides one technique of managing the dilemmas created by the avoidance of the issue of death. . . . The staff also use the medium of humor to communicate about the prospect of a patient's death, predictions of the time of death, their possible responsibility for patients' deaths, and the possibility of a staff member dying. At the same time humor allows the patients to express their protest, fears, and doubts about the physician's competence. Most important of all, humor reinforces a detached attitude toward dying patients.

The problem of communication is one in which definitive answers applicable in all situations are not likely to be found. Much depends upon the unique characteristics of the patient and the physician and the special conditions existing at the time of dying, such as the availability of members of the family, chaplains, or priests to give support to the patient and to help if special problems arise.

It is of some importance to recognize that the professional people dealing with illness and death receive their professional training on top of and much later in life than their early socialization and thus share with patients and other members of the public the early experiences, beliefs, ethical values, and attitudes of the culture. Glaser and Strauss (1968:151–159) urge greatly improved training for terminal care in schools of medicine and nursing. Within this framework of additional training it would appear that emphasis should be given to the issue of communication to prepare physicians and nurses better for dealing with crises. This might include effective ways of dealing with survivors, considering possible application of the findings of Lindeman, Klein, and others regarding the importance of providing an early outlet for grief after the death of a loved one to avoid serious emotional problems that may later develop if grief is not expressed (Volkart, 1957).

Conclusion

Death and dying remain taboo topics in Western society and perhaps also in most human societies. We have not yet learned "how to help the patient to be an individual human being even though he is gravely ill and dying." If human life could be made more meaningful and rewarding, would death and dying become less taboo?

Although our society has developed defenses to avoid discussing death with the dying person, it seeks means of communicating with persons after they are dead. A search for contact with life after death is reflected in public ventures reminiscent of Ponce de Leon's search for the fountain of youth. Occultism, mysticism, and spiritualism continue to receive support.

Death, the ultimate unknown, continues to serve man in stimulating new, creative projections. Most of mankind appears unwilling to accept death as an inevitable, final separation, and, for large segments of humanity, religions remain strong in orienting man's life on earth to eternal life. Major scientific efforts are focused toward extending life through animal and human experimentation, applications of new treatments, the use of prosthetic aids and vital transplants. Cryonics offers the opportunity of postponing death by freezing in hopes that new discoveries may permit cure and rejuvenation. Some attempts are being made to redefine death in ways likely to soften its traumatic effects. Meanwhile, the themes of death and eternal life continue to provide stimuli for the creative development of the arts.

REFERENCES

Aronson, Gerald J.
    1959 "Treatment of the dying person." Chapter 14 in Herman Feifel (ed.), The Meaning of Death. New York, Toronto, London: McGraw-Hill.

Becker, H., and D. K. Bruner.
    1931 "Attitudes towards death and the dead." Mental Hygiene 15:828–837.

Emerson, Joan P.
    1963 "Social functions of humor in a hospital setting." Ph.D. dissertation, University of California, Berkeley.

Farberow, Norman L. (ed.).
    1963 Taboo Topics. New York: Atherton.

Feifel, Herman (ed.).
   1959   The Meaning of Death. New York, Toronto, London: McGraw-Hill.
   1963   "Death." Pp. 8–21 in Norman L. Farberow (ed.), Taboo Topics. New York: Atherton.

Glaser, Barney G., and Anselm L. Strauss.
   1965   Awareness of Dying. Chicago: Aldine.
   1968   Time for Dying. Chicago: Aldine.

Howard, Alan, and Robert A. Scott.
   1965/66   "Cultural values and attitudes toward death." Journal of Existentialism 6(Winter):161–174.

Jakobovits, Immanuel.
   1959   Jewish Medical Ethics. New York: Bloch.

Jung, Carl G.
   1934   "The soul and death." Pp. 3–15 in Herman Feifel (ed.), The Meaning of Death (1959). New York, Toronto, London: McGraw-Hill.

Kalish, Richard A.
   1968   "Life and death: dividing the indivisible." Social Science & Medicine.

Kalish, Richard A., and Robert Kastenbaum.
   1968   Bibliographical notes of ongoing studies, Omega.

Knutson, Andie L.
   1967a   "The definition and value of a new human life." Social Science & Medicine 1(April):7–29.
   1967b   "When does a human life begin? Viewpoints of public health professionals." American Journal of Public Health 57(December):2163–2177.
   1968a   "Body transplants and ethical values: Viewpoints of public health professionals." Social Science & Medicine.
   1968b   Preliminary unpublished findings.
   1968c   "The definition and value of a human life in public health practice." Presented at the Canadian Public Health Association Program in Vancouver, British Columbia.

Lester, David.
   1967   "Experimental and correlational studies of the fear of death." Psychological Bulletin 67(January):27–36.

Saphir, O.
   1938   "Religious aspects of the autopsy." Report of the Committee on Necropsies of the American Hospital Association, Bulletin No. 163. Chicago: American Hospital Association, 89–96.

Scott, C. A.
   1896   "Old age and death." American Journal of Psychology 8:67–122.

Shneidman, Edwin S.
   1963   "Suicide." Pp. 33–43 in Norman L. Farberow (ed.), Taboo Topics. New York: Atherton.

Sudnow, David.
   1967   Passing On. Englewood Cliffs, N.J.: Prentice Hall.

Volkart, E. H. (in collaboration with S. T. Michael).
   1957   "Bereavement and mental health." in A. H. Leighton, J. A. Clausen, and R. N. Wilson (eds.), Explorations in Social Psychiatry. New York: Basic Books.

Williams, Mary.
   1966   "Changing attitudes to death." Human Relations 19 (November): 405–423.

PART TWO

How Doctors, Nurses, and Hospitals Cope with Death

4

The Prognosis of Death

Louis Lasagna

SINCE WE ARE ALL moving at variable paces toward death, one might conceivably look upon all of life as a terminal illness from which only death can liberate us. Whether such a definition is excessively lugubrious can be debated; for the purposes of this chapter it is not a workable one. Operationally, therefore, I shall define "terminal illness" as a disease state whose presence raises in the mind of physician, patient, or family an expectation of death as a direct consequence of the illness. "Prognosis" will be used in its classic sense of forecasting, of predicting outcome, in this case the estimation both of the likelihood of death as a result of a specific medical condition and the time at which such death will occur. Sudden unexpected death, since it provides no opportunity for prognosis, will be considered only insofar as it may be the specific mode of termination of some disease states.

Variations in Medical Competency

A variety of factors will modify both the frequency of prognostication and its accuracy. To begin with, there is the element of diagnostic skill. Obviously, the physician who does not recognize that a patient's life is threatened will not manifest behavior contingent on such appraisal. Every doctor quickly begins to acquire a mental dossier of horrible mistakes of this sort, perpetrated by himself and by his colleagues—the meningitis that is treated for several days as a "flu headache," the perforated appendix passed off as "a little indigestion," the premonitory angina pectoris dismissed as "root pain from pinched nerves." I can still recall vividly the young woman brought to the hospital one night when I was the admitting resident. She had the classical story, physical signs, and chemical signs of severe diabetic acidosis, but had been misdiagnosed as appendicitis by her physician.

Important differences between doctors exist in regard to other determinants of behavior. In addition to diagnostic acumen, the physician needs to possess the relevant information concerning the "natural life history"* and management of the disease. It will serve little purpose for him to diagnose correctly if he then does not know how to treat or does not know what the outlook is, with and without treatment. Malignant melanoma, for example, is usually diagnosed readily because of the distinctive nature of the lesion clinically and histologically. Unfortunately, however, the prognosis is not simple, despite firm opinions to the contrary held by many doctors. Traditionally, medical students used to be told (and perhaps many still are) that malignant melanoma—its very name bodes ill—is one of the most lethal cancerous growths, rapidly leading to the demise of its unlucky victim. Yet this is only true for some—perhaps half of the patients who have a melanoma removed will still be alive and apparently well five years later, and at least some of these are permanently cured.

Even the most competent of doctors, however, will be hampered in his prognostication and in his management of the patient with potentially fatal disease if the state of our knowledge is defective, if there are not reliable data available to allow accurate guesses to be made. Feinstein (1967a) has eloquently pointed out how hampered medicine has been by the archaic classification of disease that is the heritage of the nineteenth-century preeminence of Virchowian cadaveric pathology. There is still preoccupation and satisfaction with such inadequate labels as "myocardial infarct" or "cancer of the lung," and not enough concern for the details of anamnestic, physiologic, and biochemical stratification of disease that will ultimately permit the elucidation of prognostic indicators. The utility of such "staging" of disease in the delineation of empirical correlations will be discussed later.

Variation in Therapeutic Efficacy

An important variable is provided by the available therapeutic modalities—pharmacologic, surgical, mechanical, nursing, or others.

---

* In this age of surgical derring-do and widespread use of drugs, prescribed and self-prescribed, almost no disease can be said any longer to have a "natural" history.

The Prognosis of Death

These present multiple opportunities for improving the outlook, or for deleteriously affecting it. A life-saving drug may be withheld either because the diagnosis is in error or because the doctor in charge is unaware of the appropriate treatment. The injudicious application of a drug or a surgical procedure that is not indicated may shorten life.

Unfortunately, there is marked disagreement about the proper therapy of many medical conditions where life is at stake. In the condition known as hereditary polyposis of the colon, there is a general consensus that the risk of developing colonic cancer is so high that prophylactic colectomy is probably indicated. But in other potentially malignant colonic lesions there is no suggestion of consensus. The single colonic polyp is considered by some to be malignant until proved otherwise, and thus a candidate for surgical removal in all patients; by others the colonic polyp is looked on as a generally benign lesion which deserves to be managed conservatively and optimistically (Baker *et al.*, 1966). In chronic ulcerative colitis, the prognostic picture is also unclear. An analysis of nearly two thousand German-Czech cases of ulcerative colitis by Henning (1967) yielded only three instances of colonic cancer, whereas "Anglo-American experience unequivocally identifies ulcerative colitis as one of the conditions that predispose to cancer of the colon" (*New England Journal of Medicine*, 1968). Despite the latter statement, few American and English physicians advise patients with ulcerative colitis—even the highest risk group, that is, those with disease having its onset prior to the age of 20 and continuing for over ten years—to have a prophylactic total colectomy, with its sentencing of the patient to a lifetime of ileostomy drainage.

There are few topics more controversial in medicine than that of anticoagulant therapy for patients with documented myocardial infarctions. In August, 1965, *Prescribers' Journal*, a periodical distributed to all English doctors by the National Health Service, reported a survey of forty-one physicians chosen from among the panel of examiners for membership in the Royal College of Physicians (London) (*Prescribers' Journal*, 1965). In response to the question "Do you use anticoagulants in treating acute myocardial infarction?", twelve doctors said that they prescribed such drugs for all patients with acute cardiac infarction, twenty-one prescribed them for selected patients only, and eight never used them! The article concluded: *"Prescribers' Journal* clearly hesitates to offer advice where the eminent disagree."

Early in 1968 a British study reported a serious rise in mortality from asthma (*British Medical Journal*, 1968). Mortality had increased two and a half times between the ages of 5 and 34 years from 1959 to 1966 in England and Wales and eight times between the ages of 10 and 14. The period coincided with increasing use of both corticosteroid drugs and pressurized bronchodilator aerosols, especially of isoprenaline (isoproterenol). There is increasing suspicion that excessive use of the latter drug may actually make asthma worse in some patients, and alarm now exists about the possibility that this time-honored therapeutic technique may actually be the cause of death in many patients.

Since 1962, three separate prospective studies of prophylactic portacaval shunt surgery for cirrhosis of the liver (Conn and Lindenmuth, 1962; Garceau *et al.*, 1964; Jackson *et al.*, 1965) have suggested that this formidable operation, in use for many years, may not prolong the life of the patient with cirrhosis who has never hemorrhaged from his dilated esophageal veins. The most recent report (Jackson *et al.*, 1968) indicated that hemorrhage from these varices developed among shunted and nonshunted patients at an equal rate, but that when bleeding occurred after shunt surgery it was invariably fatal. Deaths from liver failure and bleeding peptic ulcers among shunted patients were significantly more frequent than in the unoperated group and were primarily responsible for the fact that at twenty-four month's follow-up 77 per cent of the medically treated patients were still alive, whereas only 53 per cent of those surgically treated survived. The investigators concluded that this traditional surgical technique "is not recommended in the non-bleeding . . . cirrhotic patient with recent ascites, jaundice, or encephalopathy," but in the discussion following the paper's presentation the lead author still held that ". . . in a patient with no history of liver failure but with non-hemorrhaging esophageal varices, I probably would advise the operation if there were no other extenuating circumstances. . . ."

The field of cancer and allied malignant diseases has been characterized by a number of attempts to classify clinical data in such a way as to improve prognostication. As Feinstein (1967b) has pointed

The Prognosis of Death

out, some cancer patients are asymptomatic, their cancer having been discovered during a routine physical examination or as the result of an X-ray taken during a check-up or during a mass screening drive. Others have only symptoms attributable to the cancer at its site of origin or to surrounding inflammation, infection, or obstruction, with no evidence (at least on history-taking) of anatomic dissemination of the cancer. (Thus, spitting blood may be a "primary" symptom of lung cancer, rectal bleeding of colonic cancer.)

The Variable of Time

Still other patients may have symptoms that imply metastatic spread, such as jaundice in a patient with cancer of the stomach or bone pain in someone with breast cancer. Finally, there are "systemic" symptoms that do not arise from the locale which is the origin of the cancer, but which do not necessarily imply spread of the growth. Such symptoms are weight loss, fatigue, or loss of appetite. A patient may, of course, present any combination of primary, systemic, and metastatic symptoms.

There is, as well, the variable of time. How long have the symptoms been present? Symptoms of short duration do not, of course, imply that the tumor has been present for only a brief period of time. On the other hand, a patient with "primary" symptoms of long standing presumably has a slowly progressive cancer. The asymptomatic cancer detected accidentally might be anticipated to be more benign and slow-growing than other tumors.

Feinstein retrospectively analyzed the records of 678 patients with cancer of the lung and 279 patients with cancer of the rectum. The five-year survival rates, regardless of therapy, are shown below, stratifying patients on the basis of symptomatic history:

SYMPTOMS	LUNG CANCER	RECTAL CANCER
None	18%	64%
Primary, of long duration	16	45
Primary, of short duration	9	34
Systemic	6	20
Metastatic	0	0

Since laymen are constantly being warned to seek medical counsel at the earliest symptom of cancer, it may seem paradoxical that patients who have primary symptoms of long standing do better than those who see a doctor because of symptoms of short duration. These data are explainable, however, if one subscribes to the theory of "biological predeterminism" of cancer, which postulates that cancers have an intrinsically determined rate of growth and malignant potential, with some destined for explosive growth (and poor prognosis) and others destined to grow slowly (and to have a good prognosis) regardless of therapy.

Stage of Disease

Feinstein has lumped together the asymptomatic group and those patients with primary symptoms of long duration as "indolent," the "systemic" group and those patients with primary symptoms of short duration as "obtrusive," and he has called patients with "metastatic" symptoms the "deleterious" category. This grouping acknowledges the hierarchy of survival figures shown above, and also has the advantage of providing fewer subcategories with larger numbers of patients per new category. Feinstein has then restratified these symptomatic groups on the basis of anatomic stages, that is, whether there was anatomic evidence of local growth only, evidence of regional invasion, or evidence of distant dissemination. The figures on five-year survival rates are shown below:

Lung Cancer (all types of treatment)

	ANATOMIC EVIDENCE			
SYMPTOMS	LOCALIZED	REGIONAL SPREAD	DISTANT SPREAD	TOTAL
"Indolent"	24%	10%	4%	17%
"Obtrusive"	15	5	1	7
"Deleterious"	0	0	0	0
Total	16%	4%	1%	7%

It is clear that both the anamnestic and anatomic forms of staging contribute to prognostic accuracy. For those cancers with anatomic

The Prognosis of Death

evidence only of local growth or regional spread, there is a significant difference in survival between the various symptomatic categories. For rectal cancer, for example, all patients with anatomic evidence of localized cancer have about a fifty-fifty chance of living five years. Yet patients in this group who have symptoms suggesting metastatic spread will all be dead in five years, whereas almost three-fourths of those who are asymptomatic or have primary symptoms of long duration will survive for five years.

Rectal Cancer (after surgical resection)

SYMPTOMS	ANATOMIC EVIDENCE			TOTAL
	LOCALIZED	REGIONAL SPREAD	DISTANT SPREAD	
"Indolent"	72%	40%	6%	52%
"Obtrusive"	49	19	7	33
"Deleterious"	0	0	0	0
Total	57%	26%	6%	38%

These patients have also been analyzed by Feinstein for the relative efficacy of radical and conservative surgery. For this purpose, patients with either symptoms or anatomic evidence suggesting distant spread are labeled Class D. Those with anatomic evidence only of localized tumor plus "indolent" symptoms constitute Class A; those with "obtrusive" symptoms and evidence of regional spread are in Class C. All others are labeled Class B. The figures for five-year survival are as follows:

Type of Surgery for Cancer of Lung

CLINICO-ANATOMIC STATE	PNEUMO-NECTOMY	LOBECTOMY
A	34%	29%
B	20	29
C	15	14
D	8	11
Total	21%	25%

Type of Surgery for Rectal Cancer

CLINICO-ANATOMIC STAGE	ABDOMINO-PERINEAL RESECTION	ANUS-PRESERVING RESECTION
A	63%	67%
B	63	56
C	19	25
D	7	7
Total	41%	40%

There seems little evidence in these figures that the amount of tissue removed has any effect on life span, but there is obviously a good deal of prognostic information in the clinico-anatomic staging. (It is conceivable that the more radical surgery has a higher intrinsic operative and postoperative mortality which roughly counterbalances a certain advantage in terms of tumor eradication, but the practical consequences remain the same: The radical procedure is no more effective than the conservative one.)

Cancer of the breast is another type of neoplasm concerning which there is a great deal of controversy over whether radical and simple surgery (that is, mastectomy) differ in their therapeutic implications. There is a paucity of evidence on how long breast tumors are present before medical consultation is sought, but there is evidence that prognosis is related both to the histologic "wildness" of the tumor and its degree of spread. A decade ago, the Mayo Clinic published a survey of 8,488 case reports (Berkson et al., 1957). The five-year survival rate for women without metastasis was 78 per cent, whereas it was 36 per cent for those with metastasis. In patients without metastasis and with malignancy Grade 1—the most benign histologic stage—the survival rate was 96 per cent. For patients with malignancy Grades 2, 3, and 4, the percentages fell to 86, 76, and 74 per cent if metastasis was not present, and to 61, 43, and 30 per cent if metastasis was present.

Reality Versus Illusion

The act of prognostication is beset by numerous obstacles. The examples just cited are impressive enough, but too often precise in-

The Prognosis of Death

formation is not available, because it has not been systematically collected or analyzed, or it is not available to the practicing physician. (Nor is this solely a problem of the isolated rural doctor. I remember some years ago when a distinguished professor of surgery was shocked by the fact that a group of university clinics reported a 20 to 25 per cent mortality within thirty days in patients subjected to surgery for cancer of various sites. On analyzing the data for his own clinic, however, he was surprised to discover just as poor a performance in his own department, despite long-standing conviction to the contrary.) In the absence of such knowledge, the doctor will have to rely on statements in texts (often hoary clinical clichés too long unexamined for validity), on his own experience (often limited), and on the opinions of colleagues.

The competence of the doctor, as already indicated, will also affect the prognosis. So, in all likelihood, will the hospital and the allied health personnel caring for the patient. A recent nationwide retrospective analysis of death rates following general anesthetic, for example, found wide variations among the thirty-four cooperating institutions (Moses and Mosteller, 1960). The death rates ranged from 0.27 per cent to 6.40 per cent, a twenty-four-fold ratio. Adjusting these rates for sex, year, previous operation, physical status, age, and operation reduced variations but left substantial differences. Two well-known statisticians who reviewed the data concluded that "there are real differences in institutional death rates for which neither the data ... nor sampling error furnish an explanation."

Impact of Progress

Still another difficulty is the changing course of many diseases. Prognosis is "disease-bound," but it is also "time-bound."* Not many years ago, patients with pernicious anemia or Addison's disease (hypoadrenalism) were doomed to an early death; today such individuals are relatively easily maintained in good health. Before the advent of antibiotics, patients with infections of their heart valves almost always died of this ailment; at present 70 to 80 per cent of such patients can

---

* *The Baltimore Sun* carried an item last year in which it reported that in 1828 the city's health commissioner listed the following causes of death: "teething—16; drinking cold water—10; *coup de soleil*—1; mortification—14."

be cured, although serious residual scarring of the heart valve remains a problem. In Osler's day, lobar pneumonia was fatal to 20 to 40 per cent of adult patients, whereas few such patients die in 1969. Meningitis due to the meningococcus used to claim the lives of 70 per cent or more such patients; today only 5 to 15 per cent of those adequately treated die. Typhoid fever in the preantibiotic days killed perhaps 20 per cent of affected patients; with the availability of chloramphenicol treatment, most of these patients now survive.

In my medical school days, acute leukemia was a "diagnosis that called for philosophy and sympathy, not science," in the words of one of my teachers. With the advent of new drugs, prolonged remissions and even apparent cures are seen with some regularity in children, and occasionally in adults. The advent of the "artificial kidney" has dramatically altered the prognosis of patients with various poisonings as well as those with bilateral acute and chronic renal disease. Advances in organ transplantation are rendering old prognostic indicators obsolete: It has already been suggested that death be redefined as the irreversible loss of function of an organ that is vital to life and cannot be replaced with a transplant.

In the management of hypertension, there for a long time has been general agreement that "malignant hypertension," a rapidly progressive and dangerous variant or stage of hypertensive disease, should be vigorously treated with anti-hypertensive drugs. Only relatively recently, however, evidence has appeared, in the form of suitably designed trials, to support those who have alleged that such drugs should also be routinely used in patients with more modest levels of hypertension. It now appears reasonably clear that the outlook for such patients will be modified by treatment, just as the formerly grim prognosis for malignant hypertension has been ameliorated (Veterans Administration Study Group, 1967).

The management of hypotension, on the other hand, continues in some respects to remain both controversial and unsatisfactory. Those cases of cardiovascular shock due to fluid or blood loss for some years now have been reasonably well managed by simple replacement of body fluids. "Cardiogenic shock" and "septic shock," on the other hand, remain enigmas. Although the advent of techniques for monitoring central venous pressure have improved the situation somewhat, there is still great disagreement about whether to use sympathomimetic amines (and if so which ones), sympatholytic drugs, cardiotropic glycosides, or the like. A few years ago, for example, norepinephrine was in great vogue; at present isoproterenol is in the ascendancy but without clear-cut evidence that the prognosis on the average has been greatly altered.

Influence of Available Treatment

In what way do prognostic considerations affect the doctor in his choice of treatment? There is not much hard fact on this point, although some general observations probably can be safely made. There are two extreme ways of reacting to the possibility that one's patient has a potentially fatal disease. One is to pull out all the therapeutic stops—to use any and all measures that might prevent or postpone death. The other is to resign oneself (really the patient) to a fatal outcome, make the patient as comfortable as possible, and wait for the end. In between these antipodes lies an infinitely graded set of responses. What determines which type of response it will be?

One important basis for decision lies in the availability of effective therapy. A physician is not likely to withhold an assuredly curative drug or surgical procedure from a patient who appears ready to die within hours if untreated. This situation, however, is rarely the one that obtains in clinical practice. More often one is faced with an individual whose demise is not so precisely predictable, and for whom available therapy offers only slight hope of success, coupled with the distinct chance of harm, even of hastening the moment of death. For instance, most drugs available for treating disseminated cancer are highly toxic, and some doctors are sufficiently unimpressed by their efficacy to avoid prescribing them in most cases. The Whipple procedure for cancer of the pancreas is a formidable bit of surgery, with high mortality and morbidity rates and scant chance of success; it is not often applied at present. Cardiac transplant is still so chancy, and the precision of prognosis for cardiac patients so poor, that most doctors probably would not elect to be the recipients of heart transplants.

In making such judgments, the personality of the physician will certainly affect the decision. Some are "aggressive" therapists, eager to use new or old drugs or surgical procedures, frustrated by inability to adopt a healing posture (even a spurious one). Others are "conservative," fearful of drugs and their side effects, dubious of success in seriously ill patients, unconvinced that frenzied doctoring is anything but *furor therapeuticus* in the patient with terminal cancer or intractable heart failure. (In our surveys, there is evidence that doctors fall into at least two therapeutic groups—those that select the most powerful drug available, and those that are happy to sacrifice potency in return for less toxicity.)

Telling the Patient

How much do doctors tell their patients about the prognosis? Again, data are not generally available on this point. Medical education at the formal level provides little or no training in handling the problems of death. Surveys of physicians (Lasagna, 1968) show that they rarely believe that their approach to the dying patient owes anything to medical training. Furthermore, they disagree markedly in what such patients should be told. Most doctors probably do not tell dying patients, in so many words, that their end is in sight, even though *they* would wish to be told if in that position. This reluctance is probably due to several facts.

First, the doctor may consider it both pointless and cruel to tell the truth to a dying patient. Second, it is disturbing to many doctors to go through such a discussion with the patient—it is likely to be both awkward and abrasive to the doctor's ego to concede his helplessness, as well as his relative ignorance about just when death will take place. Third, the doctor may know his patient (and the family) less well today than in the past; if so, he will be in a less satisfactory position to know how best to handle the total situation.

Telling the Family

The family, on the other hand, is usually told—at least some member of the family is told the prognosis. There are both professional and legal traditions that make such discussion almost mandatory, despite the fact that most of the problems discussed in the preceding paragraph apply equally well to communication between the doctor and the relatives of the patient. One standardized hospital procedure that helps to achieve this disclosure is the "critical list." Every hospital has a list of patients who are deemed in imminent danger of death. Although instructions to the staff about what qualifies a patient for such a list are generally vague, and the decision is essentially a matter of medical judgment, once the decision is made certain administrative wheels are set promptly in motion—next of kin are notified by whatever means required to achieve contact, even when relatives are in distant places; pastoral visits may be arranged for administering last rites; and so on.

For less critically ill patients, the prognosis of terminal illness may set other administrative machinery into action. The terminal patient who is not too sick to be moved but who requires continued hospitalization will be transferred, when possible, from an "acute" hospital to a "chronic" hospital or nursing home. Such patients are often resented by the house staff of an "acute" hospital because they take up beds that could be used for more acutely ill (or "interesting") patients who will better allow the doctor to fulfill his preferred role of dramatic and effective healer. Arrangements of this sort are often tedious and complex, since adequate terminal facilities are in short supply, and there are both medical and economic details to be investigated by the agencies involved.

Reactions of Patients

The patient's response to knowledge (or unjustified fear*) that he possesses a terminal illness is highly variable. Some will take such information stoically, and make arrangements in regard to business affairs, family matters, and so on in a highly efficient manner. Others will sink into paralytic despondency, withdrawing from social intercourse with friends, family, and physician. Some will adopt the protective device of denying the fact that they are seriously ill. Many will, however, be aware of their impending demise, will discuss it freely and wish only to be kept free of distressing symptoms, such as pain and insomnia (Hinton, 1964).

The patient and his family may take the news of terminal illness

---

* The doctor must be alert to the possibility that his patient erroneously believes himself to suffer from a terminal illness; effective reassurances to the contrary can achieve great benefits.

as the signal for anxious (and often guilt-laden, in the case of relatives) searching for other medical opinions that will contradict the diagnosis and prognosis or at least offer new hope in the form of pharmacologic, surgical, or other treatment. This is always a touchy situation—some doctors take such behavior as a personal affront, others view it with disfavor because of an honest belief that the family will only spend a great deal of money to no purpose. Since all doctors are fallible, a happy compromise is often to suggest obtaining an additional opinion, but to discourage lengthy "shopping" for good news that is not really to be had except from a quack or fraud.

Mortality of the Bereaved

For some patients and families, the last weeks or months are better spent at home rather than in the hospital. This is a decision which must be made in consort, since it involves medical issues as well as psychological, social, and economic ones.

One interesting recent study (Rees and Lutkins, 1967) has described "the mortality of bereavement" in the area around the small market town of Llanidloes, Wales. Almost all the residents were patients of a single group practice. A total of 5,184 patients lived in the survey area. During the period of study, 488 residents died. Of these, 108 were excluded from further analysis because they had no close relatives living in the area. Nine neonatal deaths were also excluded.

It was found that 4.76 per cent of "bereaved" close relatives died within a year of the death in the family, whereas the control group showed a rate of 0.68 per cent. During the second year after bereavement, the figures were 1.99 and 1.25 respectively, a statistically insignificant difference. The risk for male relatives was greater than for female, 6.4 per cent versus 3.5 per cent. Widowed people in the bereaved group showed a higher mortality rate than widowed in the control group, 12.2 per cent (in the first year) as contrasted with 1.2 per cent. Again, the risk was higher for widowers than for widows.

The risk of a bereaved relative dying within one year of bereavement was twice as high if the first relative died in hospital than if he died at home. The risk of bereaved relatives dying was even greater when the relative died at sites other than hospital or home, such as roads, fields, a cemetery, chapel, bowling-green, or pond. Such deaths were invariably sudden, with presumably greater shock to the relatives. Grief and distress were often increased by the need for necropsy and inquest.

These data, while they require confirmation, suggest the need for further attention to the somatic as well as the psychologic impact of terminal illness on family as well as on the patient. They suggest that the suddenness of death, the place of its occurrence, and the way in which social customs and laws impinge on the survivors may be important determinants of health.

REFERENCES

Anonymous.
    1965 "Anticoagulants and myocardial infarction." Prescribers' Journal 5(August):33–34.

Baker, J. W., et al.
    1966 "Malignant potential of colonic polyps." Sec. 8, pp. 207–229 in F. J. Ingelfinger, A. S. Relman, and M. Finland (eds.), Controversies in Internal Medicine. Philadelphia: W. B. Saunders.

Berkson, J., et al.
    1957 "Mortality and survival in surgically treated cancer of the breast: a statistical summary of some experience of the Mayo Clinic." Proceedings of the Staff Meetings of the Mayo Clinic 32(November):645–670.

Conn, H. O., and W. W. Lindenmuth.
    1962 "Prophylactic portacaval anastomosis in cirrhotic patients with esophageal varices. A preliminary report of a controlled study." New England Journal of Medicine 266(April 12):743–749.

Editorial.
    1968 "Increasing deaths from asthma." British Medical Journal 1(February 10):329–330.

Editorial.
    1968 "Risk of cancer in ulcerative colitis." New England Journal of Medicine 278(April 18):907.

Feinstein, A. R.
    1967a Clinical Judgment. Baltimore: Williams and Wilkins.
    1967b "A new staging system for cancer, and a re-appraisal of 'early' treatment and 'cure' by radical surgery." Transactions of the Association of American Physicians 80:111–119.

Garceau, A. J., et al.
    1964 "A controlled trial of prophylactic portacaval shunt surgery." New England Journal of Medicine 270(March 5):496–500.

Henning, N.
    1967   "Carcinoma of the colon in ulcerative colitis: What is the risk?" German Medical Monthly 12(August):402.
Hinton, J.
    1964   "Problems of the dying." Journal of Chronic Diseases 17(March): 201–205.
Jackson, F. C., et al.
    1965   "Clinical investigation of the portacaval shunt. I. Study design and preliminary survival analysis." Archives of Surgery (July): 43–54.
    1968   "A clinical investigation of the portacaval shunt. II. Survival analysis of the prophylactic operation." American Journal of Surgery 111(January):22–42.
Lasagna, L.
    1968   Life, Death, and the Doctor. New York: Knopf.
Moses, L. E., and F. Mosteller.
    1960   "Institutional differences in postoperative death rates. Commentary on some of the findings of the National Halothane Study." Journal of the American Medical Association 203(February 12):492–494.
Rees, W. D., and S. G. Lutkins.
    1967   "Mortality of bereavement." British Medical Journal 4(October 7):13–16.
Veterans' Administration Cooperative Study Group on Antihypertensive Agents.
    1967   "Effects of treatment on morbidity in hypertension. Results in patients with diastolic blood pressures averaging 115 through 129 mm Hg." Journal of the American Medical Association 202(December 11):1028–1034.

5

Physicians' Behavior Toward the Dying Patient

Louis Lasagna

THE BEHAVIOR OF THE doctor toward his seriously ill patient is inevitably affected by the physician's biases and prejudices about the patient and his disease. What are some of the important determinants of this behavior?

One important variable is the age of the patient. Our society tends at present to worship youthfulness (although not immaturity) and to equate aging with mental and physical deterioration. There is no compelling reason to believe that physicians differ significantly from the lay public in their orientation to aging. Accordingly, one would anticipate that total medical care for the moribund young patient will be more vigorous, extensive, and sustained than the attention accorded the dying oldster. The younger patient's "premature" death will often be considered more tragic, a candle abruptly snuffed out when it had just begun to burn, an example of unfulfilled promise no less to be mourned merely because its quality and quantity are unpredictable.

Dislike for the Aged

The poet W. P. Snodgrass, in a poem from *After Experience* recalling his days as an orderly at a Veterans' Administration hospital, has captured the essence of resentment of the aged and infirm, the useless social driftwood demanding attention from younger, productive members of society who grudgingly provide a sustenance they do not consider justified. The last stanza, with its terminal attempt at conciliation, somehow does not ring true, and fails to balance the harsher, more candid verdict contained in the preceding sections:

A FLAT ONE

Old Fritz, on this rotating bed
For seven wasted months you lay
Unfit to move, shrunken, gray,
No good to yourself or anyone
But to be babied—changed and bathed and fed.
    At long last, that's all done.

Before each meal, twice every night,
We set pads on your bedsores, shut
Your catheter tube off, then brought
The second canvas-and-black-iron
Bedframe and clamped you in between them, tight,
    Scared, so we could turn

You over. We washed you, covered you,
Cut up each bite of meat you ate;
We watched your lean jaws masticate
As ravenously your useless food
As thieves at hard labor in their chains chew
    Or insects in the wood.

Such pious sacrifice to give
You all you could demand of pain:
Receive this haddock's body, slain
For you, old tyrant; take this blood
Of a tomato, shed that you might live.
    You had that costly food.

You seem to be all finished, so
We'll plug your old recalcitrant anus
And tie up your discouraged penis
In a great, snow-white bow of gauze
We wrap you, pin you, and cart you down below,
    Below, below, because

Your credit has finally run out.
On our steel table, trussed and carved,
You'll find this world's hardworking, starved
Teeth working in your precious skin.
The earth turns, in the end, by turn about
    And opens to take you in.

Physicians' Behavior Toward the Patient

*Seven months gone down the drain; thank God
That's through. Throw out the four-by-fours,
Swabsticks, the thick salve for bedsores,
Throw out the diaper pads and drug
Containers, pile the bedclothes in a wad,
And rinse the cider jug*

*Half-filled with the last urine. Then
Empty out the cotton cans,
Autoclave the bowls and spit pans,
Unhook the pumps and all the red
Tubes—catheter, suction, oxygen;
Next, wash the empty bed.*

*—All this Dark Age machinery
On which we had tormented you
To life. Last, we collect the few
Belongings: snapshots, some odd bills,
Your mail, and half a pack of Luckies we
Won't light you after meals.*

*Old man, these seven months you've lain
Determined—not that you would live—
Just to not die. No one would give
You one chance you could ever wake
From that first night, much less go well again,
Much less go home and make*

*Your living; how could you hope to find
A place for yourself in all creation?—
Pain was your only occupation.
And pain that should content and will
A man to give it up, nerved you to grind
Your clenched teeth, breathing, till*

*Your skin broke down, your calves went flat
And your legs lost all sensation. Still,
You took enough morphine to kill
A strong man. Finally, nitrogen
Mustard: you could last two months after that;
It would kill you then.*

*Even then you wouldn't quit.
Old soldier, yet you must have known
Inside the animal had grown
Sick of the world, made up its mind*

> To stop. Your mind ground on its separate
> Way, merciless and blind,
>
> Into these last weeks when the breath
> Would only come in fits and starts
> That puffed out your sections like the parts
> Of some enormous, damaged bug.
> You waited, not for life, not for your death,
> Just for the deadening drug
>
> That made your life seem bearable.
> You still whispered you would not die.
> Yet in the nights I heard you cry
> Like a whipped child; in fierce old age
> You whimpered, tears stood on your gun-metal
> Blue cheeks shaking with rage
>
> And terror. So much pain would fill
> Your room that when I left I'd pray
> That if I came back the next day
> I'd find you gone. You stayed for me—
> Nailed to your own rapacious, still self-will.
> You've shook loose, finally.
>
> They'd say this was a worthwhile job
> Unless they tried it. It is mad
> To throw our good lives after bad;
> Waste time, drugs, and our minds, while strong
> Men starve. How many young men did we rob
> To keep you hanging on?
>
> I can't think we did you much good.
> Well, when you died, none of us wept.
> You killed for us, and so we kept
> You, because we need to earn our pay.
> No. We'd still have to help you try. We would
> Have killed for you today.

Listen now to a British neurologist as he expressed his sentiments about the age factor:

> For many patients the stroke has replaced pneumonia as the "old man's friend" by terminating a life which had already become a burden. The enthusiastic investigation of such patients is misplaced; their lives should be allowed to move to a peaceful and dignified

close. But strokes increasingly afflict younger patients . . . and the possibility that something may be done, to minimize the damage already done or to prevent further damage, justifies investigation [in such patients] (Marshall, 1967).

Age and Response to Treatment

To be sure, the physician has good reason to anticipate that his therapeutic ministrations may be less effective in the elderly patient. Old age, with its accumulated physical insults to the body, is often associated with a decreased resiliency, a diminished reserve, a lessened ability to bounce back from a new assault. The youngster who is critically ill is likely to suffer from one illness; the geriatric patient's illness is often just one of many ailments that plague him concurrently. Whatever the reasons, it is painfully evident that the treatment of a disease like acute leukemia is remarkably more successful in children than in adults.

Gofman and his colleagues (1966) have drawn certain important conclusions about aging with reference to the process of atherosclerosis, on the basis of certain data. Gofman believes that the loss of predictive value of blood lipid measurements for *de novo* ischemic heart disease at 55 years of age is dictated by the evolution of atherosclerosis. When the process is advanced, these lipid variables are no longer important, he reasons, and the modification of blood lipids will not alter the risk of developing new coronary artery disease. ". . . The life expectancy at 55 years of age and beyond will not be materially altered, so far as coronary heart disease is concerned, by moderate reductions in blood lipid levels . . ."

A considerable controversy erupted in 1967 in northwest London because of the following notice placed on the bulletin board of Neasden Hospital:

> The following patients are not to be resuscitated: very elderly, over 65; malignant disease. Chronic chest disease. Chronic renal disease.
> Top of yellow treatment card to be marked NTBR (i.e., Not to be Resuscitated).
> The following people should be resuscitated: collapse as a result

of diagnostic or therapeutic procedures—e.g., needle in pleura (even if over 65 years). Sudden unexpected collapse under 65 years—i.e., loss of consciousness, cessation of breathing, no carotid pulsation.

The notice, addressed to physicians and ward nurses, was signed by Doctor W. F. T. McMath, the hospital's medical superintendent. McMath was criticized by a board of inquiry appointed by the British minister of health for his blunt wording and for publicly displaying the notice (where a BBC TV team had discovered it). The minister's advisers quickly suggested that no person should be excluded from resuscitation by reason of age alone, but a number of British doctors publicly supported Doctor McMath. In a cartoon in the *Evening Standard,* one elderly patient asked another: "Is this one of those hospitals where one daren't stop breathing?"

Rank Has Its Privileges

A second variable is the estimate of "social worth" placed on the patient's life by the culture, both in general and specifically, and by the doctor in charge. A president, king, or prime minister will receive more attention than a drunken derelict. There will be more personnel mobilized, more equipment used, more expense tolerated to save the life of a famous artist or scientist than to preserve a demented vagrant.

In 1962, on an icy Moscow highway, the brilliant theoretical physicist Lev Davidovitch Landau was crushed in his car by a truck. A Czech neurologist announced that the injuries sustained were not compatible with life. The base of Landau's skull was fractured, his brain lacerated and contused. He suffered fractures of nine ribs, his pelvis, and leg, had air and blood in his chest cavity, severe abdominal contusions, and a ruptured urinary bladder. The left arm was completely paralyzed, the other arm and both legs partially so.

The scientist was deaf, blind, and speechless, and without reflexes. For two months he was in a state of coma, but the more than one hundred physicians who had come to Moscow to treat him did not give up. Four days after the accident, Doctor Landau "died": his pulse and blood pressure disappeared, and his electroencephalogram became flat. But the physicians in attendance refused to turn off the respirator; instead, they transfused blood into his radial artery, and gave intravenous adrenaline and digitalis. Life gradually returned. During the next week, death threatened on three more occasions.

Five weeks later, Landau recognized a close friend and collaborator. Eleven months after the accident, he was able to sit up in bed and smilingly accept his Nobel Prize. Landau never fully recovered, but lived another six years, a testimonial to the vigor and persistence of the international medical team that treated him and to the value placed by society on a brilliant and creative mind.

Death and Ability to Pay

There is a relation between income and the quality of medical care, but it is not a linear function. People who are so economically disadvantaged as to be forced to go without medical attention will of course be medically disadvantaged as well. Many indigent patients, however, receive care in teaching hospitals that is of a caliber often unobtainable by middle-class patients in small private proprietary hospitals.

While there is little or no systematically collected information on what may be the deleterious effects of physicians' racial or minority group prejudices on the care given to patients, it is not inconceivable that doctors, who are human beings as well as professionals, will treat less compulsively and thoroughly a patient whose sex, color, religion, or political affiliation for some reason raises unseemly passions in the doctor. (One famous example in drama is the case of the amoral artist Louis Dubedat, in *The Doctor's Dilemma,* who is denied treatment by a famous physician who both detests Dubedat and covets his wife.) The Negro in America is clearly at greater risk in terms of maternal and fetal mortality than the white, but it is not clear how much of this is simply attributable to poorer housing, poorer nutrition, lessened access to hospitals, or other factors. It may comfort the physician's conscience to believe (and it may well be true) that these other variables are primarily responsible, even if the net result for the Negro is unchanged.

One would like to think that the ability of a terminally ill patient to pay would not enter into decisions about medical care, but it would be unrealistic to propose such a generalization. To begin with, access to certain physicians and surgeons will be limited for the poor, who will not have the freedom of the rich to travel far and wide to see specialists (or to have them visit the patient), or to pay the fees of such specialists. In one kidney dialysis center, ability to pay the not inconsiderable costs of weekly dialysis is a prerequisite to enrollment in the program. The new heart transplant operations are fantastically expensive, and one wonders who would foot the bills for the indigent if and when the surgery were to become generally available.

The activities of relatives and friends of the patient can be either helpful or harmful. A proper degree of concern for a critically ill relative may result in seeking out additional consultation, or a change in physician or nurse when the patient seems to be receiving poor care. On the other hand, relatives may harm the patient by well-meaning but disastrous meddling in a case where good care is being provided. At the very least, such concern, if expressed in unpleasant or insulting terms, may alienate the doctor. (Unfortunately, some doctors childishly resent *any* suggestion of the need for consultation, even when meekly and courteously proffered by the family.) But another result may be to transfer the patient to less capable hands.

The Unattractive Patient

The physical characteristics of a patient may also result in his receiving suboptimal care. The incontinent old patient whose body, bed, and room often reek of urine and feces despite the attempts of the nursing staff to keep him clean may provoke an avoidance reaction in the doctor, who consciously or unconsciously may forego examining the patient as frequently as he would if the patient were an alluring young female with diaphanous bed garments and a penchant for heady perfumes. An aversion may also be displayed for the whining, complaining patient.

The alcoholic patient frequently suffers in this regard. Scorned by society, disheveled, dirty, and obstreperous, demanding of attention and a disruptive influence on the ward, he often antagonizes nurses, orderlies, and doctors, who resent his appearance, behavior, and demands on their time. Such patients require much more personal attention than most patients, but they often end up mummied in hospital swaddling, tied down and immobile. Such treatment, while expedient for the staff, may be disastrous medically as well as inhumane.

The decrepit "bum," in addition, may conjure up in the minds of his doctors the presence of communicable diseases. I remember a resident physician telling me once that he could not bring himself to give mouth-to-mouth resuscitation to such a person, for fear he would contract tuberculosis. (The fact that the person administering the resuscitation—which requires the doctor to exhale into the patient, not inhale—probably runs little risk in this situation did not seem to affect his opinion.)

Another way in which patients can affect their own prognosis lies in their propensity for following directions. There are many reports in the literature indicating that large numbers of patients do not take medications as prescribed. A few do not even bother to fill prescriptions; many more take their drugs less frequently than recommended, or for shorter periods of time than recommended. The reasons for such failure have not been adequately investigated, but one can at least postulate possible reasons: poor memory; low intelligence; a feeling that one is getting better and the pills are no longer needed; the (opposite) feeling that the pills are "not working"; the occurrence of side effects that are unpleasant enough to dissuade the patient from adherence to instructions; lack of hope in the patient, so that he sees no reason to take any medication. It would seem highly desirable to study these variables so that patient behavior could be modified in the appropriate direction. Unfortunately, many doctors seem unaware of the fact that the problem even exists; most seem convinced that their patients usually follow directions reasonably well.

Appealing and Unappealing Diseases

The approach to the patient is also affected by the disease from which he suffers. Cancer, for example, still arouses in many people the image of hopeless, horrible disease. Surveys of the lay public aimed at investigating the delays shown by patients in seeking medical advice for signs or symptoms suggestive of cancer reveal that the word cancer is associated with ideas of mutilation, death, and suffering. The physician shares some of these notions, since many cancers still defy treatment. As a result, a patient who is known (or suspected) to be ill with advanced metastatic disease may be "written off" as someone whose demise cannot be delayed and who will be better off as soon as he passes on.

Heart disease, on the other hand, is a different matter. There is, for the physician, no automatic cerebral reflex signifying "no hope." Patients who enter the hospital with the most severe cardiac decompensation are known to be able to leave the hospital looking and feeling remarkably well. Most patients with heart attacks leave the hospital alive, and many will be essentially normal after discharge. In addition, the *pace* of development of critical cardiac illness may condition the physician to act with speed and vigor. One minute a man is well, and the next he is lifeless, the victim of a heart attack. The contrast between health and death is startling. There has been no time for becoming conditioned to death, to expecting and accepting it. As a result, full resuscitative activity is mobilized. Since there is "nothing to lose"—the patient is dead unless the heart can be restarted—the doctor is likely to go through the full armamentarium available to him, in rapid succession. The efforts may not be successful, but the doctor also knows that, if they are not, they will not be excessively prolonged in any case.

This element of duration of treatment brings up the deleterious effect of chronicity. Doctors who receive satisfaction from providing months or years of care to a patient without much in the way of evidence that the patient is improving (and with perhaps a reasonable amount of complaining from the patient about the lack of progress) are in the minority. Most doctors relish the role of the effective therapist; they do not fancy the role of the impotent, frustrated physician. The patient with intractable pain, for instance, is a constant reminder to the doctor of his limitations, just as is the patient with intractable edema, or arthritis, or psychosis.

Bright Side and Vice Versa

Another variable affecting physicians' attitudes toward the care of the seriously ill patient is the relative position of the doctor on the optimism-pessimism continuum. At times this position is primarily determined by the basic personality of the doctor—he may be a person who looks ahead in a hopeful fashion in most situations, no matter

Physicians' Behavior Toward the Patient

how desperate the problem really seems to be, or he may be attracted to the gloomy view ("We're limited in what we can do for most patients," "Everybody's got to go sometime," and so on). It might be predicted, for example, that physicians who are depressive psychologically would tend to see their patients' problems in a pessimistic light, and to be less able to cope with them.

But the doctor's attitude—again along a pessimistic-optimistic continuum—about a given disease or group of diseases may be based not only on his basic personality but also on the profession's general semantic misconceptions. "Senility," to illustrate, can hide everything from dementia to drug intoxication. This awful word trap may preempt certain diagnostic or therapeutic maneuvers, and deceive the physician, causing him to miss the correct diagnosis of melancholia, excessive sedation, or simple neglect.

"Atherosclerosis" is another such wastebasket term, still associated in the minds of many with aging and irreversibility. For a long time, vascular disease of this kind was considered a "wear-and-tear" phenomenon, an inevitable concomitant of advancing years. Today there is no certainty about its causation, and reason to believe that it is related to exogenous influences such as dietary fats, and that dietary modification, or drug treatment, can alter its progression. Obviously the doctor's philosophy about atherosclerosis can affect his management of the aged patient suffering from serious atherosclerotic disease.

It has already been indicated that cancer is usually viewed pessimistically. Metastatic brain tumor, for many doctors, carries such a poor prognosis that its diagnosis tends to paralyze attempts at therapy. Although unrelieved gloom about such lesions is often justified, there is some evidence that this is not universally the case. A British study (Deeley and Edwards, 1968) reported that in a quarter of the cases in a necropsy series of individuals suffering from lung cancer the brain was the only site of secondary deposits of cancer. Almost half the patients who received full treatment (whole brain X-ray therapy) were able to return to a relatively normal life for at least one month, 15 per cent for more than six months, and 7 per cent for more than one year. At three years, 4 per cent of the patients with treated cerebral metastases were still alive. There was no way of predicting response to therapy; such factors as initial level of consciousness or duration of cerebral symptoms were not prognostically useful. Before treatment most of these patients were described as "drowsy," "ill," "inattentive" or "uncooperative"; some were in coma.

Conservatism or Radicalism?

An aggressive, optimistic outlook toward Hodgkin's disease and related lymphomas also seems to pay off. More vigorous and extensive X-ray therapy, for example, is apparently associated with a significantly improved prognosis in some groups of patients with these ailments (Kaplan, 1968).

It is not clear whether doctors who are "conservative" about one general form of therapy (such as drugs) are conservative about other forms of therapy (such as X-ray or surgery). Some physicians pride themselves on their slowness to adopt new drugs (one neurologist used to brag that he would not prescribe a drug until it had been on the market for eight years—"Let the other guys make the mistakes with those flash-in-the-pan drugs that turn out to be toxic or not effective"). The use of "unproven" remedies, such as dietary fat restriction to decrease atherosclerosis, will be espoused by those doctors whose attitude is: "Why not try it? What harm can it do?" It will tend not to be recommended by doctors who believe: "There's no evidence that it works. Why should I radically upset the eating habits of my patients —and perhaps of their families—because of a hope that may be unjustified, and without being sure that the new diet may not cause unpredicted troubles?"

Are there doctors who are "heroic" by nature, and attracted to the dramatic personal act, such as may be required in cardiac resuscitation, or passing an endotracheal tube to assist respiration? Contrariwise, are there "mousy" doctors who are repelled by such heroics? (I am convinced that anesthesia and surgery tend to attract the former type more than the latter.) There are many decisions in regard to surgery for the critically ill patient where aggressive or conservative therapeutic attitudes will affect the cause of therapy. A recent medical article stated the opinion of one British physician: "No patient with valve disease should be considered too ill for surgery, assuming that a skilled surgical team . . . is readily available" (Emanuel, 1968). An editorial in the same journal a week before, discussing another type of heart surgery—for a defect in the septum between the ventricles —pointed out: ". . . a prognosis of 20 years for the untreated patient often has to be weighed against an immediate operative risk of more than 15 per cent" (*British Medical Journal*, 1968a). Some surgeons acquire a reputation for willingness to operate on anyone who is desperately ill but whose life might be saved by an operation; others seem unwilling to acquire a "bad operative mortality record" in patients whose hopes are slim.

The physician's personal habits may also affect his therapeutic preferences, or at least his therapeutic efficacy. The doctor who is a "jogging" enthusiast is more likely to push this form of exercise in his recovered coronary patients than the doctor who abhors exercise. The obese doctor is going to be less effective than the lean physician in advising low-calorie diets to his overweight patients. (He may also have a higher threshold for the diagnosis of "overweight.") The physician who has not been able to stop his own cigarette smoking is not likely to act the role of the evangelist crusader against tobacco.

Quality as Product of Intensity of Care

There are objective evidences of "corporate" optimism or aggressiveness in therapy that may also affect the care of the terminally or seriously ill. I refer to the "teams" or "units" whose existence is based on the assumption that careful arrangements (for equipment, personnel, and so on) made in anticipation of the entry of patients with life-threatening illness will favorably affect prognosis. This may take the form of a cardiac arrest team, a coronary care unit, a burn unit, a trauma unit, an intensive care ward, a renal dialysis team, or an organ transplant facility. It is beyond contention that the life-span of at least some patients who enter the jurisdiction of such teams will be extended through expert use of up-to-date treatment modalities.

The units just described are usually set up on a more or less permanent basis to fulfill "service" functions. But there is another way in which prognosis can be affected that is related to research. An institution may decide, for instance, to develop a cancer chemotherapy research program where none previously existed. Although it is true that the experimental nature of the drugs or surgery or X-ray regimens to be used may at times deleteriously affect the course of some patients, it is more often the case that the marshaling of manpower and the accumulation of expertise through having a large volume of clinical material focused in the hands of a small number of doctors results in a net increase in the quality of care for these patients. Indeed, the very existence of protocols calling for the systematic recording and analysis of information about research patients often brings to light either new facts about the disease under study or a more accurate quantification of facts previously known or suspected.

A recent example of this sort is the "suicidology" program concept, where special teams are created to deal expertly with the problems of individuals who threaten to take their own lives. The existence of such a program seems to provide not only medical advice in terms of specific crisis, but also the opportunity to collect data that will presumably ameliorate the future handling of such patients by generating answers to such questions as: How can we improve diagnosis of depressive states so as to predict suicidal risk? For which patients are drugs justified (with their slower onset of action) and for which should electroconvulsive shock be instituted without delay? Which patients should be hospitalized, which treated on an ambulatory basis? How can one predict which patients may attempt suicide with the very drugs prescribed for their depressions? How can one mobilize family and other extra-hospital support to tide patients over periods of severe stress?

Therapeutic Enthusiasm

The care of the terminally ill will be subject to vagaries associated with fads and fashions in medicine. At times such medical attitudes are clearly related to solid evidence in favor of a new therapeutic posture, such as in the case of agranulocytosis (the disappearance of circulating white blood cells). Here the advent of antibiotics changed the prognosis radically. Before antibiotics, many of the patients died and there was little one could do for them; since antibiotics, most of them survive. A similar situation was created when arteriography of the cerebral blood vessels made it possible to diagnose treatable brain lesions that previously could only be suspected on clinical grounds.

At other times, the change in therapeutic posture is no less dramatic, but the enthusiasm generated seems out of proportion to the actual clinical results. An example of the latter would be the discovery of cortisone and ACTH as a treatment for the severely ill patient with rheumatoid arthritis. Before cortisone, arthritis was a generally unexciting clinical field for most doctors. Treatment of many forms of arthritis was limited in efficacy, and the chronicity of the ailments tended to frustrate doctors. After cortisone, the field of arthritis was revolutionized. It is now an extremely active area of investigation, with all aspects of arthritis under scrutiny. While part of the revolution was due to the admittedly dramatic effects of cortisone in some patients, it is more likely that the continuing enthusiasm is due to the opening up of new areas of research interest into the basic nature of rheumatoid arthritis, and the luring of capable investigators into the field. Today, cortisone is acknowledged to be of definite but limited use in the treatment of rheumatoid arthritis, with serious potential toxicity contingent on its long-term use; nevertheless, the approach to the arthritic patient is more optimistic and aggressive than in the past.

Euthanasia, Yes or No?

The attitude of the profession toward euthanasia will obviously affect the care of the terminally ill. So long as our society continues to look upon the purposeful shortening of life as murder, euthanasia will not be as important a consideration as it will become when the culture accepts mercy killing as ethical and desirable for some. There have now been several cases which seem to set important precedents in this area (Lasagna, 1968). In two Swedish cases, for example, the doctor and the relatives agreed to stop treatment that was maintaining life in two elderly patients. The judge ruled that the physician acted properly. It would seem logical to take the next step, and "actively" to cut short life (with drugs, for example) in other cases where continued existence seemed meaningless.

It is unfortunate that such enthusiastic attempts are made at times to keep alive individuals who should not be deprived of their "right to die." The following letter appeared in the correspondence column of the *British Medical Journal* (Letter to Editor, 1968):

> Sir,—A doctor aged 68 was admitted to an overseas hospital after a barium meal had shown a large carcinoma of the stomach. He had retired from practice five years earlier, after severe myocardial infarction had left his exercise tolerance considerably reduced. The early symptoms of the carcinoma were mistakenly thought to be due to myocardial ischaemia. By the time when the possibility of carcinoma was first considered the disease was already far advanced; laparotomy showed extensive metastatic involvement of the abdominal lymph nodes and liver. Palliative gastrectomy was performed with the object of preventing perforation of the primary tumour into the peritoneal cavity, which appeared to the surgeon to be imminent. Histological examination showed the growth to be an anaplastic primary adenocarcinoma. There was clinical and radiological evidence of secondary deposits in the lower thoracic and lumbar vertebrae.
>
> The patient was told of the findings and fully understood their import. In spite of increasingly large doses of pethidine, and of morphine at night, he suffered constantly with severe abdominal pain and pain resulting from compression of spinal nerves by tumour deposits.
>
> On the tenth day after the gastrectomy the patient collapsed with classic manifestation of massive pulmonary embolism. Pulmonary embolectomy was successfully performed in the ward by a registrar. When the patient had recovered sufficiently he expressed his appreciation of the good intentions and skill of his young colleague. At the same time he asked that if he had a further cardiovascular collapse no steps should be taken to prolong his life, for the pain of his cancer was now more than he would needlessly continue to endure. He himself wrote a note to this effect in his case records, and the staff of the hospital knew his feelings.
>
> His wish notwithstanding, when the patient collapsed again, two weeks after the embolectomy—this time with acute myocardial infarction and cardiac arrest—he was revived by the hospital's emergency resuscitation team. His heart stopped on four further occasions during that night and each time was restarted artificially. The body then recovered sufficiently to linger for three more weeks, but in a decerebrate state, punctuated by episodes of projectile vomiting accompanied by generalized convulsions. Intravenous nourishment was carefully combined with blood transfusion and measures necessary to maintain electrolyte and fluid balance. In addition, antibacterial and

antifungal antibiotics were given as prophylaxis against infection, particularly pneumonia complicating the tracheotomy that had been performed to ensure a clear airway. On the last day of the illness preparations were being made for the work of the failing respiratory centre to be given over to an artificial respirator, but the heart finally stopped before this endeavour could be realized.

This case report is submitted for publication without commentary or conclusions, which are left for those who may read it to provide for themselves.

W. St. C. Symmers, Sen.

The advent of organ transplants is beginning to change the way critically ill patients are managed. The potential recipient of a heart transplant will be looked upon more optimistically now than in the past. Paradoxically, the potential *donor* of a heart transplant may have his existence cut short, since there are exigencies in regard to time that will put a premium on cardiac removal and transplantation before post-mortem degeneration has set in. (Since "young" hearts will make better transplants than "old" hearts, this may become one area where the present inclination of doctors to favor the young patient in prolonging life may be reversed.)

Should the Dying Be Told?

There are all too few data on the extent and manner of discussions of impending death between patient and doctor (or physician and relatives) and the effect of such discussions. Surveys suggest that doctors do not learn how to handle this problem in school or hospital training, and that many physicians do not look on it as a researchable question (Oken, 1961). Although doctors in general affirm that they would personally want to be told if critically ill, they usually withhold such information from their own patients (Aldrich, 1963). There is a great deal of lip service given to the concept that "some patients should certainly be told," but it is never made clear just how the choice is to be made.

In most instances, discussion of death is treated as something to be shunned. Children dying on a hospital ward are treated furtively, and with secrecy, rather than with dignity, in the belief that the other children would be "upset" if the truth were known. In fact, it appears that dying children often fear death, and have fantasies about it which can be dispelled with simple reassurance (Yudkin, 1967). The whole area badly needs more data and less repetition of clichés.

How are we to identify those patients who should be told "all"? How much do we tell relatives? (It is often assumed that telling a relative is tantamount to shielding the patient from the knowledge, despite evidence to the contrary. People who are close to each other may readily betray their emotions to each other.) Is the doctor the best person to break the news? Would the minister be better? How technically is it best done? What of the other patients on the ward or floor? What is the impact of another patient's death on them? Should *they* be told in advance? What is the most dignified and humane way of handling the body and effects of a deceased patient in a hospital environment?

The above considerations have been discussed not in an attempt to confer an air of spurious scientism upon the problems of the dying patient, but rather to list some important areas of interaction between doctor, patient, family, and institution. I am sure there are many others that I have neglected, and that there are errors (albeit unintentional) in what has been said. The important points are that the care of the dying patient is complicated by many factors other than those usually considered, and we have for too long failed to study this important problem with the precision and compassion it deserves.

REFERENCES

Aldrich, C. K.
   1963   "Dying patient's grief." Journal of the American Medical Association 184 (May 4):329–331.
Deeley, T. J., and J. M. Rice Edwards.
   1968   "Radiotherapy in the management of cerebral secondaries from bronchial carcinoma." Lancet 1 (June 8):1209–1212.
Editorial.
   1968   "First British heart transplant." British Medical Journal 1 (May 11):315–316.
Emanuel, R.
   1968   "Too ill for cardiac surgery?" British Medical Journal 1 (May 18):400–402.

Gofman, J. W., W. Young, and R. Tandy.
   1966   "Ischemic heart disease, atherosclerosis, and longevity." Circulation 34(October):679–697.

Kaplan, H. S.
   1968   "Clinical evaluation and radiotherapeutic management of Hodgkin's disease and the malignant lymphomas." New England Journal of Medicine 278(April 18):892–899.

Lasagna, L.
   1968   Life, Death, and the Doctor. New York: Knopf.

Letter to Editor.
   1968   British Medical Journal 1(February 17):442.

Marshall, J.
   1967   "The use and abuse of cerebral angiography in the diagnosis of strokes." American Heart Journal 74(August):145–148.

Oken, D.
   1961   "What to tell cancer patients. A study of medical attitudes." Journal of the American Medical Association 175(April 1):1120–1127.

Snodgrass, W. P.
   1968   After Experience. New York: Harper.

Yudkin, S.
   1967   "Children and death." Lancet 1(January 7):37–41.

6

Innovations and Heroic Acts in Prolonging Life

Robert J. Glaser

THE REMOVAL OF THE heart from one person and its substitution for a diseased organ in another is an enormously dramatic procedure. It is not surprising that Christiaan Barnard's first cardiac transplantation in man, performed in December, 1967, was one of the most highly publicized events of our time. While many applauded this medical first, there were those who expressed less enthusiasm, and a few were indignant because of the moral and ethical implications that were inevitably brought to the fore. To me, however, the fact that attention should be focused on certain extramedical considerations of heart transplantation in man did not come as a surprise because almost ten years earlier, when I was the chief administrative officer of another university medical center, where a detailed experimental study of liver transplantation was underway, I was involved in a decision as to whether that previously untried procedure should be attempted in man.

The circumstances were as follows. A man who had shot himself through the head in a suicide attempt was brought into the emergency room of the university hospital. The clinical signs indicated massive, irreversible brain damage, and death seemed imminent. My surgical colleagues, who had been working over a long period of time on the problem of liver transplantation, had carried out a carefully planned series of laboratory investigations; these had eventuated in the definition of a surgical technique for transplantation of the liver, one that had

Innovations, Heroic Acts in Prolonging Life

been successfully carried out repeatedly in dogs. A number of animals had survived the procedure and the transplanted livers had functioned well. My colleagues now reasoned that their experience in the laboratory had brought them to the point where a human trial was justified. Further, a potential recipient, a man in the terminal stages of liver failure, was in the hospital.

The importance of successful liver transplantation in man was obvious to me as it would have been to any physician. One need consider only one statistic, namely, that annual deaths in the United States from cirrhosis of the liver alone are in excess of 26,000, to appreciate the promise of successful liver transplantation for such patients; indeed, it would represent the only chance for their survival.

But the issues raised by the proposal were awesome. Because the liver, like the heart, is unpaired and necessary to life, its removal makes death a certainty. In the strict legal sense, therefore, extirpation of this organ from a still-living patient could be viewed as a homicidal act, even though the donor was doomed to death from an unrelated cause. The moral, ethical, and legal issues involved had not hitherto been confronted and were of such magnitude that we concluded that the transplantation should not be undertaken. Thus, what would have been the first transplantation of an unpaired organ in man was postponed, although the same surgeons successively carried out the procedure a few years later.

Others holding responsible administrative posts in medical centers undoubtedly have faced similar questions in the last few years, although in remarkably short order the performance of numerous single-organ transplantations has apparently constituted enough of a precedent to lessen the gravity of the decision.

The episode I cite is of some historical interest, now that heart transplantation has become relatively commonplace. At least it is less of a sensational event these days even though we are a long way from achieving long-term success. The episode also illustrates the dilemmas that we face as the result of progress in biomedical science. At the same time, it emphasizes the fact that today, even as was the case a century or more ago, medicine involves art as well as science. In a wide spectrum of illnesses, ranging from a simple upper respiratory infection to a life-threatening affliction, the physician often faces complex decisions that cannot be made wholly on the basis of exact knowledge. The constant acquisition of new information improves the overall situation but much remains to be learned.

The intent of this chapter is to examine certain of the problems and issues that we confront as a result of our acquiring the means to extend the lives of "dying," or at any rate, critically ill, patients through heroic intervention. We shall not directly be concerned here, for example, with the prevention of disability and/or death through such measures as immunization against poliomyelitis, or with the reduction by drugs of the death rate from hypertensive heart disease, important though these both be. Rather what does concern us are the new, potentially important additions to the physician's armamentarium whereby diseased organs, vital to life, can be replaced by physiologically effective ones. Replacement per se brings to mind, consciously or subconsciously, the concept of immortality, something that has a powerful appeal for most men. The quest of Ponce de Leon centuries ago, and the more recent claim for rejuvenation of sexual function exploited so successfully by the late quack John Brinkley, testify to man's continuing search to avoid aging and death. Of course, the element of drama that characterizes organ transplantation gives it special attraction.

It is not fair to criticize the surgeon because his act of intervention in transplantation is so newsworthy. That there are those who can perhaps be criticized for utilizing the public media for reporting what more properly should be communicated via learned journals is difficult to deny. But in our society, one must recognize that dramatic aspects of medicine inevitably provoke interest, which may be disproportionate in terms of the importance of the specific underlying stimulus. Nonetheless, the subject of transplantation, particularly of a single unpaired organ, is obviously a fascinating one, bound to attract the public's attention. In the succeeding sections, I will present a brief review of the field, and then move to an examination of the following aspects: the rise of organ transplantation; its impact on the definition of death; the problem of the supply of organs; the significance of tissue rejection; the status of professional competence, and the costs of heroic procedures; the shaping and misshaping of public opinion; the quality of prolonged life; the need for criteria for prolongation and termination of life; and a final note on the rational basis of hope.

Rise of Organ Transplantation

The development of the artificial kidney as a substitute for badly diseased natural ones provided a means whereby the vital excretory function of the kidneys could be maintained for prolonged periods. In turn, this scientific advance contributed significantly to the performance of kidney transplantation in patients with advanced chronic nephritis and other diseases that culminate in complete failure of both kidneys. The artificial kidney constituted an effective means of life support for patients with renal failure until transplantation could be performed. It also made it possible for such patients to come to surgery in a relatively more normal physiologic state, and thus made them better risks. In December, 1954, Doctor Joseph E. Murray and his co-workers at the Peter Bent Brigham Hospital in Boston performed the first kidney homograft to result in a long-term success. Their patient lived for eight years, succumbing to the same disease in the transplanted organ that had destroyed his own kidneys. The latter fact is of great medical interest itself although it cannot be discussed here.

Initially, kidney transplantation depended on, and was also restricted by, two essential conditions. The first is that man has two kidneys but can live normally with only one, so the healthy living donor accepts as an *immediate danger* in providing one of his two kidneys only the tiny statistical risk of surgical mortality. The second factor is that transplantation between identical twins completely circumvents the fundamental problem of rejection, that is, the process by which one living being treats the introduction of tissue from another, even from his own mother or father, as an invasion and marshals defenses to repel it. Another and more precise way of defining the phenomenon is to say that the body develops antibodies as a potent immunologic defense against the antigens of foreign proteins, unless the relationship between the latter and the host's own tissues is so close as to be unrecognized by these defenses as being "foreign."

The obviously stringent restriction of renal transplantation to the unusual circumstance where donor and recipient were identical twins was largely eliminated as a result of the fundamental studies of Sir Peter Medawar; his work on the nature of immunity and of the mechanisms for its inhibition, particularly by means of immuno-suppressive drugs, opened the way for kidney transplantation on a broad scale. It became apparent that the transplantation of a kidney from a related individual or even an unrelated one could be successfully accomplished. Indeed, it was soon found that kidneys taken from cadavers immediately after death were capable of normal function when introduced into a recipient.

As a direct consequence of the foregoing studies, more than twenty-five hundred kidney homografts have been performed in the last fifteen years. The one-year survival rate has been 75 per cent or better, and the two-year life expectancy is of the order of 50 per cent. The longest survival to date of an identical twin has been more than twelve years and, in a patient who received his graft from a nonrelated person, about ten years. In fact, life with a borrowed kidney has been sufficiently durable that in a very few cases—less than one-half of 1 per cent of the total—patients have survived long enough to develop cancer and die of this cause instead.*

As with kidney transplants, the advent of heart transplantation depended on a combination of technologic advance and the further accrual of immunologic knowledge. The heart-lung machine, the development of which some years earlier made open-heart surgery for certain congenital and acquired cardiac defects a routine procedure in many medical centers, also was a *sine qua non* for cardiac transplantation. Although not as efficient as the artificial kidney, which in a sense has a simpler function to perform, the heart-lung apparatus does provide for oxygenation and circulation of the blood for three to six hours at a time; a period of this duration, with the heart and lungs out of the circulation, is adequate for the surgeon to perform a cardiac transplantation.

Because heart transplantations in human patients were initiated much later than kidney transplants, our observations are far more limited. It is clear, however, that results have not been as good to date. The longest survival has been that of Barnard's second patient, Doctor Philip Blaiberg; he was operated on in January, 1968, and survived at least one crisis due to hepatitis and possible rejection. Blaiberg died in August, 1969, more than nineteen months after receiving

---

* Recently it has been suggested that the risk of malignancy may be enhanced because of the use of immuno-suppressive measures.

a new heart. The second longest survivor was Father Charles Boulogne of France, who died in October, 1969, slightly more than seventeen months after operation. The results as of May, 1969, are reviewed in Table 1.

TABLE 1
Three-month Survival Rate of Recipients of Heart Transplant Operations, by Period When Operation Was Performed

PERIOD WHEN OPERATION WAS PERFORMED	PERCENTAGE OF RECIPIENTS SURVIVING FOR THREE MONTHS		
	ALL OPERATIONS	U.S. AND CANADIAN OPERATIONS	FOREIGN OPERATIONS
December, 1967–May, 1968	16%	20%	11%
	N(19)	(10)	(9)
June, 1968–November, 1968	38%	46%	22%
	N(78)	(55)	(23)
December, 1968–May, 1969	23%	28%	10%
	N(35)	(25)	(10)
Total	31%	38%	17%
	N(132)	(90)	(42)

Although new cases were continuously being added, the number of persons with someone else's heart beating in their chests tended to stay at about 50 per cent of the total who had had the operation, but significant numbers died within days or weeks. The three-month survival rate in 132 operations proved to be one in three (Table 1). Two patients have had a second heart transplant, but neither did well.

The first attempts to transplant the spleen, liver, and lung were made in 1963. The results have so far been unimpressive. Of the first seven replacements of the spleen, there was one five-year survival and two one-year survivals, but the operation remains at best a controversial one. About sixty liver transplants have been performed to date; at this writing, one survivor is doing well after twenty-one months, and a second sixteen months, after operations. Since July, 1967, one-third of Starzl's patients have survived over a year. It should be noted that the surgical procedure for liver replacement is technically considerably more difficult than for cardiac transplantation, and the immediate postoperative mortality is consequently much higher.

Of the first eight whole lung transplants, the longest survival was eighteen days. Three patients in Japan received a single lobe and survived, but in each case the grafted lung tissue had to be removed from one to three weeks after transplantation. A patient in Belgium died in 1969, ten months after acquiring a whole lung graft, a new record for this organ. The interruption of the involuntary nervous system incident to removal of the lung is a major problem and so is primary infection (as contrasted to secondary infection due to the use of immuno-suppressive agents).

Efforts to transplant the pancreas, attempted first in 1966, have been unrewarding.

Definition of Death

Even with only a relatively small number of surgeons undertaking the procedure, the advent of heart transplantation created a brisk demand for hearts. Because those involved in transplantation stated publicly that the donor's heart should be beating at the time it was removed, a considerable degree of concern was generated on the part of the medical profession as well as the public. Hearts from potential donors who have been dead for more than a few minutes offer little or no promise of survival to prospective recipients. The imagery conjured up was by and large unexpressed, but at one point Barnard found it necessary to protest, "We are not vultures."

Practically speaking, if a donor's heart is to be used, it is necessary to maintain artificially the circulation of the donor, who has "just died" or is "about to die," by means of the heart-lung apparatus until the recipient is ready to receive the transplant. On the other hand, to describe as "dead" a patient who is still breathing and whose heart is still beating creates new issues. Thus, it becomes a matter of great urgency to define death in a way that (a) gives the "dying patient" every possible protection in terms of his rights; (b) protects the cardiac surgeon from allegations of violating moral, civil, or criminal law; and (c) does not preclude a potentially life-saving operation for the patient desperately in need of a new heart.

The Hippocratic Oath obliges the physician not only to help, but also "never to harm," a patient, "nor to give advice which may cause his death." The ancient pledge applies well to what may be described as the modern doctor's dilemma.

Innovations, Heroic Acts in Prolonging Life [109

Twenty-five years ago, when I was concluding my residency training, the decision as to when a patient was dead was a relatively uncomplicated one. When a patient's heart stopped beating and he ceased to breathe, he was pronounced dead. Death might be verified by electrocardiogram—the absence of electrical impulses on the tracing was considered decisive. Under certain circumstances, the injection of such drugs as epinephrine (adrenalin) was carried out as a heroic measure but rarely produced more than a few additional spasmodic cardiac beats.

Since those days, however, medical science has developed new methods for support of both cardiovascular and respiratory functions. Thus, prompt cardiac resuscitation can restore a normal heartbeat in a significant percentage of patients stricken with coronary occlusion and/or a lethal cardiac arrhythmia, such as ventricular fibrillation. Combined with mouth-to-mouth breathing or mechanical assistance from a respirator, cardiac resuscitation has in fact produced a marked reduction in the immediate mortality from acute myocardial infarction, and has improved the immediate prognosis of this common, life-threatening affliction.

Unfortunately, even short periods of circulatory failure, associated as they are with inadequate oxygenation of the blood, can result in irreparable brain damage. In such instances, despite the return of a normal heartbeat and subsequent adequate circulation of oxygenated blood, the patient no longer can function intellectually. In short, he is doomed to a vegetative existence. As measured by continued circulation and respiration, machinery can maintain life in such a person for long periods.

In our inquiry into the meaning of death, we must differentiate between cardiac death and brain death. Because we are often slow to give up old concepts for new ones, this question may be debated for some time but, practically speaking, the answer is already in hand. Life and death, like day and night, are not absolute qualities but move one into the other. Thus, death comes at different times to different tissues and organs, affecting cells of the brain in only a matter of minutes but less rapidly altering skeletal muscle and bone.

Insofar as it involves organ donors and their rights, the technical question of death has been resolved, by popular consensus, in the recognition that the brain and not the heart is the seat of human life.

In August, 1968, thirteen transplant surgeons met in the Cape Town Conference on Heart Transplants. Following this meeting, Doctor Denton Cooley of Houston, Texas, who at that point in time had performed the largest number of cardiac transplants, reported: "On the sticky question of how to determine the donor's death, there was no heated controversy, probably because all of us had answered this question for ourselves a long time ago. We agreed that neurological examination and electroencephalograph tracings should show no signs of cerebral activity, but did not define the length of time this should be so. In most heart transplants performed to date, this period exceeded two hours. In two of my donors, there was a flattened EEG for four days prior to transplantation . . ."

In due time, an authoritative opinion was set forth by a Harvard Medical School *ad hoc* committee, which provided a definition of irreversible coma, or so-called "brain death syndrome." A relatively simple series of clinical tests to substantiate irrevocable loss of intellectual function was defined: the absence of a response to outside stimuli, such as pain; the absence of spontaneous movements or breathing; the absence of reflexes, and presence of fixed dilated pupils; and the failure of spontaneous breathing when the respirator is turned off for up to three minutes at a time (Beecher, 1968).

Meanwhile, the House of Delegates of the American Medical Association issued a policy statement intended to safeguard donors against overeagerness in behalf of recipients: ". . . When a vital single organ is to be transplanted, the death of the donor shall have been determined by at least one physician other than the recipient's physician. Death shall be determined by the clinical judgment of the physician . . ." In this connection, in a number of medical centers, where transplantation has been performed, independent evaluation teams made up of physicians uninvolved in the program had already been established to certify the appropriateness of both the donor and the recipient for their respective roles. For example, in the Stanford University Hospital, donors are evaluated by several neurologists or neurosurgeons, and recipients by several cardiologists. In each instance these physicians are not part of the transplantation team.

There the matter now rests. Although the beating heart remains for some a symbol of life and love, its role has been put into perspec-

Innovations, Heroic Acts in Prolonging Life

tive scientifically. The brain is our master control; the heart is just a pump.

The Problem of Supply and Demand

Surprisingly, the definition-of-death issue has been much easier to resolve than other items on the heart transplantation agenda. The next questions deal with demand and supply; they begin with, "Who gets a new heart?" followed by, "Where do we get hearts?"

Specific criteria for selection of recipients have been difficult to establish, but most medical scientists believe that heart transplantation should be limited to patients with so-called end-stage heart disease, mainly those with advanced coronary artery disease. These are persons who have usually had multiple myocardial infarcts, have markedly impaired blood-pumping action, cannot work, and often cannot even get out of bed—in short, patients for whom the outlook is not only hopeless but also extremely limited in time.

People with end-stage heart disease form a substantial group. In the United States, more than a million people die each year of cardiovascular-renal diseases, nearly 750,000 from diseases of the heart itself and nearly 600,000 from arteriosclerotic diseases, including coronary arteriosclerosis. Heart transplantation mainly concerns this last group, but in reality only a minor fraction of it, because half or more of the total number succumb to sudden death from myocardial infarction. Meanwhile, those who respond to medical management of their disease cannot be considered candidates, even though a fatal attack may overtake them at any time. Estimates of total potential heart recipients in the United States have ranged from 5,000 to 80,000 per year, with 40,000 as a probably realistic number.

Selection of patients for heart transplant so far has depended primarily on the clinical judgment of the surgeon and the consent of the patient and his family. As noted, however, in most centers independent cardiac experts have been involved in approving the selection. To date no serious effort has been made to displace the seat of clinical decision. In 1968, Senator Walter Mondale of Minnesota introduced a bill calling for the establishment of a national commission to represent the public in exploring the ethical and social implications of health science research and development, and to set policy goals, but not to regulate specific health activities. In hearings on the bill before the Senate Committee concerned, Doctor Barnard appeared to testify against the bill and engaged in a sharp exchange of views with Senator Abraham Ribicoff of Connecticut. Barnard described the Mondale proposal as an "insult to doctors." Several American heart surgeons and anesthesiologists favored the proposed legislation, however.

Ideally, the donor heart should be free of disease; preferably it should come from a young adult, for coronary sclerosis is very common in older adults, especially males, even though they may be asymptomatic. In practice, heart donors for the most part have been persons suffering fatal head injuries in automobile accidents, or those dying from massive strokes or other irreversible brain disease. The combined annual toll within these categories is about 250,000. There are about 60,000 prospective donors between the ages of 15 and 49. Victims of homicide and suicide are also potential heart donors, but in these cases, and particularly in the former, the medico-legal requirement of an autopsy is apt to be a major obstacle. Further, if the heartbeat is restored, a vexing question arises: Can murder be charged? In one instance to date, an assault victim who suffered irreversible brain damage served as the donor of a heart; because his heart was removed while it still was beating, attorneys for the donor's assailants have claimed that murder was not committed.

There is considerable interest on the part of physicians as well as laymen in developing the legal and technical means to make available beating hearts and other functional organs for transplantation. A few states have enacted versions of a Uniform Anatomical Gift Act, a model law modifying the nearest of kin's traditional legal right to dispose of the remains and instead giving the individual himself the right to will what shall be done with his body. Many thoughtful citizens have designated that their bodies should be made available to medical schools and teaching hospitals for teaching and/or research purposes; indeed, in some instances, there is an oversupply of such bodies. In any case, most bodies received via this route are those of elderly persons who have often succumbed to debilitating diseases, and their organs are of no potential use for transplantation.

Many persons have offered their organs for transplantation after death. Nevertheless, the number of heart transplantation operations

Innovations, Heroic Acts in Prolonging Life [113

performed has been limited both by a shortage of appropriate donors, and by the high costs involved, especially in terms of aftercare, which demands constant surveillance and repetitive technical observations. The number of willing and appropriate recipients in medical centers where transplants are being done is large, but donors are few, and the rather poor results of cardiac transplantation to date appear to have discouraged the families of prospective donors.

It may be that transplantation of a heart from one human being to another will never be a wholly accepted practice. Among all the other reasons, including the need for the donor to be free of heart disease, cancer, infection, or any other transferable disease, is a subtle question of logic. That one person must lose his life in order that someone else may live probably is, at least to some idealists, an offensive idea. In any event, the net saving in terms of human life is zero.

Substitutes for Human Hearts

What about a mechanical heart? It is natural that attention should be directed toward the possibility of constructing an artificial device as a first alternative. The artificial kidney, the heart-lung machine, and a world of automated gadgetry provide examples of the incredible things that machinery can do; a truly effective artificial heart would have enormously wide application.

Efforts to develop a mechanical heart are in progress, but the best estimates suggest that it will be years before such a device will be available for clinical trial. It is reasonable to predict that with the expenditure of sufficient funds and the enlistment of the talents of skilled engineers and other scientists, it would be possible to develop a mechanical heart that is relatively foolproof and, therefore, useful for the replacement of diseased hearts. But such a machine should not be confused with the various pacemakers, boosters, or pumping devices currently available, some of which are described in the press as artificial or mechanical hearts. The latter are intended to assist the heart or, at best, take over its function for brief periods of time.*

---

* As this chapter was being written, Cooley implanted a mechanical heart in a patient with end-stage heart disease, but emphasized that the device was only a "standby," and could be expected to function only for a week or ten days at most. He stated that he introduced the prosthesis in the hope that a heart from a human donor would become available, and one did after several days. The prosthetic device was replaced but the patient died on the third postoperative day.

The tremendous difficulties confronting those who attempt to build a mechanical heart should not be overlooked. Not much larger than a man's fist, the human heart beats regularly, approximately seventy times a minute from birth to death, a period that often extends seventy years or more. As if this fact were not phenomenal enough, the heart has an inherent regulator that enables it to speed up and meet the body's greater need for oxygen in exercise, and conversely to slow down when the body is at rest. The best of machines do not have this degree of reliability combined with such remarkable flexibility; the finest mechanical machines so far invented get out of order and require servicing at intervals.

An artificial heart would not only have to be relatively small and extremely efficient in both structure and function, but it would also have to be absolutely "fail-safe" in terms of its power source. As we have noted, brain function, on which meaningful human life is totally dependent, in turn requires uninterrupted cardiac function. Failure of the circulation for only a matter of a few minutes produces irreversible brain damage. The development of a system for energizing such a pump so that it will beat steadily and also respond to increased physiological demand is a task of gigantic proportion.

Further, we must also learn how to prevent damage to red blood cells as they course through the artificial organ. One of the unique and essential features of the human heart and blood vessels is the presence of a nonwettable lining, which permits the oxygen-loaded red cells—themselves quite fragile—to move through rapidly without being bruised or broken. One of the limitations of the present heart-lung machine is the significant destruction of red blood cells that occurs. Because destruction of red cells proceeds at an unremitting rate, the use of the existing apparatus as a stand-in for the heart and lungs is limited to a period of a relatively few hours; beyond this time, the hemolysis of red cells and the resultant release of hemoglobin become so great that the procedure must be discontinued.

It will become even more apparent, when we discuss tissue rejection, that we have at hand no quick route to dependable single-organ transplantation. Is there a long-term solution that is both practical and relatively simple? If the answer is yes, it eventually may lie in the utilization of organs from higher mammals. The hearts and livers of such animals as sheep, baboons, pigs, and calves represent a supply that is almost unlimited and free of many of the drawbacks inevitably involved in the use of human organs.

The hearts of a number of mammals are anatomically quite similar to that of the human. A few abortive attempts have been made to transplant animal organs into humans; for example, the heart of a chimpanzee has been implanted in a man. Although none of these attempts has been successful in any significant sense, and the surgeons responsible for undertaking them have been subject to censure in some quarters, the actual surgical procedure has been successfully carried out and the function of the transplanted organ has been maintained for brief periods of time.

While chimpanzees, having many features comparable to man, suggest themselves as organ donors in preference to other mammals, they are in fact not a practical source. There are probably no more than five hundred in captivity in America, and estimates suggest that it costs about $10,000 to raise a chimpanzee. Baboons, on the other hand, are available in larger numbers, and any number of sheep or pigs could be provided if the market demanded.

Tissue Rejection

The steady progress that has characterized biomedical research in the past few decades suggests that the problem of tissue rejection will be solved. But it is, of course, not possible to predict accurately how soon control of the rejection process will be achieved. Until it is, animal organs cannot be used in transplantation, and success with human donor hearts will be limited at best. So far, rejection is the major roadblock to human organ transplantation. The surgical procedure, especially in the case of heart replacement, is not in itself an obstacle. No one has been more enthusiastic about cardiac transplantation than Christiaan Barnard, but Barnard himself has said that ". . . rejection of the transplanted heart is inevitable . . ." and that what the transplant surgeon offers is "palliation and not cure." This, in other words, confirms what immunologists pointed out early on —that the state of the art (surgery) has outrun the state of the science (immunology).

Clearly, the future of organ transplantation lies in the precise definition of the rejection phenomenon and the development of means whereby rejection can be prevented. Although there may be differences in some aspects of rejection in animals as contrasted to man, it is likely that understanding of the basic phenomenon, once achieved, may well apply to all higher animals as well as to man. It is on this basis that I suggest the possibility of our ultimately being able to use animal tissues in man. In any case, once we gain full understanding of the rejection process, the knowledge should be applicable not only to transplantation of the heart, but also to transplantation of the lungs, liver, kidneys, and other organs.

The introduction of drugs, such as imuran, capable of suppressing antibody formation, as noted earlier, has made possible much of the progress to date. In addition, the corticosteroids, in combination with immuno-suppressive agents, appear to enhance tolerance. Recently, anti-lymphocyte globulin (ALG) has been useful in inhibiting antibody production by lymphocytes. Thus, ALG has the effect of inhibiting a key factor in the natural defense system, an action that is at best a mixed blessing. While the agent aids in temporarily blocking tissue rejection, it also weakens the host's defense against infection. The same is true of imuran and the corticosteroids. Hence, although the massive use of drugs inhibits rejection, bacterial infection almost inevitably results. While antibiotics effectively control many bacterial infections, in the face of significantly depressed host defenses infection is apt to overwhelm the patient. Thus, a number of cardiac transplant patients, including Barnard's first one, Louis Washkansky, have succumbed to secondary bacterial infection.

Surgeons have sought to reduce the chance of tissue rejection by tissue typing, that is, by establishing compatibility of donor and recipient tissues. The procedure is analogous to the typing and cross-matching of blood for transfusion, but huge gaps in our understanding of tissue matching persist. The inadequacy of our knowledge is perhaps best shown by the fact that some of the poorest results in heart transplantation have been recorded in instances when tissues from donor and patient appeared well-matched. Conversely, limited evidence of rejection has been found in other cases where the tissue matching was poor. The science of tissue typing is probably about twenty to thirty years behind that of red blood cell typing.

Professional Competence

Initially, it was feared that cardiac transplantation would be carried out on too large a scale, considering the problems of postoperative management. This possibility might well have been strengthened by the enthusiasm of some cardiac surgeons; for example, following the Cape Town conference already mentioned, Cooley made this statement: "In the spirit of extreme optimism and goodwill, the panelists reviewed the heart transplants performed to date and concluded that transplantation was no longer an experimental procedure. For the patient with end-stage heart disease, it has become an effective therapeutic measure to prolong and improve life."

In my view, heart transplantation must still be regarded in large measure as an experimental procedure; certainly the results to date cannot possibly justify classification of the operation as a form of established treatment. As a matter of fact, the number of operations to date does not constitute a sufficiently large sample to enable adequate analysis and comparison of the several variables. I believe the procedure should be limited to a few centers where the presence of competent surgeons as well as immunologists will insure the collection of valid data and their subsequent evaluation.

In fact, there has been no eagerness on the part of most American cardiac surgeons to "hop on the bandwagon." As cases have accumulated, there has been a distinct and admirable tendency on the part of many able surgeons to take a wait-and-see position; some have even suggested a moratorium on cardiac transplantation until immunological knowledge has had a chance to catch up.

The latter proposal drew the fire of Doctor Owen Wangensteen, Professor of Surgery Emeritus at the University of Minnesota, a distinguished surgical leader, who has been called "the mentor of a thousand surgeons" (including Barnard, Doctor Norman Shumway of Stanford University Medical School, and Doctor Walton Lillihei of the Cornell University Medical College). Wangensteen urged that competent surgeons be allowed a free hand, and opposed a moratorium or outside supervision of their efforts by groups of experts.

Following the earliest heart transplants, Wangensteen said: "Heart transplants are an important development and they must be given their chance. All of the surgeons who did the work are men of conscience as well as great skill and enormous courage. They have demonstrated tremendous ability and a lot of originality."

Later, testifying before the Senate Subcommittee on Government Research on the Mondale proposal, Wangensteen recalled that there was similar criticism of the first open-heart surgery at Minnesota and said: "The mandate that researchers in medicine already have from Congress, through the National Institutes of Health, constitutes a sufficient guideline to insure against abuse, to lend encouragement and support for the dedicated, experienced, and knowledgeable persons engaged in innovative therapeutic surgical procedures, including heart transplantation."

Not all medical scientists would, of course, agree entirely with Wangensteen's viewpoint. There would, however, be substantial concurrence with the position recommended by the American Medical Association's Judicial Council (1968) viz., that transplant procedures be carried out only by physicians with special knowledge and training in this area, in medical institutions with facilities designed to protect the welfare of the parties concerned. (See Peterson, Chapter 12, "Control of Medical Conduct.")

As I have noted, most American surgeons have by and large approached the problem conservatively. Heart transplantation has been carried out in about fifteen major medical centers out of at least a hundred in the United States, and in a number of these centers only one or two operations have been done.

I would reemphasize my own view that given the limited state of our knowledge, cardiac transplantations should be done only in the relatively few centers where there is not only the surgical competence available but as well the immunologic expertise and interest. Further, detailed protocols should be followed so that our understanding can be enhanced to the maximum.

Costs of Heroic Procedures

Cost is one deterrent to the popularization of heart and other organ transplants, quite aside from the many other issues, including the key consideration of benefit to the patient. Shumway's first patient, Mike Kasperak, spent the last sixteen days of his life in 1968 in the Stan-

Innovations, Heroic Acts in Prolonging Life [119

ford University Hospital. In this period, his hospital bill totaled $28,845.83; the various charges are listed below:

Ward bed	one day at $55	$ 55.00
Intensive care unit bed	fifteen days at $151	2,265.00
Operating and emergency rooms		990.00
Anesthesia supplies		223.50
Medical-surgical supplies		4,584.90
Drugs		1,782.28
X-ray		643.75
Laboratory		6,947.00
Physical Therapy		833.40
Blood, 288 units		7,200.00
Transfusions		3,256.00
Miscellaneous personal services		65.00
		$28,845.83

It is only fair to point out that the costs in Kasperak's case were even higher than they would have been otherwise because Kasperak suffered from a number of major complications that reflected the ravages of long-standing heart failure. But even without these, the costs in his and other transplant cases have been very high.

It should also be noted that inasmuch as Doctor Shumway and the members of his team are salaried, full-time academicians, no bill was submitted for their professional services. To our knowledge, surgeons in other centers who have performed transplantation of the heart and liver have likewise not submitted professional fees, and only rarely has any professional charge been made for kidney grafts. Thus the total costs do not include what might properly be substantial professional fees.

Generally, the costs of these heroic operations have been paid out of research grants from the National Institutes of Health or from funds supplied by voluntary health organizations or foundations. Blue Cross Hospital Service paid most of Kasperak's hospital bill, but did not cover the $7,200 worth of blood he needed during the sixteen days following surgery.

The National Heart Institute has estimated the minimum cost of a heart transplant at $20,000 for the period of hospitalization, plus several hundred dollars a day thereafter for the management of the patient's postoperative course. The latter phase is most demanding because it involves the task of balancing potent therapeutic agents against the rejection phenomenon.

Obviously, these are sums that even families of upper-middle-class income cannot afford. If the operation were to have wide acceptance, it would even be a burden on the United States Treasury. To do 5,000 heart transplants a year at $20,000 would cost $100 million; to do 80,000 (the upper estimate of potential recipients) would require $1.6 billion a year. The latter amount is approximately equal to the entire budget of the National Institutes of Health for 1968–1969.

From the point of view of economics, it is difficult to see how cardiac transplantation, or for that matter, other types of organ transplantation can be performed in large numbers at these rates. Medical economists state the theoretical problem simply enough. There is an upper limit on financial resources, public and private. To spend more on one thing means spending less on something else. Hard choices, the equivalent of placing a dollar value on human life, eventually have to be made in the course of maximum efforts to prolong life.

We must ask ourselves a difficult question: Is it better to spend a large portion of our financial resources for the benefit of relatively few persons or to put these same large sums into services for a great many people? For example, millions of persons, particularly those in lower income and poverty groups, seriously lack primary medical care and public health services. These groups are notable for higher mortality and morbidity rates. Here the savings in lives, through application of knowledge already available, could be measured in thousands.

We are accustomed to placing a high value on each life; the physician is educated to think in terms of his individual patient. When we broaden our concern from the individual to the general populace, we face a distinct conflict: decisions that are made on the basis of the greatest good for the greatest number inevitably bypass the needs of given individuals.

Public Opinion: Its Shaping and Misshaping

What may properly be called "instant reporting" made the first human heart transplantation in South Africa probably the most widely publicized medical event of our time. "This is the first time a scientist has been more popular than a pop singer," said Barnard. "I think this is progress." The way in which the public took the idea of new hearts for old to its bosom was as amazing as the feat itself. A public opinion poll in London showed that 70 per cent of laymen endorsed the use of heart transplants as a means of alleviating serious heart disease, this at a time when the total number of operations performed was less than fifty. Similarly, a Gallup survey indicated that 70 per cent of Americans stood ready to donate their vital organs after death.

We live in an age, among other things, of high-speed, high-pressure communication of every sight, sound, feeling, and idea that appears capable of arresting attention. It is an age that Greer Williams (1968) has aptly described as one of "information overkill." People are getting too much information too fast—faster than they can digest it and adjust to it, and faster than they can relate it to what they already know.

The public relations and advertising experts apparently have so convinced us of the need to communicate and sell ourselves that anyone who does not seek the attention of his contemporaries, who does not talk and write, orate and publish, is apt to be thought of as old-fashioned, if not peculiar. As Marshall McLuhan so clearly saw, the medium is the message.

Heart transplantation may be considered a case in point. Following the first two operations in South Africa, the procedure was heralded in glowing terms around the world. An enormous amount of attention was suddenly focused on the subject although in fact the underlying experimental work had been going forward, quietly and systematically, devoid of public attention for a matter of years.

Shumway and his colleagues, over a period of eight years, had devised surgical techniques for transplantation and had carried out the procedure successfully in dogs. Indeed, some time prior to Barnard's first case, Doctor Shumway had stated his intention to perform cardiac transplantation in man as soon as the appropriate combination of donor and recipient were identified. As is now well known, following Barnard's first case, the pace of cardiac transplantation increased rapidly, both in the United States and abroad; a number of the attempts were sporadic, but in a few centers major programs were pursued.

The publicity attendant on cardiac transplantation underlines the complex relationships between science and public policy, and the need, in a period of great technical advances, to consider the broad implications of these advances as well as the relatively narrow scientific ones.

Fundamentally, reliable, objective public reporting of science is in the interest of all—physicians, patients, and the population at large. Only if the news media exhibit the highest sense of responsibility can we have a well-informed population. The public, if well informed, will certainly support science, so that the research on which progress is dependent can be continued. But overemphasis of spectacular procedures or methods that have extremely limited payoffs can lead not only to bitter disappointment and heartbreak among patients and their families but as well to disillusionment and loss of confidence by the public at large. Given the limitations of available resources, a situation that is presently especially aggravated by the multiple demands of the military, urban blight, and race problems, it is mandatory that decisions be made as wisely as possible and not on the basis of improper emphasis on some dramatic event of little long-term importance.

Doctor Irvine H. Page, a distinguished research scientist in the cardiac field, has addressed the question of how to divide available resources: "I suspect the usual turn of events is occurring; the plumber surgeons are cutting in because we neither know how to prevent nor how to cure atherosclerosis." Page urges that funds for research into the nature and prevention of heart disease be protected from the competition of more glamorous but wasteful and superficial efforts to forestall end-stage heart disease.

In the present state of knowledge, the greatest potential opportunity for reduction of death and disability from heart disease lies in changing the eating, smoking, and exercising habits of our citizenry. This uphill struggle against self-indulgence lacks appeal. It is neither innovational nor heroic, and from what we know about human motivation, it is not very promising. Yet this kind of self-discipline is likely to remain the only chance for really significant reductions in total mortality and morbidity for some time to come.

Quality of Prolonged Life

Earlier I mentioned the increasing problem of vegetative, non-intellectual existence in patients with irreversible massive brain damage. This brings us logically to the issue of euthanasia. The doctor is caught between two contradictory positions: (a) to do everything possible to keep the patient alive, but (b) to do nothing to prolong pain and suffering uselessly. Practically speaking, it is easier to start heroic life-saving measures than it is to stop them. The objective of medical practice is to conserve life. Not only medical ethics but the law admonish the doctor against any conscious, deliberate, willful act to shorten life.

In days gone by, the problem of outliving one's usefulness was far less common than it is today. Before the introduction of antibacterial agents, bacterial pneumonia—"the old man's friend"—often brought a prompt and merciful end for the patient with chronic, incurable disease. Take, for example, the patient with severe atherosclerotic blood vessel disease who suffers a massive stroke but survives it. Fifty years ago, such a person was a prime candidate for fatal pneumonia. Today he is treated with appropriate antibiotics, and, while these drugs are not infallible, the odds favor their being effective. What may result is a seriously handicapped patient with no hope of rehabilitation. There may be imposed an untold amount of emotional trauma and financial burden on his family or on society.

In addition to the antibiotics, a number of measures contribute to the maintenance of life today; most of these are recent additions to the physician's armamentarium.

Parenteral Medication Various physiologic fluids, including those containing amino acid mixtures, vitamins and other purified foodstuffs, plasma, and whole blood can be administered intravenously to maintain the body's fluid and nutritional balance for protracted periods of time. Such fluids combat negative nitrogen balance, shock, blood loss, and other potentially lethal conditions. Massive blood transfusions have been particularly important in reducing the mortality from trauma and some forms of major surgery.

Super-Voltage Radiation and Anti-Tumor Chemotherapy These two forms of treatment have improved the outlook in various forms of malignant disease. With certain cancers, cures are achieved, but in a far larger number improvement is of significant degree, though palliative. Surgery is sometimes combined with these treatments. Often successive remissions occur as the result of more vigorous therapy, although in the long run the patient may succumb. Death is postponed, as are the attendant problems of decline in the quality of remaining life, but the problems are inescapable.

New Forms of Surgery This chapter has been largely devoted to one such new form—organ transplantation. In the modern era, new surgical techniques have been continuously devised and older ones improved; more radical forms of surgery have been rendered possible because of better anesthesia and/or pre- and postoperative support. The impact of the heart-lung machine, making open-heart surgery possible, already has been discussed. The fields of neurosurgery, vascular surgery, orthopedic surgery, and general surgery have also been broadened in significant ways.

Life-Assisting Devices In addition to the heart-lung machine and the artificial kidney, other means have been added to make it possible to maintain life where it was hitherto impossible to do so. Improved cardiac glycosides, vaso-pressor substances, and anti-arrhythmic drugs are of major importance. Our hold on life also has been strengthened by development of measures for cardiac resuscitation, especially external cardiac massage and electrical stimulation of the heart. Because cardiac massage is easily carried out, even by laymen, it has been possible to lessen the immediate mortality following acute coronary occlusion. On the other hand, resuscitators and respirators may merely serve to keep alive patients with advanced, degenerative, and incurable diseases although no tangible benefit can be expected.

Cardioactive agents and mechanical apparatus to maintain respiration can prolong life—if life is measured by breathing and heartbeat —for long periods in individuals who have suffered overwhelming central nervous system injury or disease with loss of intellectual function. Such injuries, particularly if they are traumatic in origin and have occurred in relatively young people, serve as a strong stimulus to physicians to do everything possible to sustain physiologic function if there seems to be even a remote chance that there may be reversal of the disability. Once the attempt to prolong life is initiated, it becomes progressively more difficult for the physician

Innovations, Heroic Acts in Prolonging Life [125

to stop the machinery and terminate life, even though it is clear that intellectual function is irretrievably lost.

For many years, thoughtful persons have pondered the issue of euthanasia. The pain of watching a loved one suffer unmercifully has led relatives to resort to "mercy killings." But the latter are obviously no solution in the context of our legal structure. Now, with innovational and heroic measures available to maintain life, at least non-intellectual life, for long periods of time, reexamination of the issue is definitely in order.

The public is reasonably well informed on the availability of the life-saving measures listed above. In many areas, systematic campaigns have been conducted to educate laymen in the use of mouth-to-mouth respiration and external cardiac massage as emergency measures. It is not surprising, therefore, that the same public generally expects these measures to be applied to hospitalized patients in a terminal state. Such attitudes make it all the more difficult for physicians not to employ them, even when they promise only a useless prolongation of the vegetative state.

We have, at the present time, no very good data as to the practices of physicians in prolonging or terminating life in the face of a hopeless prognosis. Undoubtedly, there is wide variation. One can speculate that in our teaching hospitals, where more sophisticated techniques are generally available, and where the staffs include physicians in training (interns, residents, and fellows) the use of heroic measures is more common. The presence of large numbers of personnel, including residents, interns, and medical students, may well also complicate the decision-making process. It is quite likely that in these settings some physicians might find it more difficult to withhold antibiotics, fluids, or other life-supporting medication, lest they be criticized by their colleagues. Steps that allow differentiation between heart death and brain death will in time make it easier to develop a rationale for termination generally acceptable to the medical profession and the public and, therefore, make termination under appropriate conditions finally supportable in ethics and law.

Moving from individual to social values, we must emphasize again the enormous economic and emotional costs of prolonging life in the presence of irreversible disease, especially if intellectual function is lost. A significant number of hospital beds and many more nursing home beds are today occupied by patients in the latter category.

Needed: Criteria for Prolongation and Termination of Life

At this point in medical history, where we can look to further development and perfection of life-prolonging measures, we must attempt to define in more specific ways the criteria for their employment, and particularly the criteria for their discontinuation. These definitions will be difficult at best to achieve and they will be imprecise. In evolving them, physicians, lawyers, behavioral scientists, and clergymen must participate. The final judgment does not lie, as some may argue, only with the doctor of medicine.

Agreement on principles will be difficult to obtain. Yet the lengthening of life expectancy and the increasing number of patients presenting problems of the sort we are discussing make this issue one of major consequence for our society. As a first step, the kind of information provided in this book or pinpointed by the research questions it raises should help answer some of the following questions:

1. What are the numbers of patients suffering from incurable illnesses where prolongation of life is feasible even though intellectual function has been lost? What are the financial implications of prolongation?
2. What are the current practices employed by physicians?
3. What are the attitudes of physicians, nurses, and other hospital and health personnel toward prolongation and termination of life?
4. What are the attitudes of various segments of the lay public?
5. What are the legal implications?
6. How should these issues be dealt with in the education of physicians, nurses, and other health personnel?

We must develop a set of guiding principles that in the long run will benefit all of society, enabling the application of the knowledge and skills of medicine where they can be beneficial, and avoiding their use when no benefit, and sometimes disservice, to the patients and their families results.

In the evolution of such policies, it is mandatory that adequate safeguards be established. It is unlikely that policies can be defined that are so specific as to obviate subjective decisions on the part of health professionals. Human nature being what it is, there is no room for wrong decisions in issues of this magnitude, whether they are based on inadequate evidence, poor judgment, or malicious intent.

Just as we have made great progress in the battle against disease, let us hope we can make comparable progress in the wise application of new knowledge.

Any Day, a Cure May Be Found

An understandable basis for the effort to prolong the life of patients with an incurable disease is the hope that a cure may be found any day. While we all recognize the desirability of keeping hope alive, we may at times tend to dismiss such a statement as an exercise in wishful thinking, which in fact it usually is.

Yet the value of keeping an intellectually intact, socially useful person alive as long as possible will not be questioned by anybody who knows the thrilling story of Doctor George R. Minot (Rackenmann, 1958). Minot shared the Nobel Prize for his role in the demonstration that liver extract was an effective treatment for pernicious anemia, a disease that was classified as a malignant blood disorder, ultimately fatal.

It is improbable that Minot would have lived long enough to demonstrate the remarkable effectiveness of liver therapy in pernicious anemia if Frederick Banting and Charles Best had not shown that the hormone, insulin, was a specific treatment for diabetes. Minot was found to have diabetes in 1921, at the age of thirty-six. He fought a losing battle for the next two years to control his disease by means of diet, the only therapeutic measure then available. Insulin became available for general use in 1923, and Minot received treatment. He responded dramatically and favorably, and was able to live an essentially normal life for a good many years thereafter.

It was this turn of events that enabled Minot to continue a series of experiments that culminated in his now famous 1927 report that feeding of large quantities of liver produced regeneration of red cells in the bone marrow, and controlled symptoms of experimental anemia in dogs. The liver treatment, promptly shown to be equally effective in the treatment of human beings with pernicious anemia, won for Minot the Nobel Prize in 1934.

The number of instances in medical history that are as inspiring as the one just related are few. But both the discovery of insulin and of liver therapy undoubtedly saved the lives of hundreds of patients who were near death from one or the other disease. More recently, the introduction of penicillin in the treatment of bacterial endocarditis, another entity that had hitherto been almost always fatal, led to cures in a high percentage of cases, and provides another example of the justification for prolonging life in patients who appear to be doomed. As Cervantes pointed out in *Don Quixote*, "While there's life, there's hope."

For those of us in medicine, the preservation of life remains a noble goal; but in seeking this objective we must more and more concern ourselves with the quality of the life we preserve. For in ways undreamed of by Cervantes, the definition of life is today a far more complex problem than it was a few decades past.

REFERENCES

American Medical Association Judicial Council.
    1968 "Ethical guidelines for organ transplantation." Journal of the American Medical Association 205 (August 5) :89–90.

Beecher, H. K., *et al.* (Ad Hoc Committee of the Harvard Medical School).
    1968 "A definition of irreversible coma." Journal of the American Medical Association 205 (August 5) :85–88.

Rackenmann, F. M.
    1958 The Inquisitive Physician. Cambridge, Mass.: Harvard.

Williams, G.
    1968 "Needed: a new strategy for health promotion." New England Journal of Medicine 279 (November 7) :1031–1035.

7

Patterns of Dying

Anselm L. Strauss and Barney G. Glaser

PROBABLY LESS THAN one-third of all deaths in the United States now take place outside of a hospital or other institutional setting. Changing health practices and medical technology seem destined to bring about still further institutionalization of dying. That people elect to die in such institutions—or that their families make such choices for them—means that outsiders to the family have been delegated responsibility for taking care of the dying during their last days or hours. This delegation of responsibility, whether partial or total, is of immense importance for everyone concerned: for patients, families, and for the hospital staffs.

The last take their responsibilities with the utmost seriousness, in accordance with the directives of professional practice and the dictates of conscience. But close scrutiny of terminal care suggests that only the more strictly medical or technical aspects are professionalized. The training of physicians and nurses equips them principally for the technical aspects of dealing with illness. The psychological aspects of dealing with the dying and their families are virtually absent from training (Quint, 1967; Becker *et al.*, 1961). Hence, although physicians and nurses are highly skilled at handling the bodies of terminal patients, their behavior toward them otherwise is more or less outside the province of professional standards. Much, if not most, nontechnical conduct toward, and in the presence of, dying patients and their families is profoundly influenced by commonsense assumptions, essentially untouched by professional considerations or by current knowledge from the behavioral sciences.

It is significant that while technical aspects of terminal care are planned, carried out explicitly, reported in writing or orally, and reviewed either by responsible superiors or by colleagues, in contrast most other actions of personnel toward and around dying patients are nonaccountable (Strauss et al., 1964:73–87). Personnel do and say many things that only incidentally or accidentally reach the ears and eyes of other personnel. The psychological and social aspects of terminal care may be good, but are carried out on the basis of private initiative and judgment rather than as part of accountable decision-making.

Institutional Differences

The research results incorporated in this chapter* underscore how strikingly different are the modes and courses of dying on different types of wards in hospitals. The organizational efforts at each locale differ, in consequence, as the staff copes with the patterns of dying characteristic of their particular ward. Although staffs are well aware both of the dying patterns and the organizational patterns, they take very little cognizance in their planning and review of related matters that are not strictly "nursing" or "medical." Traditionally only these latter matters are accountable, and only these are emphasized in schools of medicine and nursing.

All except very small hospitals are sharply differentiated internally among types of wards or medical services. On some wards there is little dying (obstetrics), but even on intensive care wards or cancer wards, not all patients are expected to, or do, die. Each type of service tends to have a characteristic incidence of death and tempo of dying. On many emergency services, for example, death is frequent and patients tend to die quickly. The staff, therefore, is geared to perform urgent, critical functions. Modes of dying also affect interaction between patient and staff, as well as the organization of the staff's work. For instance, on many intensive care wards, some patients are expected to die quickly if they are to die at all; others need close

---

* This chapter is taken with some modifications from the various chapters of our *Time for Dying* (Chicago: Aldine Publishing Company, 1968). See also our *Awareness of Dying* (Chicago: Aldine Publishing Company, 1965), and the book by Jeanne C. Quint, our associate—to whom we are much indebted—*The Nurse and the Dying Patient* (New York: The Macmillan Company, 1967).

attention for several days because death is a touch-and-go matter; still others are not likely to die but do need temporary round-the-clock nursing. Most who die here are heavily drugged or past consciousness. Nurses or physicians do not need to converse with these patients. This is in contrast to what is typical of medical wards, where some patients are likely to die lingering deaths, fully conscious at least in the earlier phases of dying, and ready or eager to talk with the staff.

Patterns of Death

The course of dying—or "dying trajectory" (Glaser and Strauss, 1968:1)—of each patient has at least two outstanding properties. First, it takes place over time: It has duration. Specific dying trajectories can vary greatly in duration. Second, a trajectory has shape: It can be graphed. It plunges straight down; it moves slowly but steadily downward; it vacillates slowly, moving slightly up and down before diving downward radically; it moves slowly down at first, then hits a long plateau, then plunges abruptly to death. Dying trajectories themselves are perceived, rather than the actual courses of dying. This distinction is readily evident in the type that involves a short, unexpected reprieve from death. On the other hand, in a lingering death, bystanders may expect faster dying than actually occurs.

Since dying patients are defined in terms of when and how they will die, various patterns are commonly recognized by the hospital personnel and, if possible, terminal care is organized accordingly. For instance, there is the abrupt, surprise trajectory, as a patient who is expected to recover suddenly begins to die. Fast action is needed, and often a ward is not organized for this particular type of emergency. For an expected lingering death, however, with great pain expected at the end, the staff is likely to organize drug-giving with that end in mind.

Ordinarily there are certain events—let us term them "critical junctures"—that appear and are directly handled by the organization of hospital work. These occur in either full or truncated form: (1) The patient is defined as dying. (2) Staff and family then make preparations for his death, as he may do himself if he knows he is dying. (3) At some point, there seems to be "nothing more to do" to prevent death. (4) The final descent may take weeks, or days, or merely hours, ending in (5) the "last hours," (6) the death watch, and (7) the death itself. There may be announcements that the patient is dying (by physician to staff, by staff to family members, by kinsmen to each other, much less often to the patient himself) or that he is entering or leaving a phase. Death itself must be legally pronounced and then publicly announced.

When these critical junctures occur as expected, on schedule, then all participants—sometimes including the patient—are prepared for them. For instance, the nurses are ready for a death watch if they can anticipate when the end will come. When, however, critical junctures occur unexpectedly, staff members and family alike are somewhat unprepared. For instance, a patient expected to die quite soon may vacillate sufficiently often for the patient to cause stress among kinsmen and hospital staff. Whenever he fades, the nurses may call the family, for, as one nurse said, "If you do not call the family and the patient dies, that's wrong." The family members arrive for their last look at the dying man, but he lingers. They finally leave, saying: "Please call us again." Such a cycle affects changes in the activities and moods of the various participants—including the physician.

Staff's Sentimental Mood

When the staff can predict the course of the patient's dying, its work with other patients, as well as with him, is made easier. Critical junctures can be planned so that manpower will not be withdrawn suddenly from scheduled tasks with other patients. Miscalculations in forecasting can play havoc with the organization of work and affect even the probabilities of his dying right then and there. When such crises occur, the staff attempts to regain control over the disrupted organization of work as quickly as possible. Since a revised notion of the patient's condition may necessitate new procedures of additional time spent at his bedside; considerable reordering of work, even changes in the division of labor, may be involved.

A disruption of the ward's organization of work is paralleled by a shattering of its characteristic "sentimental mood" or order (Glaser and Strauss, 1965). For instance, in an intensive care unit where cardiac patients die frequently, the mood is relatively unaffected by one

Patterns of Dying

more speedy expected death; but if a hopeless patient lingers on and on, or if his wife, perhaps, refuses to accept his dying and causes "scenes," then both mood and work itself are profoundly affected.

Another important variable that affects what goes on during the course of dying is the intersecting of experiences people have had with illnesses or with hospitals. Thus, chronic patients, having lived with their symptoms, often are experienced in reading them, sometimes more so than some staff members, especially when the latter have had little experience with the specific disease. A heart patient who had been strapped into a certain position before being X-rayed once told a nurses' aide that she had better move him quickly into another position, lest his lungs fill up with fluid. She refused. To her horror, he soon began to pass out, and only by dint of quick action did the staff save him. By contrast, when a staff understands that its patients may know much about the specific symptoms of their fatal illnesses—and even about the courses of their illnesses—terminal care is unmarked by such incidents. Renee Fox's study of a chronic hospital provides many examples (1959). Patients may complain about their care, reviewing it against the background of stays at other hospitals. Personal careers may also greatly affect responses. For example, a dying patient who happens to be a nurse is likely to be upsetting to the attending nurses and even to others on the ward. A female patient who reminds a nurse of her own mother can be disturbing.

Quick Dying

Before turning to "slow dying," let us look at quick trajectories. Modern American hospitals—at least the more progressive ones—are, above all, set up to handle the latter. On the intensive care units, emergency wards, operating rooms, and medical wards, medical technology and highly trained staff are concentrated, on constant call, and in a relatively constant state of readiness to meet the challenge of saving ("heroically"), if it makes sense to do so, a patient who is dying quickly. As defined by staff, this may mean within minutes, hours, or a few days.

Three general quick types are as follows: In the "expected quick death," it is clear to the staff that the patient will almost certainly die in a few hours or, at most, a day or two. The case of "unexpected quick dying, but expected to die" differs in that the staff are certain that the patient is dying, but do not anticipate the early turn for the worst. In a case of "unexpected quick dying, not expected to die," a patient who has been expected to recover suddenly starts to die quickly, completely surprising staff, family, and other persons involved. In general, unexpected and expected quick deaths have differential impact on the staff and family. The former types are much more disturbing, since the basis of medical work and ward sentiment toward the patient is changed abruptly and drastically.

Even the expected quick trajectory has a fair degree of complex behavioral accompaniments. Consider only the family-staff interaction. Expected quick death usually or often means there are family members in the nearby waiting room or hallway waiting for news. In the beginning, a nurse or doctor may tell them "Everything is going to be all right," but "They know it's not and you know it's not." But time moves fast, and family members must have some explanation to prepare them for the worst. As the patient worsens, the family is briefed by the doctor or a resident; they receive a preannouncement of impending death. This carries a tacit agreement, sometimes made explicit, that the staff will keep the family posted as often as possible on the patient's condition; and so some family members feel no need to ask questions while waiting. Others may want to ask questions as the time plods on, but may be afraid. Others simply ask whenever they see any staff member. A frequent answer, until the patient has died is, "He is still not out of danger" or "He's still with us."

The proximity of the family to the dying patient raises the possibility of the staff's having to manage scenes (such as public and loud crying), and also, since a quick death is expected, having to manage the family's desire to be present at the death or to take a last look at him before or after death. In some cases, the last look or witnessing of death is allowed and turns out to be no problem to the staff. In other cases, family members faint and must be revived. Some are given a corner of privacy, so that they may cry and gain control of themselves.

The presence of the family at the bedside during death must be carefully handled by staff since a scene or tantrum is very disrupting to the sentimental order of the ward—including the reactions of other patients. Moreover, there is a danger that a relative might upset bedside equipment or the dying patient. Staff members may also feel embarrassed and helpless in this situation because there is, they feel, nothing to say—unless they are simply to tell the family it is hopeless.

When an obviously soon-to-die patient arrives on a ward and when there is no time to try anything to save him, the usual maneuver is to put him in a room by himself. When there is time, yet clearly no chance of saving the patient, the staff watches, waits, and gives comfort care until death. They time their efforts according to his downhill progression, all the while remaining unusually alert for a cue that would indicate the possibility of redefining his outlook to "has a chance." Should this critical juncture occur, they stand ready with skills and, hopefully, equipment to try to save the patient. Staff members frequently refer to the frustration and helplessness they feel while they wait, holding their power in abeyance for a change in the patient that would give them a chance to act.

Unexpected Dying

On the other hand, simply because a patient has been given no chance and shows no sign of a change in condition, the staff does not, *ipso facto*, do nothing. If there is time, the effort may nevertheless be made to save, or perhaps only to prolong, his life, even in the face of little chance of success. Hence, when there is time, they may create a chance where there was none, and organize their last-ditch heroics accordingly, sometimes successfully. Last-ditch heroics may be encouraged by several factors. One is that the patient is of such high social value that his loss must be averted at all costs, if possible (Glaser and Strauss, 1964). A medically interesting patient may also stimulate last-ditch heroics. When there is time for the family or even the patient to participate in a decision of last resort, especially in surgery, the choice often hinges upon the relative likelihood that, if saved, the patient will be able to live a normal life. Neither the family nor the patient typically wishes to reverse the outcome if they recognize that it will unquestionably result in prolonged ordeal or pain.

In contrast to expected quick deaths, the unexpected have surprise as a main feature, and surprise may vary from relatively little to complete. It makes a considerable difference whether the surprise comes as an emergency or as a crisis. An emergency situation almost always implies that the facilities for mobilization of life-saving action are at hand and that action can be initiated at a moment's notice. In the crisis situation, adequate preparation is often lacking, so that the need to act immediately more or less immobilizes the staff. In the emergency situation, they tend to recover quickly from surprise, mobilize immediately, and promptly achieve a solid feeling about what is happening. In the crisis situation, the relative disarray of work and sentiment requires a much longer period of resolution before the organization of work and the sentimental order are both solidly reestablished.

When a patient is expected to die, but not quickly, the staff attempts to anticipate the timing as specifically as possible. They then develop sentiments according to the stages of the trajectory. On medical wards, when an unexpected quick death begins in a lingering patient, expected stages may be entirely left out of the dying. For example, the family, as yet unprepared, must be found and told their relative is almost dead, an often shattering task for the nurse or doctor as well as for the family. Staff work and sentiments lose their customary tempo and continuity. Sudden procedural shifts may be required. Facilities must be obtained quickly and the right physician found, or the patient must be moved to the intensive care unit. Or if he remains, extra nursing staff may have to be found to help with other patients until the crisis can be turned to an emergency.

Having become personally involved with the patient and his family, the nurses may suffer some shock at the dying. They may expect the lingering patient to be alive each day as they arrive on the ward. For the time being they forget he is dying. On the other hand, the unexpected quick trajectory may be well received on the medical ward. If a patient has been lingering in pain, has been degenerating, has been comatose for months, is draining his family of all their money, has clearly reached the point of "nothing more to do," with nothing much to make his last weeks and days socially meaningful or even comfortable, the staff may wish that he die or be allowed to die.

Wards with a greater frequency of deaths tend to temper staff for the surprises as well as for the expected. A surprise can be warded off: "We generally lose them anyway." Protection against surprise is sustained by other facets. The dying patient would have lasted only a few days anyway, so the temporal loss is not great. The unexpected quick dying may be welcome relief from bearing even a few more days of an ordeal painful to all. The quicker death also maintains the ward personnel's motivation to rescue patients, by relieving them of a "no-chance" patient sooner than expected and opening a bed for a patient who can be saved. The intense work and intense focus on medical aspects of saving also provide buffers. Staff have less time to dwell on the surprise and the sad fact of imminent death. Rather they must concentrate on mobilizing for the emergency and preventing crisis. Part of this intensity in medical care involvement is induced by closer collaboration with the physician than on wards where slower dying is more typical.

Slow Dying

Among the more complex types of dying trajectories are those that are quite properly thought of as "slow"—whether the time of death is certain or uncertain, and whether the patient dies sooner or earlier than expected. One main property of lingering death is its potential unpredictability, with regard to both the biological and human aspects of dying. To be sure, many a patient slowly declines, or lingers on plateaus between several declines or abrupt deteriorations, without unexpected important events occurring. But in a decline of any considerable duration, a number of special events are probable. Any one can begin to make a special story of the dying. Despite the death, the story may have happy endings for its main characters. Or it may be a very sad story indeed.

The slow decline, then, is fraught with both hazard and opportunity. On the hazard side: the dying may take too long, the bodily deterioration may be unexpectedly painful or unpleasant, the patient may discover he is dying when he is not supposed to know, and so on. On the other hand, slow decline may allow a man time to make his will, round off unfinished business and family affairs, and even permit him to patch up differences with his spouse or other members of the family. Slow dying also furnishes the setting for courageous or tranquil endings, and a participation that buoys the staff. All these consequences are less likely to occur with swift or sudden dying.

Slow dying, then, is likely to be accompanied by an evolving story, stretching over weeks or months; or perhaps stories, since staff members do not always agree with each other's versions. If dramatic enough, patients' stories are long remembered by people who participated in them. Even trajectories that are fairly uneventful right down to the last phases can produce memorable stories. An interesting feature of the continuing story is that people who have never seen or been involved in the care of a patient sometimes react to it. Dying patients may become personages not only for personnel who care for them, but also for those who work elsewhere in the hospital. Thus one patient whom we observed set such difficult problems for the nursing and medical staff, involving the management of her pain, that she provoked persistent discussion extending, during periods of crisis, far beyond the ward. Personnel were discussing her story on other floors, in the hospital's restaurant, and even in the classrooms of the associated school of nursing.

Effects of Patient on Staff

Strangers may react to a dying patient's story, but the reactions of those in prolonged, direct contact with him are necessarily more complex. They cannot simply react to the story or to the person lying in the bed. When the patient groans, requests something, complains, or grows angry at them, their answering actions are not toward isolated behaviors but toward elements of a continuing story. A reverse logic implies that a patient's reactions to staff members can be directed toward altering or sustaining the story that they have constructed about him; indeed, a patient may, from his first days at the hospital, deliberately attempt to shape the staff's collective story. Patients who die quickly can produce dying stories, but patients with slow trajectories are much more likely to have stories that are consequential for their nursing and medical care. One important consequence of any patient's story—one we dare not overlook—is its influence on the efforts made in his behalf, and thereby (whether we wish to admit this or not) on whether his life will be shortened or prolonged and to what purpose.

Unless a person dies abruptly, with virtually no warning, the dying trajectory includes a stage of "last days" and perhaps even "last weeks." The hospital staff usually finds itself engaged in a complex juggling of tasks, people, and relationships. Its juggling consists, first, of organizing a number of potentially shifting treatment and care tasks. As a patient becomes visibly sicker and weaker, the staff typically stop certain activities and simultaneously initiate new ones. The comfort care activities may become very detailed and may now require considerable nursing skill; the medical care necessary to keep him alive may remain quite complex, although different from earlier medical care.

The Family's Concerns

Meanwhile, the staff must also juggle people and relationships whose existence can cause great disruption to the ward's work and sentimental order. If the patient is visible to other patients, their reactions to his last weeks and days must be taken into account, particularly insofar as they may see his dying as a rehearsal of their own. And both the family and the patient present problems of management.

With families, problems tend to center around four issues: (1) the family needs to be prepared for the forthcoming death; (2) they may need to be persuaded to delegate responsibility for the dying person to the hospital; (3) they may require coaching in proper modes of behavior while at the hospital; and (4) they may need to be helped in their grieving, either for their own sake or for the sake of preventing disruption of ward activity. The nature of these central problems suggests that the personnel may be considerably engaged in working with the family during the patient's last days. Such problems do not arise if there is no family or no one close enough to visit the hospital. In American geriatric hospitals, for example, family-handling problems are minimal.

If a family is to be prepared for a patient's death, it first must be forewarned. Lingering trajectories allow the physician great latitude in timing his notice to the family. Indeed, he does not know exactly when the patient will die and may not be able to predict whether there will be temporary reprieves, plateaus, and even reversals. His first tidings may be long delayed; they may consist initially of cues to stimulate a gradually growing awareness; these may be repeated. Ineffective pacing of forewarnings—or insufficient trust by the family—

may result in their shopping around for a "better" doctor, one with a "cure," even though cure is really not the issue. Usually, the physician first communicates with the "strongest" family member, who then has the responsibility of disclosure to the other relatives.

During the last days, family members may ply the staff with queries about how long the patient has to live and whether he will die peacefully. Those queries must be handled. If they are not, scenes are likely to erupt on the ward.

Some families can accept the forthcoming death of a relative, but others need help in coming to terms with the event. The staff then offers rationalizations or supports those of the kinsmen: "Yes, it will be a blessing if he goes soon." "Yes, he is lucky that he has no pain at all." If the last days stretch into weeks, the staff can sustain the relatives' acceptance by displaying equanimity and by giving undiminished comfort care to the patient. They can give reassurances that he will die peacefully. They can correct unfounded expectations about how he will die. When reprieves occur, staff can signify quietly that death is still on the way without encouraging false hopes. If need be, the nurses can put pressure on the physician to "explain again" to a relative who will not face the facts.

Relatives' acceptance of a forthcoming death may relate to whether they already partly have overcome their grief. Virtually everybody may be fairly well "grieved out" if the end comes slowly, especially if the patient's social value is relatively low (for instance, if he is a very old person). If at all possible, a tactful staff allows close kinsmen plenty of time with the dying person, especially during the last days, so that they can quietly live through their grief. Sometimes personnel do not recognize grieving as such—it has many individual and cultural variants. But by and large they do understand that a wife must be with a dying husband, children with a dying parent, that separation would be more painful than participation in the dying. Some hospitals have convenient rooms where relatives may wait when they cannot stay at the bedside.

When it seems advisable that the dying person should remain ignorant of his forthcoming death, family members must not display their grief before the patient. Staff members may have to warn kinsmen about this danger or take steps to prevent its occurrence. Since

Patterns of Dying

grieving may begin the instant that close kinsmen are forewarned of death, the staff may immediately begin giving support.

Grief-Workers

Nursing personnel often find their role as sympathetic listener or comforter a major one during the final days. They are especially moved when they see the patient's death as a grave social loss, or when they associate it with their own personal past, or, sometimes, when a family member has behaved admirably. Social workers may tend especially, with self-consciousness, to become "grief-workers," attempting with professional deliberateness to "work through" the grief of relatives; this is perhaps most noticeable on pediatric wards. Priests, chaplains, and nuns also engage in such activities; indeed, they may be called on by a desperate nursing staff afraid of the disastrous effects of death and unable themselves to help the relative. Psychiatrists may also be called in to work with family members.

The staff's problem of getting suitable behavior from the family members is linked closely with whether the family is adequately prepared for the death and does its grieving on schedule. A wife may cause upsetting scenes, for instance, if she is not prepared for her husband's death when it finally draws near. A relative who grieves too early and too openly may disturb the patient; even if the latter is quite aware of his forthcoming death, he may not be sufficiently resigned to it.

The staff may also have to coach relatives in appropriate bedside behavior. If family members visit in too great numbers, a rule may be laid down that only close kin may visit "from now on"—especially as death becomes imminent. A family that is too noisy may need to be reprimanded; the staff may forbid access to the ward to all but the closest kin. In rooms with several patients, visitors may be especially careful not to disturb nearby patients with chattering or sobbing. When a patient has a private room, kin still may need to be taught not to "get in the way." Often a nurse will ask someone to leave the bedside or the room when she suspects that a nursing or medical procedure may disturb the onlooker. Visitors may also harass the staff by making what the latter considers unjustified, overanxious, or just plain fussy demands. Various tactics are used to make the offending person behave properly. What is considered inappropriate depends not only on the patient himself, but also on how attached the personnel have become to the patient, how well they have come to know the family member, or the nature of the patient's evolving story. The staff, however, may call on other family members to restrain the overdemanding person or one who offends in other ways.

Jurisdictional Disputes

The staff's final problem is that the kinsmen may not willingly delegate the patient's care during his last hours. Such unwillingness may vary in seriousness. At its most extreme, the patient simply is withdrawn from the hospital, usually against professional advice. (This is much more prevalent in countries like Malaya or Greece, where the hospital is less accepted as a place to die than in the United States.) Sometimes an American family takes a patient home during his last days because it believes it can provide adequate care there; the family may discover its error and return him to the hospital.

Even families who know very well that their dying kinsman should remain in professional hands may try to interfere with the staff, suggesting or demanding that certain things be done differently. The staff require and develop counter tactics to cope with this behavior. More generally, however, hospitals allow close kin to carry out routine comfort care while the nurses and physicians give the more difficult or professionalized care. As life draws to a close, sometimes the staff tactfully allows a mother or wife to take over the comfort care almost totally if this is possible.

Neither the severity of problems that a family will present to the hospital staff nor the degree of success the staff will have in managing a family during the last weeks and days are entirely predictable. (The reverse of the question is the problems the family will have with the staff.) Among the structural conditions that militate against the relative tranquility and success of the interaction are the number of visiting relatives, the distance from which they have come, the experience they have had with hospital customs and rules, the amount of trust they have in the professionals, and the amount or kind of ward space.

Leave-Takings

As the last weeks become days, and the days become hours, a critical juncture arises. It comes when close relatives say final farewells to the dying patient or—if he is not aware—when they take their last looks at him alive. Told that he has not long to live or warned by their own senses, they take leave. These leave-takings are likely to be awesome ceremonies, even when the dying man is comatose, has been socially dead for some time, or is elderly. Each day's separation implies the possibilities that *this* may be the last time visitors will see the patient alive. When family members travel considerable distances to visit at the hospital, they may be able to come only on weekends or at several-day intervals. They must make each farewell not knowing whether they will "ever see him again." The anguish may be shared by some staff members. Where "final" leave-takings are frequent and anguished, the disruption of scheduled work and sentimental order is sometimes devastating to the staff.

As for the patient himself: He is much more likely than his family to be the center of the staff's attention, unless he is comatose, scarcely sentient, or so ill as hardly to be reacting as a person. Under these latter conditions, the staff's juggling of its work around him need only be minimal. When last days stretch out interminably on wards organized for faster turnover of patients, or when mode of dying is so extraordinarily unpleasant as to disturb staff members, the personnel face major problems.

If the dying person is sentient but unaware of his impending death, then the staff's problems may be associated with keeping him unaware, or at least keeping his suspicions sufficiently damped down. If his pain is great, he can be "snowed" with drugs during his final days.

If he has become aware that he is dying, he must come to terms with dying. If he has had many months to face his mortality, he has probably entered or reentered the hospital better prepared than if his period of awareness has been short or sudden. If he is not elderly and has not already come to terms with the inevitability of death, a quick decline is likely to precipitate crises of awareness for the sentient patient and his family.

Even in slow dying, the breakthrough of awareness during last days can be traumatic. The staff sometimes has little control over the structural conditions that determine the impact. For instance, a patient may know he has an extremely serious illness, but not regard it as fatal. Then he suddenly is told, intentionally or not. We observed, for example, the first days of a teenager who had learned of his imminent death from a friend who had learned of it from another friend, whose parents in turn had received the information from the patient's parents. The blinding news, combined with a deep sense of his parents' betrayal, resulted, as the staff members put it, in the boy's almost complete "withdrawal" and "apathy." Consequently, the staff could not be of much help.

Transactions with Death

The patient may come to terms with his own mortality if his awareness and understanding develop sufficiently early so that he can confront his dying. Coming to terms involves two separate processes. The first consists of facing the annihilation of self, of visualizing a world without one's self. The second process consists of facing up to dying as a physical, and perhaps mental, disintegration. Some people are fearful of dying in great pain, or with extreme bodily disfiguration, or with loss of speech, or of "just lying there like a vegetable." Others think hardly at all about these aspects of dying, but tremble at the prospect of the disappearance of self. Moreover, some patients who have come to terms with the idea of death may only later focus on dying, especially when they are surprised, dismayed, or otherwise affected by bodily changes. On the other hand, someone who lives with his dying long enough may become assured that he will "pass" peacefully enough, and only then fully faces the death issue.

Most frequently, perhaps, patients come to terms by themselves or with the help of close kin. Nurses, however, may be drawn into the processes. The patient typically initiates the "death talk"; the nurse tends to listen, to assent, to be sympathetic, to reassure. The nurse may even cry with a patient. Occasionally, a patient repeatedly invites nurses into conversations about death or dying, but they decline his invitations. Their refusals tend to initiate a drama of mutual pretense:

Neither party subsequently indicates recognition of the forthcoming death, although both know about it.

Other parties, too, sometimes play significant roles in such processes. In one such situation, an elderly patient was rescued from the isolation of mutual pretense by a hospital chaplain who directly participated in his coming to terms; eventually the chaplain also persuaded the wife, and to some extent the nurses, to enter into the continuing conversation. Patients sometimes rely on members of the clergy to move their spouses to faster acceptance of the inevitable and thus ease their own acceptance.

A Hard Thing to Talk About

On the whole, American nurses and staff physicians seem to find it difficult to carry on conversations about death or dying with patients (Quint, 1967). Only if a patient has already come to terms with death, or if staff can honestly assure him he will die "easily," if he is elderly, do they find it relatively easy to talk about such topics with him. Unless a patient shows considerable composure about his dying, nurses and physicians lose their composure, except when they are specially trained or specially suited by temperament, or have some unusual empathy with a patient because of a similarity of personal history. When the patient's conversation during the last days is only obliquely about death and dying—consisting, for instance, of reminiscences of the past—and is not unpleasant or unduly repetitious, he has a better chance of inducing others, including the nurses, to participate in his closing of his life. Clergymen also are expected to play major roles in this phasing-out of patients. Psychiatrists sometimes perform analogous functions during the phasing-out of more secular-minded patients. (See Ross, Chapter 8, "The Dying Patient's Point of View.")

The closing-off of various aspects of everyday business is important. These include material and personal matters, like the drawing up of wills and the settling of quarrels. Physicians may allow a businessman to close his affairs, though the patient may have to insist on his right to do so. The physician may permit distraught families to urge reluctant patients to draw up, alter, or sign wills. A lawyer is sometimes brought in by the family or physician to help persuade the patient. A chaplain or priest sometimes considers that his professional duties include bridging relationships between the dying person and an alienated spouse or offspring.

Sometimes the patient accepts his forthcoming death even before the staff. Moreover, the patient's "social willing" may shock his family or the staff precisely because he has imaginatively reached his life's end before they have. One patient, for instance, relied on the intervention of his sister (who happened to be a nurse) to will his library to a neighboring college; his wife would never discuss the matter with him. A more extreme instance of social willing, which shocked a hospital's personnel, was when a patient, during his last days, insisted on signing his own autopsy papers.

Dying Versus Work Schedule

Still another great barrier may block even the best-intentioned staff from providing adequate help to a patient when he faces his demise: the immense difference between the staff's and the patient's conceptions of time. The staff operates on "work time." Their tasks are guided by schedules usually related to many patients, both dying and recovering. But a dying patient's personal sense of time often undergoes striking changes once he becomes aware of his impending death. The future is foreshortened, cut out, or abstracted to "after I am gone." The personal past is likely to be reviewed and reconceptualized (Kavinovsky, 1966). The present takes on various kinds of personal meanings. Things previously taken for granted may now be savored as unique but unfortunately transitory. Occasional reprieves, recognized as only reprieves, evoke temporally significant reactions running from, "Oh, God! take me, I was prepared and now will not be prepared" to gratefulness for unexpected time.

The important point is not so much the variability of temporal reconstructions as the difficulty, and sometimes complete inability, of outsiders to grasp these personal reconstructions. One cannot know about them unless privy to the dying person's thoughts. He may keep them to himself, especially in a situation of mutual pretense. He may not be able to express them clearly, especially when he becomes less

Patterns of Dying

sentient. A busy staff may have little time to listen or to invite revealing talk, particularly if patients are competing for attention. In many American hospitals nursing aides spend more time in patients' rooms than the nurses do, even during last days. When aides manage to grasp a patient's temporal reordering of his life, they may be unable to pass along this knowledge to the nurses, or not feel free to do so, or assume that the information is unimportant. And they are not ordinarily accountable for reporting such information.

When the patient's personal time and the staff's work time are highly disparate, considerable strain may be engendered. Nor is the source of the trouble necessarily evident to either. Sometimes, of course, the staff does sense something of a patient's reconceptualizations, without necessarily realizing their deep import, and may somewhat adjust its own work time to his requirements.

Alone with One's Death

A staff's failure in understanding a patient's attempts at achieving psychological closure in his life contributes to another process: the patient's increasing isolation, whether or not he perceives it. He may, of course, understand very well that staff members are not interested in his awesome problem, or cannot grasp its nature even if they wish to. If he has tried to communicate with the staff, he may despair of their understanding. Or he may prefer to communicate with his family or his minister, although he may actually be unable to "reach" them either (Quint, 1963).

It is not only the communications problem that produces isolation, however. In all the countries we have observed, we found strong tendencies to isolate a dying patient during his last days in the hospital. Isolation techniques—perhaps "insulation" is a better term—have their source in various structural conditions. For instance, if everyone agrees a patient should be kept unaware, then attempts to buffer him from knowledge immediately set in motion a train of insulating mechanisms. The isolating process is also called into play if the patient accepts or invites mutual pretense about his dying. The insulating mechanisms are blunted, however, if the patient is openly aware; even then, staff may avoid death talk or even the patient's room or bedside. The patient who will not accept his fate or is dying in a socially unacceptable way also arouses avoidance—sometimes by his family as well as the staff.

During a patient's last days, the staff lightens its work and increases the probability of giving good comfort care by moving him closer to the nursing station. Of course, he may be grateful for the added security of being near the staff, but the move may frighten him despite explanations. The move not only forewarns the aware patient, but it also isolates him from satisfying friendships he has made with other patients. Because of unpleasant odors or perhaps uncontrollable groans and sobbing, he may even be moved into a separate room. At the last, the staff tends to put him either into a single room or with a comatose patient. If the roommate is not comatose, he may complain about the dying patient's behavior, and this would stimulate the staff to move one or the other. Of course, when patients are moved to an intensive care ward, they are quite isolated from people other than the staff, including their families.

All these conditions contribute to the isolation of dying patients. Although a patient may welcome being alone, or alone with kinsmen, he may also fight against his insulation. He may plead successfully to be left with friends and acquaintances, and the staff will wait until he is no longer sentient before moving him. A patient who is already in a single room may devise tactics to get personnel into his room and to increase the time they spend with him, by making urgent demands and complaints or by making himself appealing. The limits of demand tactics are suggested by what happened to one woman who customarily fixed her listeners by the repeated tale of her life. This tactic drove them into nonresponse while they took care of her creature comforts.

A patient can gain more attention from the personnel if he can charm them. The better they like him, the more contact they are likely to give him anyway, unless his dying distresses them so much that they cannot bear to be around him. In slow trajectories, a staff member may pull away from a patient not just to minimize contact with him, but to minimize her own emotions and reactions. She is attempting to lessen the chances of his biography having a lasting impact on her own. On the whole then, under these kinds of structural conditions, it is much easier for patients to gain relative privacy from staff intrusions than to get attention. To the extent that patients fail in either aim, they lose the contest over the shaping of their own passing.

Manipulation of Trajectory

There are two especially critical junctures with immense potential for disturbing either the patient or the staff. The first occurs when someone decides to prolong the patient's life, although others believe he should be allowed to die quickly. The second juncture occurs when someone decides to hasten a patient's death, although others believe this intervention should not be made. These decisions sometimes involve the patient's participation—especially the decision to shorten his life.

His role in the decision not to prolong his dying, or perhaps even to hasten it, is not limited to negotiating with the physician. Patients directly shorten their own lives by various actions—by not eating, by fatally exposing themselves to cold air at open windows, or, more overtly still, by suicide. Patients who are being kept alive through intravenous feeding or machinery are less likely near the end to kill themselves by pulling out the tubes or by asking that the machine be turned off; but we have known a successful instance of each action.

Decisions to prolong or shorten life, however, usually are made by the close kin or by physicians, rather than by the patients themselves. Physicians know what patients and families often do not; life can be extended or shortened for at least a few hours or days, and sometimes longer, by various medical tactics. Several factors bear upon the physician's decision. The nature of the illness is one determinant. During the last days of certain patients—for instance, geriatric cases—physicians customarily make no great attempts to stretch out the dying. In general hospitals, physicians are more likely to keep life going as long as they judge it sensible to do so: Institutional pressures constantly remind them that this is their professional task. Indeed, if a patient unsuccessfully attempts to end his life, physicians are very likely to take steps to prevent renewed attempts.

Nurse Versus Doctor

Nurses in all countries seem to be caught in a bind over prolonging or hastening the dying process. By and large, they tend to resist prolongation. They do not always agree with the physician that a patient's life should be prolonged. "What is the sense of it?" they ask among themselves, sometimes even asking the responsible physician. Nurses may show their disagreement openly and may exert direct pressure on physicians. When they do not attempt to influence his decision, they may harbor disturbing doubts about the paradoxical power of modern medicine; it can extend life for good reason or for none at all.

Family members sometimes may have a major share in shaping this last phase of the dying. Occasionally there may be a conflict between the physician and the family over the family's desire to shorten the ordeal. Or, if the patient is dying at home, the family may rush him to the hospital in order to give him a few more days or weeks. They may ask the doctor to bring in a consultant, or shop around for another doctor, although usually he cannot prolong the patient's life. Although kinsmen may request the doctor not to prolong the dying, he in turn may force on them a direct decision as to whether to shorten life. Rather than precipitate a direct confrontation with the moral decision, he may gently ask whether there is "any more we should do," and the relative, sadly or gratefully, or with some other emotion, probably signals "no." Perhaps more often, close relatives either leave the decision up to the doctor, or are unaware that he and the staff explicitly exercise control over shortening or lengthening life.

Who Will Play God?

The essential issue in these last days is: Who shall have what kinds and degrees of influence in shaping the end of the patient's life? That issue involves not merely how the patient shall die, but also how he shall live while dying. A dying person can hold almost complete control over how he lives his last days by not entering a hospital, or can regain it by leaving the hospital (Wertenbaker, 1957). Yet his trajectory may depart radically from his expectations of it, requiring new decisions. Opinions of doctors and nurses also may need to be modified or even reversed during prelude to death.

Above all, to shape the trajectory during the last days requires juggling tasks, people, and relationships. It also requires juggling time: time for tasks, time for people, time for talk. Most subtle of all, everyone is juggling the time chance still allows; control over aspects of dying may be manageable for a time, but not forever. These various contingencies are immensely unstable: For the staff, the patient can be kept unaware just so long. His family can be kept under control just so long; the strain of waiting or of continual farewells mounts. The staff itself can stand for just so long a patient acting unacceptably in the face of death. During the last days, every major person in the dying drama operates within a context of multiple contingencies.

Disposing of the Family

Consideration of the patient ends with his death. But the hospital's work is not yet finished. It must dispose of the body; it must wind up its relationship with the family; it must write a conclusion to the patient's story. Hospitals are well organized for disposing of the body (a process we shall not discuss here), but they vary in the procedures for disposing of the family and have little or no organization for ending the patient's story—the staff does this latter task on its own, as any particular story seems to require. It is generally felt that the sooner the hospital achieves these dispositions the better, so pressure is put on the staff to expedite them.

"Disposing of" the family involves the announcing of death; it also may involve allowing the kinsmen a last look at their dead relative. Both situations involve problems of management and may, under various conditions, have untoward consequences either for staff or for family. There may be difficulties in ushering the family off the ward. The family members still must settle details of the death with the hospital.

Disposing of the Event

After the body and family are gone from the ward, there remains only the staff's disposition of the patient's story among themselves.

This disposition is a social-psychological process that brings the story of the patient's dying and death to a close in their minds. The degree to which it is necessary varies. At one extreme are the stories of patients whose trajectories and deaths are typical and expected. These stories are routine and never really bothersome; since they were accurate before death, there is no need to develop post-mortem stories. When these patients are gone, they tend simply to be forgotten.

But several kinds of patients have a strong or unusual story in death; it is difficult to forget. Some have an inaccurate pre-death story; some, none at all. The post-mortem story explains what happened and is part of the staff's bringing the case to a close, in effect erasing it from the sentimental order of the ward. Characteristics of the patient himself and of the family also help generate a post-mortem story about the patient (e.g., he was a wonderful person while facing death; a mother would not visit the dying son). The two principal factors in bringing the story to a close are the autopsy findings and the staff's discussion among themselves and with the relatives. Staff members may also have to come to terms with the patient's story through personal grieving and introspection. Sometimes all three ways are combined.

The post-mortem story is mainly developed within the ward until it is forgotten. Sometimes the manner of death is so momentous, however, especially with surprisingly quick trajectories, that the story breaks through the boundaries of the ward itself. If the patient has been on several wards, news may travel in shock waves throughout the hospital. In the surprise suicide or operating-table death, the story may become further formalized by a coroner's inquest, and perhaps then be picked up by the newspapers and spread through the community. These cases, of course, are statistically rare.

Perhaps the most positive story is the "perfect image of death" that nurses and doctors sometimes give family members who have missed the death scene and a last look. They tell such a story even when the death was unpleasant. These stories are told because it is, first of all, difficult to tell an uncomfortable story to a relative. Also, such a story might cause the family to create a scene. More important, perhaps, the staff often feels that the relative has been denied rightful participation in the death, so a vacuum remains to be filled. They fill it with the eulogy of a death occurring in comfort and peace. The family members leave the hospital with a good feeling. Such an outcome makes the nurses feel better, too.

A Set of Recommendations

We shall end with four recommendations based on our text:

1. Training for giving terminal care should be amplified and deepened in schools of medicine and nursing. The changes need to be fairly extensive. Experimentation will be necessary before faculties can be satisfied that they have provided adequate training in the aspects of terminal care—psychological, social, and organizational—now relatively neglected. How and when to teach these matters—these are questions. The most extensive initial educational turmoil is likely to come from faculty members' own attitudes toward dying and death— not only their personal anxieties and aversions to talking openly about dying in any except contemporary technical terms, but also their deep-seated professional attitudes that social, psychological, and organizational matters are irrelevant or minor in the cure of illness and the care of patients. In short: The educational reform that we advocate goes beyond merely humanizing the curriculum a little more.

2. Explicit planning and review should be given to the psychological, social, and organizational aspects of terminal care. The corrective reform called for is, again, rather radical. Hospitals need to make their personnel accountable for many social and psychological actions that currently are left to personal discretion and only incidentally are reported upward—or downward or sidewise. Personnel need to understand the characteristic trajectories of dying that occur on their specific wards, not merely as medical but also as organizational and social phenomena. All wards need to develop mechanisms for insuring a wider awareness of degrees of agreement and disagreement about what is to be done to, for, and around dying patients. Each ward needs mechanisms for discovering its patterned disagreements, and for mitigating their destructive impact on the care of patients. It also needs to understand its patterned agreements, for these can also be destructive to medical and nursing care.

3. There should be explicit planning for phases of the dying trajectory that occur before and after residence at the hospital. Most planning for phases of dying outside the hospital is strictly medical, or deals with financial aspects of the patient's life or with his geographic mobility. But the illness careers of dying patients take them in and out of hospitals, and adequate terminal care often cannot be given unless the connections between hospital and outside world are explicitly rationalized. Planning also must be done around clinic visits for ambulatory patients whose visits represent phases of dying trajectories currently regarded either as purely medical matters or as psychologically unconnected with death.

4. Medical and nursing personnel should encourage public discussion of issues that transcend professional responsibilities for terminal care. Two problems that we believe need public, as well as professional, debate are the withholding of addicting drugs until "near the end," and the "senseless prolonging" of life. About the first issue: Although there is some disagreement among staff about this matter, particularly about the pacing of such drugs, personnel generally seem to share the usual public horror of addiction. But this view is not accepted by all Americans, nor would they all be inclined to favor the withholding of addicting drugs from dying patients if this practice were more widely known. More important, perhaps, is the second issue of prolonging life, since modern technology makes it increasingly probable, beyond where patients are capable of appreciating the extra moments, days, or months. Families as well as staff members may suffer. Debates are frequent within the hospital about particular cases of prolonging life. Yet each physician, and occasionally each nurse, must make decisions about particular patients' lives, basing the decision on a sense of professional responsibility combined perhaps with standards of public conscience and sensibility. Although the physician and nurse can decide for particular patients, they cannot decide the wider issue. That must be debated, we suggest, by the general public. With some certainty, one can predict that this issue will be increasingly discussed openly as medical technology becomes increasingly efficient.

REFERENCES

Becker, Howard, *et al.*
   1961   Boys in White. Chicago: University of Chicago Press.

Fox, Renee.
   1959   Experiment Perilous. New York: Free Press.

Glaser, Barney, and Anselm Strauss.
   1964   "The social loss of dying patients." The American Journal of Nursing 64(June):119–121.
   1965   Awareness of Dying. Chicago: Aldine.
   1968   Time for Dying. Chicago: Aldine.

Kavinovsky, Bernice.
   1966   Voyage and Return: An Experience with Cancer. New York: Norton.

Quint, Jeanne C.
   1963   "The impact of mastectomy." The American Journal of Nursing 63(November):88–97.
   1967   Nurse and the Dying Patient. New York: Macmillan.

Strauss, Anselm, Barney Glaser, and Jeanne Quint.
   1964   "The nonaccountability of terminal care hospitals." Journal of the American Hospital Association 38(January):73–87.

Wertenbaker, Lael.
   1957   Death of a Man. New York: Random House.

8

The Dying Patient's Point of View

Elisabeth K. Ross

A NEW LOOK AT our care for the terminally ill has been taking place in the past decade. Innumerable papers have been published on this subject and a new Foundation of Thanatology has been created during the past year. Most articles have been written by sociologists, psychologists, and psychiatrists, the majority dealing with a philosophical, ethical, or religious aspect of the problems of the dying patient. Some literature gives statistical information about the patient and staff reactions relating to the care of the dying. Little indeed has been written about the patient's own expressions in this great crisis. The reasons for this omission are manifold. It is quite possible that the articles written are self-diagnostic; they reflect our greater comfort in philosophizing in an abstract manner about death than in entering the room of a dying human being and sitting with him until he is ready to share some of his feelings.

This chapter briefly describes what occurs when you try to get close to the dying patient, admitting explicitly that you do not know what it is like to live on borrowed time. It describes how it is when you ask your patient to be not the recipient of your services but your teacher.

As described in more detail in my book, *On Death and Dying* (1969), I was approached in the fall of 1965 by a few seminary students who were attempting to write a paper on crises in human life and wished to concentrate their attention on terminally ill patients. They asked for help as it became obvious to them that they would not be satisfied with writing a speculative or religio-philosophical essay. They seriously wondered how they could get a real and deep sense of this human crisis.

I had had a similar experience a few years before, when I was a first-year resident at Manhattan State Hospital. I remembered vividly how little help I received from reading textbooks and how instructive it was just to spend the first few months sitting and listening to these suffering human beings, attempting to make sense out of their verbal and nonverbal communications. It was easy therefore to recommend the use of the same technique. "If you want to know what it is really like to be schizophrenic, spend time with these patients, sit and listen," I suggested. "If you really wish to share and experience what it is like to have a very limited time to live, sit with your dying patients and listen."

Seminar on Death and Dying

For understandable technical reasons, I was the one elected to find a patient and we arranged the time and place of our next meeting. As I had experienced in other hospitals, such an undertaking meets a tremendous amount of resistance and often insurmountable difficulties and hostility. Suddenly this big teaching hospital did not have a single dying patient!

"Whoever had the nerve to speak with a patient about dying?" "You want to talk about dying, are you out of your mind?" These were the milder reactions, but, because of their openness, the easier ones to cope with. It was more difficult to respond to rationalizations and denial, at times a tremendous protectiveness of the patient—in the form of isolation. I mention these initial difficulties because they are an intrinsic part of our attitude toward dying patients. All who are willing to become involved in this form of learning and teaching should be fully aware of the environmental reactions toward them and their project. They should attempt to understand rather than to judge. The typical reaction is an indicator of our tremendous discomfort in facing the fact of our own finiteness and our wish to avoid it, depersonalize it, or deny it.

During the first year of this undertaking it required an average of ten hours per week to search for a patient—and to get permission from a physician to enter the room of a terminally ill patient to ask him to be our teacher.

In general, the very young physicians or the very old ones were more amenable to our requests, the nurses and nurses' aides the most interested, and the patients themselves the most enthusiastic. With few exceptions, the patients were surprised, amazed, and grateful. Some were plain curious and others expressed their disbelief that "a young, healthy doctor would sit with a dying old woman and really care to know what it is like." In the majority of cases the initial outcome was similar to opening floodgates. It was hard to stop them once the conversation was initiated and the patients responded with great relief to sharing some of their last concerns, expressing their feelings without fear of repercussions.

It was perhaps this discrepancy between the resistance and defensiveness of the staff and the readiness and appreciation of the dying patients that maintained our interest and motivation in the face of the anger and difficulties and was ultimately responsible for our present seminar on Death and Dying.

After four years of persistence and increasing support, this informal get-together, in addition to helping some students in a research project, has grown into an interdisciplinary seminar, held weekly throughout the year at the University of Chicago. A terminally ill patient is no longer interviewed at his bedside, but is seen in a screen-window interviewing room (in his own bed if necessary) with infusions and transfusions or whatever is indicated. The audience consists of doctors, nurses, chaplains, rabbis, priests, social workers, and other members of the helping professions. They observe an initial, spontaneous interview and then have an opportunity to share their own reactions, feelings, and responses in a post-interview discussion, after the patient is returned to his room. Occasionally a patient may request the presence of a relative who then sits in the interview and is questioned about his own reactions to this crisis. We have also interviewed parents of dying children in the absence of the latter. The seminar on Death and Dying is presently an accredited course for medical students and students of the theological seminary and offers a meaningful learning experience for all members of the helping professions.

The Dying Patient's Point of View

It is also the only place where the different disciplines get together and hear the other person's point of view—his innermost feelings, frustrations, and needs—and begin to realize how much our own reactions are reflected in the ultimate care of the patient.

Those participants who have attended several seminars have become increasingly sensitive to their patients' verbal and nonverbal communications and have become more comfortably involved with those patients whom they previously avoided.

The best example of the change is perhaps a woman who attended our seminar at the beginning, expressing loudly her anger about a sense of isolation and "being treated like I have a contagious disease." She left the hospital shortly after the interview and we did not expect to see her again. Nine months later, the patient requested another seminar. She shared her great relief at having been able to ventilate her anger during the first interview. She subsequently had gone into a remission. Now she returned with a new relapse of her malignancy. But she was no longer an angry, difficult patient. She said that she had to come and share with us the changes that had occurred on her old floor. "Imagine, the nurse comes in now once in a while, and actually sits down and says, 'Feel like talking?'" She experienced a sense of acceptance by the staff who felt much more comfortable with her and were able to communicate with her with greater ease. Many of the nurses made special arrangements to have their floors covered in order that they might attend the seminar. Former medical students who had taken the seminar as an elective were now interns or externs and started to refer patients to us. Once it became known that we did not break the patients' defenses down, that we followed our patients and saw them as often as they wished, referrals started to come in from many different sources. At present, we often have more referrals than we can accommodate and we follow many of our terminally ill patients without presenting them in the seminar first.

A Manpower Shortage

After about one year of struggle, it became evident that I alone was not able to follow all the patients until they died. I also ran into difficulties with very religious patients whose language I did not always fully understand. I appreciated their need to talk at times in terms of psalms, but also needed to know the deeper meaning of their communications. I thus ended in the hospital chaplain's office asking for help. For the past few years it has become a truly interdisciplinary undertaking. The interviews usually include Chaplain Nighswonger, our hospital chaplain, or one of his students. A great part of the follow-up visits are done by them if the patient's need indicates this. Since social workers and nurses as well as the doctors attend the interviews they obtain firsthand information of the patient's needs, concerns, or conflicts. The patient may vividly describe specific incidents which upset him and of which the staff is often unaware.

When the treatment team faces their own feelings and comes to grips with patient and staff problems, ways and means are discussed of helping the patient through his crisis. It becomes much easier for doctors or nurses to appreciate a patient's feelings when they hear him personally rather than read about the conflicts on a consultation sheet.

The weekly sharing of such crises brought the staff much closer together. They began to appreciate each other's needs more, too. They slowly dared to look at a dying patient, not just at his infusion. They slowly heard him and gradually began to be comfortable relating to him.

Nurses who felt "it was a shameful waste of time to spend it on dying patients" a few years ago now provide the most helpful assistance for our seminar. They are encouraged to express these feelings and gradually realize where this resistance comes from. Many of them call on us when certain types of patients stir up "untherapeutic feelings" in them. They have developed a healthy curiosity, making them much more interested and, I think, much more gratified in their work.

The initial interview is usually our first contact with the patient. We purposely do not read the chart or seek other information. We want to show our students how one can approach a stranger and get right into important things. We do not know ahead of time if a patient has been told about the seriousness of his condition. We do not regard this as relevant at all. We have learned from interviewing hundreds of terminally ill patients (half of whom have never been told of their fate explicitly) that they all know the seriousness of their condition. *They* tell *us*, not the other way around. We often simply ask them, "How sick are you?" The answer comes promptly, "I am full

The Dying Patient's Point of View

of metastasis." We got this answer from a patient described as "impossible to communicate with." The staff was sure that he did not know that he had cancer! But nobody had ever asked him.

The fact that our patients are aware of how sick they are does not mean that they share this knowledge with everybody. They depend on good relationships with their doctors and other staff. They may increasingly depend on their family. They quickly realize who is comfortable in the face of bad news and who has the need to talk about next spring when there will be no next spring. They will quietly play the game and use denial with those who need denial. They will wait, and often hope, that there is someone who takes them seriously and who can share with them the inner turmoil, the unfinished business, and respond to the great need to talk about their impending death.

The Need to Share

To talk about death and dying does not mean that the patients have a wish or a need to fantasize what it is going to be like. But they do have a need to share with someone what it is going to be like *to live* these last few months, weeks, or days. Some patients may need to keep busy, to get some help to function in some capacity when it is too difficult to give up all autonomy. Others may simply be concerned about who will take care of their children, a retarded son perhaps, or an invalid mother. That too, means talking about dying, because it takes an awareness of finiteness in order to bring the house into order. Others may need a chaplain or rabbi and may ask for reassurance about less earthly matters.

The following two examples are patients who were both young and had a short time to live. Each one of them had different needs; these we tried to understand and to meet. We met both of them only a few times, yet both became important human beings and were deeply and comfortably involved with the hospital staff.

First Case Miss T was a young woman in her thirties, black, single, and had been self-supporting. She had lost one hand in an accident, but, with the encouragement of her employer, had done a masterful job of overcoming this handicap; for example, she could type and knit. She was sent to our hospital for evaluation of a kidney condition that was found to be much more serious than anticipated.

The patient was eventually told that she needed to be signed up on the "kidney machine program" in order to live. Only two local hospitals had such programs for the indigent and both turned her down. When she was returned to our hospital, the staff had a hard time facing her. They had grown attached to this kind, soft-spoken woman and they could not comprehend that she was "condemned to death" as they referred to it. Nurses and the social worker felt the impact very deeply as they had the most contact with her. They felt both guilty and angry, raising questions about who has the right to choose who shall live and who shall die. They continued to visit her, but felt increasingly awkward and finally asked us to present her in our seminar—not so much for the patient's need as for themselves.

I interviewed Miss T a few days later. The hospital chaplain took part. Her trouble had begun, she said, with a shortness of breath about six months earlier. Doctors agreed that she had hypertension and malfunctioning kidneys. Medicine had not helped. Renal dialysis was recommended. She could not pay for treatment—it is costly—and she could not obtain it free. She felt rejected. At one of the three hospitals that she was in, the doctors were mainly of foreign extraction and she could not understand them. The food was not what she was used to. Toileting was a problem. The bathroom was down the hall. The bedpan service was poor.

She became mentally confused at this hospital, and often felt consciousness slipping away—"A little pile of smoke would come over, and I'd just fall asleep." She had repeated dreams of an operation and cure. When her sister called from California, Miss T told her she did not need to be on a kidney machine: "Everything is going to be all right."

By the time she came back to our hospital, she recognized that she was having difficulty distinguishing between her dream and reality. But she did come to face reality and it hurt her: "I was not accepted for the dialysis machine."

As her disease progressed, despite strict control of her fluid intake, her eyes began to fail. She could not crochet, knit, or read the Bible someone brought her—"So now I've taken up sleeping." Now, however, she had ordinary dreams. She did not lack for visits from friends and nephews, but her mother and sisters lived too far away to come.

The Dying Patient's Point of View

She was a Methodist and had gone to church. She had some questions about God and the hereafter: "You go to church, you hear people confess of seeing God, of God coming to them and cleansing their minds out. That has never happened to me; and I was wondering, does it really happen to people, or did it . . . just never happen to me?"

She had been a generous, giving person, and had helped persons in greater need than herself. So she was not concerned about God's judgment on that score. But she had not, as the chaplain phrased it, had a "bright religious experience," a sense of discovering God and being transformed. Was this what worried her?

"I feel that I am not getting any better, and will not get any better," she said. "I might ask now, why should I have to suffer so long? Why can't God come and get me now and take me out of misery? . . . Of course, doctors can do everything—that's their job, to try to save lives. But I just wonder, are they doing too much to save my life, since they know they cannot?"

At this point, Miss T began to tire. Within a few minutes, we drew the interview to a close. Her last comment was: "I don't know—I have a set-up in my mind like there are two gardens, a garden here on earth and a garden in heaven; and I'm just waiting on God to say which of the gardens he wants me to work in."

At the end of the week following the interview I suddenly wanted to see this patient once more. There was an unraised question still hanging in the air and I thought it would be better to attempt to bring it out in the open. The weekend was coming up and with it perhaps increased loneliness. She might feel better to discuss the "unfinished business" once more. When I headed toward her room I was not sure what to say or how to start. It was just a sense of urgency to "do it now." I invited both a priest and a social worker to attend, but neither showed up. Thus I sat by her side and shared with her the feeling that we had to talk about it once more, not knowing exactly what "it" was.

Miss T looked at me with relief and acknowledged that she too had a sense of urgency. She too felt that there was a big and important question which she wanted to ask and which needed an answer. And so we sat—almost like two children—digging in the dark and searching for something lost, not quite knowing what we had lost.

Miss T kept saying, "I know I am bad, bad, bad. . . ." and though I did not share this feeling with her, we attempted to find out what she was bad about. Was it because she was black, or single and had no children, or because she had lived with a man and was not married? We went through the whole range of things that society could condemn but nothing "felt right." Finally I was ready to give up and said something to the effect that "only God knows what you should be bad about." She looked at me with a sigh of relief and almost cried: "That's it. God! I have been calling Him for help for the last few days. God help me, God help me! And I hear Him say in the back of my mind: 'Why are you calling for help now and have never called when things were well?' What do you say to that, Doctor Ross?"

She looked at me like a frightened child now, asking, demanding, an answer. For a glimpse of a moment I wished the priest was there. He would have had an answer, I thought. She looked at me and after what seemed like an eternity, she said again, this time very quietly, "What is your answer to that?" Now I heard myself talk quietly, naturally, without struggling for words. It suddenly seemed to be a very simple question. I asked her to share with me a picture of children playing in the playground. Mother is in the house minding her own work. Suddenly a little boy falls and hurts his knees. What do you think happens?

She looked at me surprised and answered: "The little boy cries and calls for Mother."

"What happens next?" I said.

"Mother helps him back on his feet and consoles him until he is all right."

"What happens next?" I insisted.

The same surprised look came over her face, as if she wondered why I would ask such a simple, almost silly question. "The boys go back to play and Mother continues her housework."

"The children have no use for her right now, isn't that right?"

She confirmed it and I continued: "Do you think Mother resents that?"

"A mother," she said almost angrily, "wouldn't resent that!"

I looked at her very seriously and replied, "A mother wouldn't resent it, and Father would?" pointing up into the sky. . . .

The Dying Patient's Point of View

She looked with the happiest face I had seen in a long time, holding my hand lightly and smiled. She repeated almost inaudibly: "If a mother can accept that, Father will, too. How could I ever doubt that?" After a few moments of the most peaceful silence, she continued, "My time comes very close now, but everything is all right. I shared with you my concept of death, passing from this garden into the next. What is your concept?"

I thought for a while, and still looking at her face, I said, "Peace." Her last words were: "I will pass into my garden very peacefully now."

Miss T died a few hours later in her sleep.

We are often told that the attending staff has no time to get this involved with a patient, that it takes too much time. I would like to add that the only time spent with this patient was the (public) tape-recorded interview of about forty-five minutes and the dialogue just described above. Dying patients who have such a limited time do not waste precious hours. It is not the numbers of hours spent with them that counts. Counseling the dying patient is one of the most intense, most personal, perhaps the most intimate kind of encounter between two human beings. It is exhausting because of its depth and intensity but does not require many hours. It is a listening to—and at times sharing—the innermost feelings and concerns, without layers and layers of trimmings around it.

What Miss T was asking at the end was simply the question if God could accept her in His garden if the people here on earth did not find her worthy enough to continue to live—for example, to accept her in the dialysis program. Naturally, a counselor has to give his own answers and share some of his own convictions. Since I could not do that with respect to God, I had to give an answer which was both honest and understandable to myself.

When Miss T became aware of her sharing with me her innermost feelings, she asked me to do the same. We are, as counselors, so used to asking questions and become so defensive when the patient asks a question of us, that it takes a while to get used to this kind of sharing. There is no other counseling with any other type of patient where it is so important to take off one's professional white coat and just be a human being. Those who have experienced such moments will agree with me that working with dying patients is not depressing at all and can be an instructive, gratifying, and at times even beautiful experience.

Second Case Mr. L was twenty-five when he came into the hospital with acute leukemia. He was the father of three small children, all under the age of three. He was big, strong, and manly. He was not used to being pampered, washed, fed, and pushed around in a wheel chair. He had no time for denial, as his illness progressed rapidly. Within a few days it became exceedingly difficult to swallow or speak. His lips were bleeding, his tongue red and sore. He was angry and depressed, asked for a little time—all at once. He would occasionally ask me to sit down and look for words. He raised the question briefly, "Why me?" But he seemed to be too impatient even to attempt to answer it. One evening he wanted to see me, but changed his mind. He called me three times that day but felt physically so weak that he was unable to speak much. He looked desperate and struggled for words and finally gave up the attempt, asking me to return early the next morning. I left him with mixed emotions and wondered if he would make it through the night. His mother sat with him, quietly and patiently, knowing it was a question of hours.

The next morning I was informed that Mr. L had had a terrible night, was restlessly fighting with an invisible enemy, and the staff did not expect him to live until morning. He looked exhausted but almost happy when I entered the room. "Sit down and close the door," he commanded. "You would not believe it, what happened last night," he said. "There was this big train running down the tracks, faster and faster, and I kept fighting and arguing with the trainmaster that he had to stop the train a tenth of an inch short. Do you understand that?" He looked at me now with his big eyes, hoping I would grasp what he had to share.

I smiled at him and said: "Well, as I see, you won and made the tenth of an inch. The train, I guess, that runs down toward the end so fast is your life and you argued for a little bit of time and made it." He smiled now, too, as his mother re-entered the room.

I was not sure how much Mr. L wanted to share this with his mother and therefore asked him in his own words, how I could help him "during the next tenth of an inch." With the same voice of determination, he pointed to his mother and asked me to explain to her that it was all right for her to go home now. What he wanted the most was his mother's homecooked vegetable soup and a loaf of bread that his mother used to bake when he was small. He said: "I just have to have a plate of that soup and a piece of that bread once more, it smelled so good."

Mother looked at him and at me. She was obviously pleased but also worried about leaving her son after a critical night like that. We both reassured her that it was all right, both of us feeling comfortable that Mr. L would know better than anybody else what he could expect and what not.

Mother did leave and returned with a thermos bottle of her vegetable soup. The bread and the soup were the last food that Mr. L ate. He died three days after this incident. Young and strong as he was, he fought as long as he could. When he realized that his end was near, he asked once more for the things he used to enjoy. He faded away quickly after this without speaking any further about his impending death.

Mr. L talked in terms of his dreams rather than in concrete language about the awareness of dying because it was much too painful for him to say, "I have only a few hours to live." He appreciated that he was understood and answered in his terms rather than being asked, "Well, how can I help you in the short time you have to live?"

The Art of Listening

I am trying to say once again that it is an art to listen to our patients, to use their language and allow them to keep the defenses they need. It takes just a little experience and the will to sit and listen. If we do not understand what they are trying to communicate we can acknowledge that, too, and the patient will try to rephrase it if he senses that we really try to understand him.

If we are uncomfortable in the face of a young dying patient we may block out these communications and the patient may never be able to communicate what he wants to share with another human being. We deprive him and ourselves of an important experience. Though each individual patient reacts in his own way to a crisis of this nature, there are a few common denominators that are worth keeping in mind. Practically all our patients reacted to their first awareness of a fatal illness with shock and disbelief. "No, not me." Depending on the personality, the circumstances, and most important of all, the way the person was informed, this denial was soon replaced with anger and only partial denial. The statement was no longer, "No, not me," but was replaced with an angry, "Why me?"

This anger shows in many ways and is often hard to live with. We are so well trained that we should be kind to sick people, but who can continue to be friendly and cheerful when every move we make is criticized? The family who visits comes either too late or at an inconvenient time. The nurse shakes the pillows when the patient just decided to take a nap. The intern does not know how to give an injection and the kitchen sent the wrong diet. . . . We react by waiting a bit longer to respond to a call, by sticking the needle in a bit harder, by postponing our visits, and the patient feels even more deprived, isolated, rejected.

What we have not asked ourselves is why is this patient so angry? Wouldn't we be angry, too, if we had fed our little ones at home a short time ago and now have to wait for strangers to feed us? When we are in pain and dependent on the doctor to order enough analgesics, only to be told that the nurse went for a coffee break and will be back shortly with the medication? What our patients are mainly angry about are not the human shortcomings so much as the fact that we live and function and go home at night and they cannot.

If we do not react with anger, if we do not take this complaining personally but learn to empathize with our fatally ill patients and help them to ventilate their anger, they will feel less deserted and less guilty and will respond eventually with much less turmoil about their declining ability to function.

For a short time these patients may look quite comfortable and accepting of their condition. We have learned that this is often preceded by a bargaining period. Most bargaining is made with God. It is a request for some relief, some extra time, perhaps in exchange for a price. "If You give me one more year to live, I will be a good Christian and attend church regularly." Or, "If You grant me this one more wish, I will donate my eyes, my kidneys," and so forth. Another patient asked

The Dying Patient's Point of View

for only one day without pain in order to leave the hospital and attend a son's wedding. With the help of self-hypnosis this wish was fulfilled and she attended, happily, the great event. On her return to the hospital, her bargaining time was up. Before I could ask her a question she said, "Don't forget now, I have another son."

Bargaining is a temporary truce, so to speak. It is a break for the patient and the staff and family. The promises are rarely kept, but that is not important. It is important to know that these patients then function like children who want something badly and promise the impossible. Because parents, too, need a break, they let them have it, knowing full well that they will not keep the promise. We do the same with our patients. When the bargaining is over, during which time they say, "Yes, it's me, but . . ." the depression sets in.

The depression is not only over the lost ability to function, but also the sad awareness of all the things and people they soon have to leave behind. Unfortunately, we feel a need to cheer our patients up. We more often than not enter such a room and say, "Come on, now, it's not so bad." We discourage them from grieving and do not appreciate that it takes courage and strength to acknowledge that life comes to an end. Patients who are discouraged from expressing their anger and their sadness feel much more alone in their grief. They also feel ashamed and guilty or "less of a man" for their tears. By assisting them we encourage them to express their sadness. When they can say, "Yes, it is me," they are entitled to tears. I feel that it takes more strength to acknowledge it and express the grief than it does to pretend that it is all not true.

If we can accept our patients the way they are, with denial, anger, bargaining, and depression, they will work through their unfinished business and reach a stage of acceptance enabling them to die in peace and dignity.

They will ask once more to see their friends, then their children, and at the end, only a husband or wife perhaps. They will gradually separate themselves from this world and will pass peacefully "from this garden to the next," in Miss T's words, if we do not interfere and prolong a life artificially when the patient is ready to die.

Hope which is ever present even in the most realistic patient will then change from a desire to get well, or at least hope for a remission, to a hope of a death without too much suffering or, as Miss T expressed it, the hope that the end comes soon and that she might be accepted in God's garden although human beings were unable to accept her.

REFERENCES

Ross, Elisabeth Kübler.
    1966 "The dying as teacher, an experiment and an experience." Chicago Theological Seminary Register 50 (December).
    1969 On Death and Dying. New York: The Macmillan Company.

9

Consequences of Death for Physicians, Nurses, and Hospitals*

David L. Rabin with Laurel H. Rabin

"ALL THE DOCTORS!—helpless flies now, climbing across the granite face of death." With these words John Gunther, in *Death Be Not Proud*, describes his son's doctors just before the boy, after a long and brave fight, dies of a brain tumor. In such circumstances, those who would cure have always been in the position of helpless flies.

The significance of "the granite face of death" has varied from age to age, however. Just as "no other epoch has laid so much stress as the expiring Middle Ages on the thought of death" (Huizinga, 1956: 138), no other epoch has so tried to suppress it as ours. Death has become the taboo of our age as sex was the taboo of the Victorian era. After World War I, Freud (1918:41) noted, "We have shown an unmistakable tendency to put death aside, to eliminate it from life." Improved sanitation, nutrition, and housing at the end of the last century greatly reduced mortality rates, and made it easier to put death aside. A child born during the nineteenth century, for example, would probably have experienced the death of a sibling or parent before he reached manhood. Death was not hidden from life. Among the fifty-seven poems in *McGuffey's Fifth Eclectic Reader*, commonly used a century ago, twenty-seven specifically refer to death or dying and many others do so indirectly (Group for the Advancement of Psychiatry, 1965:661). The change in mortality rates has been dra-

---
* Prepared under PHS Research Grant No. CH–00158 from the National Center for Health Services Research and Development.

matic. In 1900 life expectancy was 47.3 years; in 1915 as many as one in every ten liveborn babies was unable to survive the first year of life (Lerner et al., 1963). In 1967 life expectancy was 70.2 years; the infant mortality rate was 22.1 per 1,000 (National Center for Health Statistics, 1968). With this sharp decrease in death rates and increase in life expectancy, a child born in this century might well reach adulthood without ever having experienced the death of anyone around him.

The Medical Student and Death

This is the world in which children today, including future physicians, learn about death. Never before have medical students and physicians been less able to face the reality of death, unprepared as they are by personal experience or society's teachings. Indeed, there is some evidence that physicians may have chosen their profession because of their difficulties with the concept of death. A study by Feifel (1965:634) reveals that physicians fear death much more than comparison groups of patients. Kasper (1959:263), however, noted that "as a rule, people with conscious death anxiety or overt somatic preoccupation stay away from medicine. . . ." But he also pointed out that the early histories of physicians reveal situations in which there is an unusual amount of concern about their own bodies; in psychoanalytic terms concern about one's body is equated with fear of death. For Kasper, then, fear of death is an unconscious factor in the making of a physician; he emphasizes, however, that there are many other factors influencing the choice of medicine as a profession. Even psychiatrists, physicians who study all aspects of man's nature, his fears and anxieties, have avoided an extensive study of death; also, the study of suicide has been scant in the psychiatric literature. Weisman and Hackett (1961:247) indicate that when psychiatrists do study suicide, they rarely discuss those situations in which death is appropriate or to be desired.

Medical education has, traditionally, offered little help to the medical student encountering death for the first time. In fact, discussion of death is conspicuous by its absence. "Death" is not even to be found in the indexes of most medical and surgical textbooks, nor can I recall any discussion in medical school concerning the consequences of death for the physician. Early in medical school, the student becomes

"... desensitized, not to death, but to the symbols of death such as blood, bones, corpses, and stench which disturb most people" (Kasper, 1959:261).

The medical student's first professional encounter with the dead human body comes in the anatomy course during his first year of school, often in the first week. For the student the cadaver is primarily a machine with whose pieces and parts he must become thoroughly familiar if he is to pass his anatomy examinations. When one considers the pre-medical courses to which most medical students are exposed, their reactions to the cadaver are not at all surprising. Laboratory work in animal zoology, comparative anatomy, and animal physiology require the student to kill animals and exhaustively study and dissect them. Study of the cadaver simply offers him more advanced anatomical knowledge than that which he has learned from other forms of life.

In dealing with the cadaver, Becker (1961:423) says that the students "... are not very much bothered by the fact that the cadavers they now dissect were once living human beings." It is not, however, that the students are "not very much bothered" by the cadaver's past. To them the cadavers have no past. The students do not know who they were, even what their names were. In the second year of medical school, every student studies pathology. In pathology, he observes his first autopsy. Here he can, for the first time, associate a corpse with a living person. The student sees the patient's medical record to the moment of death; often the physician who, until a few hours ago, cared for the patient speaks of the fatal illness.

The first autopsy I (DLR) attended was performed on a five-year-old boy with a congenital cyst of the liver who had died the morning following the third of a series of elective operations to drain the cyst. The surgeon, one of the most highly respected men on the hospital staff, attended the autopsy. He was obviously shaken by the child's unexpected death—the result of postoperative hemorrhage from a bleeding vessel. I later learned that he canceled all his surgery for three days following the autopsy.

This first autopsy made me painfully aware of the awesome responsibility the physician accepts and of the human limitations that constrain even the most skilled. It was also a dramatic example, to be followed innumerable times in the future, of how medicine learns from its mistakes. Even from the tragic death of a child can come knowledge beneficial to others. It was in the autopsy room that I and other students encountered our most dramatic "training for uncertainty," as Fox (1957:207) terms it. Here the medical student is ". . . struck by the fact that the pathologist cannot always explain the causes of death and that, although the 'doctors' diagnoses are often right, they can also be wrong' " (Fox, 1957:219).

In the last two years of medical school—the clinical years—the student, for the first time, is physician to the living and the dying. During the summer between my second and third years, I worked in a small community hospital in my hometown. My first dying patient was a 78-year-old unconscious woman with a brain hemorrhage and impaired circulation. I examined the patient and gave her drugs to maintain her blood pressure. I then talked with the attending physician who argued against trying to treat the patient since death was imminent and there was little to be gained from valiant efforts to prolong her life. He agreed, however, to let me try to prolong her life. Implicit throughout the medical student's education is the idea that "every death corresponds to a failure, either of the individual physician, or, more commonly, of medicine as a whole" (Bohrod, 1965:811). Since it seemed within my power to keep my patient alive, it was, I argued, my responsibility to attempt to do so; to do less was to admit failure. After three days she was still alive—though comatose and requiring increasing doses of the medicine to sustain her blood pressure. No one had visited her since her arrival at the hospital. At that point, I accepted the wisdom of the attending physician's suggestion and stopped the drugs.

Unlike this woman's wise physician, some attending physicians at university hospitals might well have advised keeping this lonely old woman alive with heroic measures, while doing extensive diagnostic testing. This, for some physicians, represents the ideal of "scientific" medicine—prolong life no matter what the circumstances. As Glaser and Strauss (1965:203) point out,

> A favorite rationale of the doctor who persists in the ideal of indefinite prolonging is an assertion that he is simply an instrument of society. He feels that society has vested in him the duty of sustaining

life and that he is therefore obliged to abdicate personal responsibility for judging the advisability of whether a particular life should or should not be prolonged.

It is argued that the medical student learns ". . . a language and point of view toward these things [death and disabling or disfiguring disease] which provide a technical and impersonal way of experiencing them. . . . He sees death not so much as human tragedy [but] as a problem in the use of medical responsibility" (Becker, 1961:273). Nothing in my medical education later prepared me for the profound responsibility of deciding whether or not I should attempt to prolong a particular life. No professor ever discussed the possibility that, given certain circumstances, death might be desirable or appropriate. Nor was it ever pointed out that I might be responsible for deciding who shall die and who shall live. Now, more than ever before, medical students must be taught to assume personal responsibility for prolonging life. They should recognize that ". . . the ways in which simple survival can be extended are now so various and so complex [for example, respirator, pacemaker, pressor medication, organ transplant] that the principle of the right to die has intervened" (Hubbard, 1968).

The Physician and Death

As the student completes his formal medical education he must make decisions about his future as a physician. At the present time, 85 per cent of medical graduates enter specialties (Coggeshall, 1965: 21). The specialty chosen dictates in large measure the physician's future experience with death; the anticipation of this future experience may, indeed, be an important factor in determining the specialty chosen. For example, the student who goes into pathology will rarely examine living patients; the student who chooses neurosurgery is going to have frequent contact with dying patients, often young people who die from trauma. The student who will practice psychiatry, on the other hand, will rarely experience the death of a patient, but he may be frequently involved with the threat of death, that is, self-destruction. Many students enter specialties that provide primary care—obstetrics, pediatrics, and internal medicine—where death is not a common occurrence. When it does occur, it can be a profoundly disturbing event.

A pediatrician in private practice for fifteen years experienced only eight deaths, excluding perinatal deaths (Seidel, 1969). He could remember with precise detail the clinical history and family situation of each child who had died. In contrast, he did not remember the total number or many details about a larger number of perinatal deaths. Death, of itself, is not necessarily profoundly disturbing to the physician. It may be disturbing when the deceased was a member of a family, a child who loved, hated, cried, laughed—someone with a brief past and a long and often promising future. The pediatrician has come to know this child and to feel affection for him and often for his family. Death, in this instance, therefore, not only ends a meaningful relationship, but seems cruel.

Internists experience many more deaths than pediatricians. Most of these deaths, however, occur among the older people in their practices. Although the internist, like the pediatrician, may have had a meaningful relationship with an older patient, he knows that, frequently, his patient has lived the expected span of years, or close to it. Though there may be grief, it is more for the loss of a relationship rather than for the reality of death. In those instances when the internist experiences the death of a younger person—someone with little children or beginning a career—he is more likely to feel frustrated and to think that medicine has failed.

The Surgeon and Death

A specialty in which death is particularly poignant is obstetrics and gynecology. The United States has a higher perinatal death rate than most other Western nations and now ranks eighteenth in the world (National Center for Health Statistics, 1967:2). As a result, there has been considerable interest in the causes of perinatal mortality. A study by Shapiro et al. (1968) on prematurity and perinatal mortality in New York City found a far lower perinatal mortality rate for private patients of board certified obstetricians than for indigent patients cared for by interns and residents. Surprisingly, the perinatal mortality rate for private patients using other physicians was lower yet. This apparent paradox is explained by the fact that a patient with a complicated problem, whose fetus has a high risk of dying, is often referred to a specialist. A high mortality rate for a physician can, therefore, reflect superior qualifications associated with a clinical practice that includes patients with complicated problems.

The surgeon, on the other hand, is constantly dealing with the possibility of death. Even the most benign of surgical procedures—appendectomy—has a death rate of 0.5 per cent (Lipworth, 1963:71). As Charles Mayo, the noted surgeon, once pointed out, "There is a lot of luck to surgery. . . . Not long ago, I had 103 consecutive cases without an operative or postoperative death. Then I had three deaths in a week" (*The New York Times*, 1968:31). Unlike the primary care physicians, however, the surgeon's relationship with the patient is usually short. He probably has seen the patient only a few times before surgery; the question of life or death is resolved within several weeks after surgery. For many surgeons, therefore, the loss of a patient may not be felt as deeply as it is by other physicians. A surgeon's success, however, is very much related to his operative mortality since it is the most visible index of success to his medical colleagues, on whom he is dependent for patient referral. Mayo, when beginning his practice, was asked by a woman to recommend a physician to operate on her gall bladder. He referred her to a surgeon who had done more than a thousand such operations, but added that the woman could choose himself. "I'm just starting," he said, "and I can't afford to lose a patient." The woman chose Doctor Mayo (*The New York Times*, 1968: 31).

Surgical subspecialists such as neurosurgeons and cardiac surgeons accept death as an everyday reality, in contrast to the general surgeons' relatively infrequent loss of patients. High mortality rates are often associated with new radical operations on vital organs. To clarify the distinction between the risks associated with the newness of the operation and the risks of the operation itself, mortality rates are often calculated separately for the first group of operations as compared with the second. Justification for high death rates for new procedures is based on the expectation of improvement over existing procedures. The surgeon further justifies using a new procedure by offering it only to those patients who have far advanced, irreparable, and imminently fatal disease. As the procedure proves beneficial and the operative mortality drops, the surgeon offers it to patients with less advanced disease who have a better chance of surviving surgery. His operative mortality rate now improves further. His experience accumulates and knowledge spreads to his surgical colleagues; the procedure is more widely used. As each surgeon begins to use the procedure, however, he, too, may have a period of high operative mortality followed by a decrease to an acceptable level. A difficult medical problem with ambiguous moral implications arises when a surgeon attempts to learn a new procedure with a high initial mortality rate, with other surgeons nearby who have great experience with the procedure.

Interestingly, patient deaths following surgery occur at widely differing rates in different hospitals. A four-year survey of death rates for surgery in thirty-four hospitals (Moses and Mosteller, 1968) indicates that the hospital with the highest death rate had a postoperative mortality twenty-four times that of the lowest. Death rates ranged from 0.27 to 6.40 per cent among the different hospitals. Adjusting the rates for each patient's physical condition, age, and type of operation reduces the variation to tenfold. Little is known about variables that affect survival in the hospitals, but the striking differences suggest that some postoperative deaths might be preventable and imply the need for inquiry into the causes of these enormous variations in postoperative mortality.

Medical subspecialists, like many surgical subspecialists, see far more death than primary care physicians. Because of the rapid increase in medical knowledge and the consequent development of medical subspecialties, patients with fatal illnesses are now more likely to be seen and taken care of by medical subspecialists. For example, a patient with a lymphoma may be referred to a subspecialist for a diagnosis and intermittent consultation. Meanwhile the primary care physician will continue to take care of the patient until late in the course of the disease. This subspecialist then will only know the dying patient and his family under abnormal and tragic circumstances. Although this physician-patient relationship may be close, it lacks the intimacy that often develops between the patient and the referring physician, a physician who, ideally, may have known the patient and his family over many years, both in health and sickness.

Coping with Death

But no matter who the physician, who the patient, or what the relationship, death is difficult for the physician to accept. Too, although death comes later in life now than in the past, the dying are with us longer. This is because of the dramatic shifts in the patterns of disease. Today people die from chronic lingering diseases rather than acute fulminating disease. This means that patients, and, therefore, their physicians, must face the prospect of death for a longer time than ever before. Each physician then must find his own way of coping with each patient's approaching death. Sadly, the physician usually copes with death in one of two ways. He may adapt a seemingly impersonal attitude toward the patient or he may avoid the patient as much as possible. Leo Tolstoy, in "The Death of Ivan Ilyich," brilliantly describes a physician's seeming impersonality as seen by his dying, middle-aged patient:

> The doctor said that so-and-so indicated that there was so-and-so inside the patient, but if the investigation of so-and-so did not confirm this, then he must assume that and that. If he assumed that and that, then . . . and so on. To Ivan Ilyich only one question was important: was his case serious or not? But the doctor ignored that inappropriate question. From his point of view it was not the one under consideration, the real question was to decide between a floating kidney, chronic catarrh, or appendicitis. It was not a question of Ivan Ilyich's life or death, but one between a floating kidney and appendicitis. . . . From the doctor's summing up Ivan Ilyich concluded that things were bad, but that for the doctor, and perhaps for everybody else, it was a matter of indifference, though for him it was bad. And this conclusion struck him painfully, arousing in him a great feeling of pity for himself and of bitterness toward the doctor's indifference to a matter of such importance.

Avoidance as a way in which physicians handle death is described in a study of patients with terminal cancer. Hackett and Weisman (1964: 308) found that "When [the patient dying from a malignancy] is pronounced incurable, the physician often asks the chaplain to make regular visits and concomitantly withdraws his presence." Obviously, the patient cannot be satisfied with impersonality and avoidance, but the physician, too, cannot be satisfied with them for they are a negation of his role as comforter as well as healer.

Aring (1968:140) tells a haunting story of the terrible consequences of avoidance: A man in his 60s entered the hospital with symptoms of a brain mass; his chest X-ray revealed a tumor that was thought to have spread to the brain.

> After the flurry of attention to the diagnosis [carcinoma], ward personnel lost interest. The patient began to be moved farther and farther from the nursing station at the front of the ward. The withdrawal that our patient experienced was not so much physical absence as uninterest.
> Our patient followed the expected course of carcinoma, reassuring us about the correctness of the diagnostic label. Despite routine feeding, he continued to lose weight, and within some weeks was as generally emaciated as might be expected. At necropsy, a meningioma of the vertex was revealed, a tumor that should have readily yielded to the correct neurosurgical attack. The lung lesion was not carcinomatous.

Fortunately this tragic consequence of avoidance is a rare occurrence, but unfortunately such treatment of the patient dying slowly from a progressive but incurable disorder is not so rare. The attention of doctors and nurses can help the dying patient as well as his family in facing the patient's death. Frequently, however, the doctor's avoidance of a dying patient extends to avoidance of the patient's family after death. As Sudnow (1967:81) points out, "With death, the patient becomes like a discharged patient, in the sense that the contractual basis for the physician's presence and interest is terminated." And yet this is a time when the patient's family may be most in need of comfort on the part of someone who knew the deceased, especially in his final hours. In a study at the National Institutes of Health of parents whose children were terminally ill with malignancies (Friedman: 1963), it was found that frequent reassurance from the physician was helpful to the parents in adjusting to their children's deaths. Sixteen of the eighteen parents who were asked to return to the National Institutes of Health after their children's deaths found the visit to the hospital and medical staff worthwhile. There seems to be value in continuing the relationship between the bereaved and the physician.

Consequences for Physicians, Nurses, Hospitals

Although the physician may try to avoid the family of a dead patient, he cannot avoid thinking about his patient. The physician may question some of his decisions about patient care. This uncertainty stems largely from the dual expectations of his two contrasting roles: member of the social order and member of the scientific community. As a member of the social order the physician responds to the patient's need for comfort, both physical and emotional, and the family's need for reassurance that the patient is getting good medical care and is not suffering unduly. The physician, if he responds only to these needs, indicates his compassion for patient and family; he accepts the unremitting progress of the disease and seeks only to keep the patient comfortable and free of pain. As a member of the scientific community, the physician responds to the ideal of "scientific" medicine requiring vigorous application of laboratory diagnostic tests, technological gadgetry, and heroic therapy in order to prolong life.

This conflict in value systems is greatest for the practitioner who cares for some of his patients in a university hospital, devoted to the development, evaluation, and application of the most advanced medical technology. To fulfill his colleagues' expectations in this situation, the physician may assent to the use of drugs and procedures for his patient which may be of little benefit and may be uncomfortable, painful, and even dangerous. An example of this would be the treatment of a person with widespread cancer of the colon with an anti-tumor drug, 5 fluro-uracil, a drug associated with a 20 per cent chance that the tumor will temporarily regress in well-selected patients. However, the drug is toxic to normal tissues and may cause mouth ulcers, diarrhea, and hair loss in many patients. For selected patients, such as a middle-aged family man with widespread cancer of the colon not affecting the liver, treatment with such a drug may be worthwhile for the slight chance of benefit. In a university hospital where learning, experimentation, and aggressive treatment of diseases is emphasized and highly valued, however, the indications for administering such a drug are often more broadly interpreted. Most patients with widespread colon cancer are considered candidates for 5 fluro-uracil. The physician caring for a patient in this setting may use the drug because of his colleagues' expectations, whereas caring for the same patient in a community hospital he might not use the drug. In the community hospital, with fewer physicians involved with the care of a given patient and less frequent conferences devoted to review of deceased patients, he would not have experienced as much of a role conflict. In the community hospital he would have been more influenced by the needs of the patient and his family.

Nurses and Death

Both university and community hospital staffs, however, see themselves as essentially life-sustaining. Nurses, who are members of the hospital staff and in the most intimate contact with patients during the terminal illness and often at the time of death, find dying patients stressful. The nurse is often the first to learn of the patient's death and she must prepare the family for the news. Because death can be legally established only by a physician, the nurse must maintain the illusion that life remains until the physician arrives and tells the family of the death. In the accompanying shock and grief, the physician comforts the family, may secure permission for an autopsy, and then hurries to other duties, leaving the nurse to help the family with the technical details of hospital discharge and with any questions about the disposition of the body. When the family leaves, the nurse must wrap the body securely, identify it, and arrange for removal to the morgue. Then she must fill out the necessary administrative papers. Her last official duty is to inform the new nursing shift of the death. All of the above duties are unpleasant, if not painful.

Where Patients Die

Hospital staffs, therefore, may look for ways to send their patients elsewhere, that is, to their own homes or to nursing homes, "... as soon as possible after the nothing-more-to-do stage starts. They wish to end his hospital [stay] . . . for several reasons. If possible, they want to spare themselves the ordeal of the last days and hours. They want to release beds for people who can recover—helping patients recover is clearly a preferred challenge" (Glaser and Strauss, 1968:183). One may question this policy. Wennberg (1967), in a study of nursing homes in Baltimore, noted high mortality rates in comparison to the annual expected mortality rate for nursing homes during the two weeks and four weeks following transfer of patients from hospital or home to the nursing homes. This suggests that the transfer of terminally ill patients is a procedure associated with considerable risk of death. Another explanation is that patients are sicker than they seem and deteriorate rapidly in nursing homes in the absence of intensive medical care. It would seem then that the physician should be careful about transferring patients in whom the balance of life is precarious.

Despite the preferences of hospital staffs, most Americans do die in institutions, whereas in the past most Americans died at home. In 1966, 71.8 per cent of deaths in Maryland occurred in institutions (Maryland State Department of Health, 1967). Institutional staffs, reflecting the general culture, try to suppress death. Hinton (1967:159) describes how, in one nursing home,

> . . . an old person about to die was often secluded in a room . . . so that residents should not become upset. [This seclusion] . . . might be successful in preventing some momentary expression of grief, but it could mean a lonely, bitter end for the dying person. It also could contribute to a pervasive atmosphere of forlorn personal unimportance. . . . They [other patients] saw that their own death was likely to be equally undignified and anonymous.

Thomas Mann in *The Magic Mountain* also describes ways of handling the dead so as to suppress thoughts of death at a tuberculosis sanitarium:

> . . . they [deaths] are very discreetly managed, you understand; you hear nothing of them, or only by chance afterwards; everything is kept strictly private when there is a death, out of regard for the other patients, especially the ladies, who might easily get a shock. You don't notice it, even when somebody dies next door. The coffin is brought very early in the morning, while you are asleep and the person in question is fetched away at a suitable time too—for instance, while we are eating.

Although the hospital is thought of as a house of healing, and although it may have preferred that people die elsewhere, it, in the past, has been a house of death. Florence Nightingale (1863, Preface) pointed out that

It may seem a strange principle to enunciate as the very first requirement in a hospital that it should do the sick no harm. It is quite necessary, nevertheless, to lay down such a principle, because the actual mortality *in* hospitals, especially in those of large crowded cities, is very much higher than any calculation founded on the mortality of the same class of diseases among patients treated *out of* hospital would lead us to expect.

Through the study of hospital deaths, however, medicine has learned from its errors and failures and added to its body of knowledge. In the 1840's Semmelweis made an important contribution that resulted in lowering maternal mortality from childbed fever among his obstetrical hospital patients. He observed lower mortality rates among mothers confined in the houses of midwives as opposed to those cared for in the hospital; he postulated " '. . . that the cadaveric material adhering to the hand can produce disease . . .' " (Semmelweis in Sinclair, 1909:50). He concluded that it could be eliminated by use of chlorine disinfectant. After the introduction of the chlorine, maternal mortality from puerperal fever in Semmelweis' clinic went from 11.4 per cent in 1846 to 3 per cent in 1847. Some years later Nightingale (1859:5) showed that mortality rates for nurses in all age groups from infectious disease were many times greater than that for the same age group in the general female population of London. Her observations, beginning with her first book on hospital mortality in 1859, helped to prepare the medical profession for the acceptance of Lister's procedures against infection, developed in 1865.

Value of the Post-Mortem Examination

Even today, a study of hospital mortality can reveal important facts which require attention. Lipworth (1963:71–76) reviewed a sample of discharge data collected from English hospitals in the Hospital Inpatient Inquiry. The study shows differences in the standardized case fatality rates for patients with ischemic heart disease, hernia with obstruction, hyperplasia of the prostate, skull fractures and head injuries, peptic ulcer with operation, and admissions of diabetes with complications. In each category the case fatality rates were lower in teaching hospitals. Even in teaching hospitals, however, there are deaths that may be preventable. Schimmel's study (1964) of the hazards of hospitalization reviews all of the hospital-induced complications on a university medical service during the course of an eight-month period. Schimmel found that of 1,014 patients, 154 died; 16 of these deaths were associated with a diagnostic or therapeutic procedure considered to be a contributory, precipitating, or primary cause of death. Duff and Hollingshead (1968) did a study of a university hospital in which they found significant variations in death rates associated with different hospital accommodations (i.e., private, semiprivate, or ward). The authors imply that the differences in death rates are linked to several factors, including differences in admission policy for each accommodation, differences in patient perception of disease, and differences in patient attitude toward hospitalization.

The study of hospital deaths through autopsy is useful as a means of teaching medical students and young physicians about disease and the problems of diagnosis. Over half the patients who die in university hospitals are autopsied. In community hospitals the percentage of autopsied deaths is less, although the percentage must be above 25 per cent in order for the hospital to maintain its accreditation. Information derived from autopsies is returned to the deceased's physician so that he can correlate his knowledge with his clinical findings. Obtaining authorization for the autopsy can be a difficult experience both for the physician and family. Rarely is instruction given in medical school on how to obtain permission for an autopsy. Frequently members of the family are divided in their feelings about permission for the autopsy; the physician must put aside his feelings, and his sensitivity to the family's feelings, to do what is expected of him—obtain an autopsy—even though he may question its value in the particular case. When one is a house officer, the director of the clinical service soon makes clear that a high rate of autopsies is expected. One noted pathologist kept a bar graph of the deaths which were autopsied from each clinical service. The clear implication was that a low percentage of autopsies indicated a second-rate service.

In 1910, Richard Cabot, at the Massachusetts General Hospital, began informal conferences with the medical house staff and the pathologist-in-chief; autopsy findings were correlated with the medical histories of patients previously treated at the hospital. These conferences marked the beginning of the clinical pathological conference.

In these conferences, a clinician reviews all the possible diagnoses that could account for the clinical history of the patient before the pathologist presents his findings. These conferences have become one of the principle means of continuing education for physicians. In addition, many teaching hospitals hold "death rounds" to discuss each death among members of the staff.

Nevertheless, in spite of this tradition, the value of the autopsy is currently being questioned. "With the contributions of molecular biology to modern medicine and the development of remarkably efficient biochemical and bacteriological laboratories which provide information essential for direct patient care, the autopsy has certainly lost its preeminence as a source of knowledge" (Davidson, 1965:814). In addition, the cost of an autopsy is estimated by Hazard (1965:805) to have increased fivefold in the past thirty years. This is particularly significant because no one pays for the cost of the autopsy! More important is the question of efficient use of the pathologist's time. With the increasing sophistication of medical science, the pathologist's laboratory responsibilities have grown enormously. Each year many more laboratory tests—which help in the diagnosis and therapy of disease—are available to physicians and utilized by them. The autopsy, however, is a lengthy procedure that leaves the pathologist less time for laboratory work. Therefore, today the medical profession must reevaluate the autopsy. The physician should save his efforts, as well as the family's feelings, for those cases where there is reasonable expectation that the autopsy examination will be of significant value.

Areas for Inquiry

In general, the medical profession seems to have little interest in the consequences of death for physicians, other medical personnel, and medical institutions. If we are to examine this problem, we must first know the circumstances under which death occurs. For example, though vast statistics about the causes of death are published routinely, none of them relate to the characteristics of physicians whose patients die in varying circumstances and of different causes. We know virtually nothing about the frequency with which death occurs in the practice of different physicians, particularly in relation to the

Consequences for Physicians, Nurses, Hospitals [187

different medical specialties. We also know little about where death occurs—home or hospital, operating room or emergency room, medical bed or surgical bed. Too, we need to know more about physician referrals of terminally ill patients. What are the consequences of such referrals, physically and emotionally? What are the consequences for the terminally ill of transfer within an institution or to an institution? Also, we have not looked at the different criteria used by physicians for hospitalizing seriously ill patients, nor have we studied the variations among hospitals in their admission policies. It is likely that there are differences and that these differences are associated with variations in the outcome of care for patients with otherwise similar diseases.

Most importantly, we should know the number of preventable deaths that occur. This will require detailed comparative studies by physicians and institutions of deaths among different population groups. Further detailed studies should be done to correlate these observations with knowledge of disease processes. The medical care process itself must be examined to be certain that current practices are not detrimental to the well being of severely ill patients. Deaths among that part of the population who find care with difficulty, who seek care late in the course of disease, and accept care with reluctance, need to be identified for special attention.

We should also learn more about the meaning and consequences of death for the physician. How does medical education with its current preoccupation with the "case" rather than the person affect the medical student's perception of death? What is the relationship between the respect given a physician by his colleagues and that physician's case fatality rates? To what extent does concern for death inhibit the development and learning of new procedures? What effect does the patient's death have upon the physician's relationship with the surviving family? Does it alter, strengthen, or sever the relationship? How do deaths occurring in the physician's practice, particularly if he practices a specialty where death is commonplace, change his way of relating to a dying patient and the patient's family? What effect does the death of a member of the physician's own family have on his relationship with terminally ill patients?

It is hoped that any inquiry into matters relating to death will help the health professions adjust better to death, to realize that all patient deaths are not necessarily medical failures, for, in the words of Ecclesiastes,

> To everything there is a season,
> And a time to every purpose under the heaven.
> A time to be born,
> And a time to die.

REFERENCES

American Medical Association.
- 1968 "Medical education in the United States." Journal of the American Medical Association 206 (November 25).

Aring, Charles D.
- 1968 "Intimations of immortality." Annals of Internal Medicine 69 (July):137–152.

Becker, Howard S. *et al.*
- 1961 Boys in White. Chicago and London: University of Chicago Press.

Bohrod, Milton G.
- 1965 "Uses of the autopsy." Journal of the American Medical Association 193 (September):810–812.

Coggeshall, Lowell T.
- 1965 Planning for Medical Progress Through Education, p. 21. Evanston, Ill.: Association for American Medical Colleges.

Davidson, Charles S.
- 1965 "The autopsy in the age of molecular biology." Journal of the American Medical Association 193 (September):813–814.

Duff, Raymond S., and August B. Hollingshead.
- 1968 Sickness and Society. New York: Harper & Row.

Feifel, Herman.
- 1965 "The function of attitudes toward death." Pp. 632–641 in Death and Dying: Attitudes of Patient and Doctor, Group for the Advancement of Psychiatry, Vol. V, Symposium 11. Publications Office, 419 Park Avenue South, New York.

Fox, Renee C.
- 1957 "Training for uncertainty." Pp. 207–241 in Robert K. Merton, George G. Reader, and Patricia L. Kendall (eds.), The Student-Physician. Cambridge, Mass.: Harvard University Press.

Freud, Sigmund.
- 1918 Reflections on War and Death, A. A. Brill and Alfred B. Kullner (trans.). New York: Moffat, Yard and Company.

Friedman, Stanley B. et al.
 1963 "Behavioral observations on parents anticipating the death of a child." Pediatrics (October) 32:610–625.
Glaser, Barney G., and Anselm L. Strauss.
 1965 Awareness of Dying. Chicago: Aldine.
 1968 Time for Dying. Chicago: Aldine.
Group for the Advancement of Psychiatry.
 1965 "Appendix." Pp. 656–667 in Death and Dying: Attitudes of Patient and Doctor.
Hackett, Thomas P., and Avery D. Weisman.
 1964 "Reactions to the imminence of death." Pp. 300–311 in George H. Grosser, Henry Wechsler, and Milton Greenblatt (eds.), The Threat of Impending Disaster. Cambridge, Mass.: M.I.T. Press.
Hazard, J. Beach.
 1965 "The autopsy." Journal of the American Medical Association 193 (September):805–806.
Hinton, John.
 1967 Dying. Baltimore, Md.: Penguin.
Hubbard, W. N., Jr.
 1968 Unpublished Commencement Address, Albany Medical School, Albany, New York.
Huizinga, J.
 1956 The Waning of the Middle Ages. Garden City, N.Y.: Doubleday.
Kasper, August M.
 1959 "The doctor and death." Pp. 259–270 in Herman Feifel (ed.), The Meaning of Death. New York: McGraw-Hill.
Lerner, Monroe, and Odin W. Anderson.
 1963 Health Progress in the United States, 1900–1960: A Report of the Health Information Foundation. Chicago: University of Chicago Press.
Lipworth, L. et al.
 1963 "Case fatality in teaching and non-teaching hospitals 1956–59." Medical Care 1 (April–June):71–76.
Maryland State Department of Health, Division of Biostatistics.
 1967 Annual Vital Statistics Report: Maryland, 1966.
Moses, L. E., and Frederick Mosteller.
 1968 "Differences in postoperative death rates." Journal of the American Medical Association 203 (February):492–494.
National Center for Health Statistics.
 1967 "International comparison of perinatal and infant mortality." Vital and Health Statistics Analytical Studies 3.
 1968 "Annual summary for the United States, 1966." Monthly Vital Statistics Report: Provisional Statistics 16 (July).

Nightingale, Florence.
   1859   Notes on Hospitals. London: Parker and Son.
   1863   Notes on Hospitals, 3rd ed. London: Longman, Green.
Schimmel, Elihu.
   1964   "The hazards of hospitalization." Annals of Internal Medicine 60 (January):100–110.
Seidel, Henry.
   1969   Personal communication.
Shapiro, Sam, *et al.*
   1968   "Further observations on prematurity and perinatal mortality in a general population and in the population of a prepaid group practice medical care plan." American Journal of Public Health 50 (September):1304–1317.
Sinclair, William J.
   1909   Semmelweis, His Life and His Doctrine. Manchester: University Press.
Sudnow, David.
   1967   Passing On. Englewood Cliffs, N.J.: Prentice-Hall.
The New York Times.
   1968   Issue of July 29:310.
Weisman, Avery D., and Thomas P. Hackett.
   1961   "Predilection to death." Psychosomatic Medicine 23 (Number 3):232–255.
Wennberg, John.
   1967   "Aspects of medical care of welfare patients in certain Baltimore city nursing homes." Mimeographed report.

10

Dying in a Public Hospital

David Sudnow

THE QUESTION in the medical profession over the definition of biological death, Robert Glaser suggests, appears to have been resolved, practically speaking, in favor of the brain, rather than the heart or lungs, as the place where human life makes its last stand. Further, medical authorities have held that, in heart transplantations, the definition must be applied by qualified persons not associated with anyone who has something to gain from seeing the owner of that life dead. Thus, medicine has moved from the traditional to a modern understanding of death and meanwhile reaffirmed the high value that physicians, and Western civilization as a whole, purport to place on human life.

Social Versus Biological Death

The biological definition, while clear-cut and apparently well adapted to safeguarding the integrity of the living human organism, does not take into account another parameter of death. This parameter, presenting quite a different set of issues and implications, deals with what I have chosen to call "social death," a phenomenon incorporating the process of mutual disengagement and rejection by which "organization man,"—more precisely, the human being as a member of society—seems prone to take his leave from the land of the living.

This view of the termination of life concerns itself not with how the biological organism expresses life, or lets go of it finally, but with how the social organization deals with this personal tragedy. A human institution, or social organization, acquires an integrity of its own, of course. It has a collection of purposes and a need to do its work and maintain itself; this need is in part consistent, but not necessarily coincidental, with the purposes and needs of individual members of society. Recognizing this much, we may speculate that the death of an individual is of about the same significance to the social organization as the death of a cell is to a biological organism. It happens all the time. Ordinarily and in small numbers, it is not considered of great moment. Other life goes on, unaffected or affected.

The cell analogy may deeply offend our sense of values, but it is useful in pointing out that death is an inevitable characteristic of life; from a logical standpoint, man is in the process of dying throughout life. We choose to overlook this technicality, and much prefer to procrastinate in accepting its ultimate reality. Thus, the statement, "He is dying," or in hospital jargon, "The patient is terminal," is acceptable for application only under a rather restricted set of circumstances. These circumstances are in essence fairly elementary. There comes a time when the seriously ill patient is not holding his own or getting better, but appears to be declining. In view of the patient's condition and his failure to respond to treatment, the physician gives up hope for recovery. He reaches the judgment that there is nothing further he can do; he may put some time limit, usually a short term, on the patient's survival.

At this point, the patient becomes a candidate for social death, in a prelude to biological death. Social death begins when the institution, accepting impending death, loses its interest or concern for the dying individual as a human being and treats him as a body—that is, as if he were already dead.*

Illustrations of Social Death

The character of this kind of living death may be quickly illustrated in a series of anecdotes. In a county hospital where I had the opportunity to study how a social organization copes with death, a nurse was observed spending two or three minutes trying to close the eyelids of

---

* This chapter is based on the author's study in two general hospitals, one public and the other private, as published in *Passing On: The Social Organization of Dying* (Englewood Cliffs, N.J.: Prentice-Hall, Inc., 1967).

a woman patient. The nurse explained that the woman was dying. She was trying to get the lids to remain in a closed position. After several unsuccessful attempts, the nurse got them shut and said, with a sigh of accomplishment, "Now they're right." When questioned about what she was doing, she said that a patient's eyes must be closed after death, so that the body will resemble a sleeping person. It was more difficult to accomplish this, she explained, after the muscles and skin had begun to stiffen. She always tried, she said, to close them *before* death. This made for greater efficiency when it came time for ward personnel to wrap the body. It was a matter of consideration toward those workers who preferred to handle dead bodies as little as possible.

Social death does not always lead to biological death, at least not in a consecutive manner. Such an instance involved a male patient who was admitted to the Emergency Unit with a sudden perforation of a duodenal ulcer. He was operated on, and for a period of six days remained in quite critical condition. His wife was informed that his chances of survival were poor, whereupon she stopped her visits to the hospital. After two weeks, the man's condition improved markedly and he was able to walk out of the hospital and go home. The next day he was readmitted with a severe heart attack. Before he died of coronary disease, he recounted his experience upon returning home. His wife had removed all of his clothing and personal effects from the house, had contemplated arrangements for his burial (on his bureau, the patient discovered an unsent letter requesting a brochure and rates of an undertaker). She no longer wore his wedding ring, and he found her with another man. The discarded husband left the house, began to drink heavily, and had a heart attack, thus placing his death in the category of a self-fulfilling prophecy, counting an assist from his spouse.

The finality that characterizes biological death is lacking in social death; more like disease, it occurs in stages—mild, moderate, severe. A mild form is imposed when the institution, for what it considers good and sufficient reasons, feels compelled to "program" a patient's death. This in effect is the case where autopsy permits are filled out prior to death. Permission of the closest surviving relative must be obtained, either by signature or telegram. Maintenance of a substantial autopsy rate is important to the hospital in maintaining its accreditation and recognition as a teaching institution. Doctors in the above-mentioned county hospital sought autopsy permits for living patients only in cases where the disease was particularly interesting or diagnostically troublesome and then only if the relative had been made well aware that the patient was expected to die shortly.

A common example of the occurrence of social before actual death in this county hospital involved the assignment of patients to beds. A patient admitted to the hospital at death's door—with extremely low blood pressure, erratic heartbeats, and a nonpalpable or weak pulse—was frequently left on the litter on which he was admitted and wheeled into a laboratory or large supply room. In such cases, a nurse explained, they did not want to use a bed and have to clean the room afterward. Since the patient would soon die, there was no need to assign him to a room. In several cases, patients were left throughout the night and died in the supply room. Those who were still alive in the morning, nurses quickly assigned to beds, before the arrival of physicians or relatives. In effect, a patient admitted in critical condition might be treated as a corpse by night and a patient by day.

When a physician abandons hope for a patient's survival, the nurses establish what they refer to as a "death watch," a fairly severe form of social death in which they keep track of relevant facts concerning the gradual recession of clinical life signs. As death approaches, the patient's status as a body becomes more evident from the manner in which he is discussed, treated, and moved about. Attention shifts from concern about his life, possible discomforts, and the administration of medically prescribed treatments to the mere activity of timing the events of biological leave-taking.

In a patient who has not yet passed into a death coma, suctioning the nasal passages, propping up pillows, changing bed sheets, and the like occur as part of the normal nursing routine. As blood pressure drops and signs of imminent death appear, these traditional nursing practices are regarded as less important; the major items of interest become the number of heartbeats and the changing condition of the eyes. On many occasions, nurses' aides in the county hospital were observed to cease administering standing-order oral medications when death was expected within the hour.

Dying in a Public Hospital [195

While there is a deep-seated feeling in our culture that a fellow man should not die unattended, the posting of a patient as being in critical condition—often meaning not expected to live—starts a mechanism of rejection arising out of procedures designed to operate for the good of the institution. While "posted patients" technically have the right to round-the-clock visitors, nurses in the charitable institution I studied strove to separate relatives from those patients about to die and whose treatment was in the phasing-out stage. They urged family members to go home and await further news there, or insisted that they wait outside in the corridors and not in the patient's room. At least part of their concern in imposing such restrictions was to expedite the handling of death within the context of other ward responsibilities. If a relative was present, then it was also necessary for someone from the staff to be present to demonstrate continuing concern. Practically speaking, to single out one of many patients for special attention created a hardship in the operation of the organization; the act was inefficient as well as futile.

At this institution physicians, too, preferred that relatives be kept away from the bedside of the dying patient, so that his doctor would be free to leave and attend to other matters. As the doctor saw it, the fact that the patient was dying did not merit his continued presence. The *raison d'être* for much of medical and surgical activity, other than research and training, is the possibility that intervention may restore health or save life. When the physician reached the point where he felt he could do nothing further to preserve life, then he symbolically signed the patient's social death warrant.

For the most part, the physician regarded the end for a dying patient unemotionally—he could hardly survive in his profession if he did not. Thus, if he had written a patient off, he felt no special discomfort if no one was on hand when death actually took place. The absence of relatives on the ward, and especially at the bedside, allowed him to wait until a more reasonable time for him to come to the ward to pronounce the patient dead and then inform the relatives of the death. In many instances, the patient was discovered dead in the middle of the night but the doctor was not informed until morning. Physicians often expressed anger at nurses who awakened them at night to tell them that a patient had died. Where such an operational pattern prevails, therefore, the physician routinely excuses himself from this final confrontation with his traditionally celebrated adversary, Death.

Death in a Coma

Most patients in this county hospital died unattended. For the most part, we may assume, they were unaware that they faced death alone. Hospital deaths are commonly preceded by a period of what is generally regarded as a coma. Of some two hundred deaths that I observed, I saw none of the Hollywood type, where the person's last sentence is interrupted by his final breath. Death in a large institution is not particularly dramatic, and every effort is made to keep it from becoming so.

The rationalization of social death, or the treatment of a still-living patient as if he were dead, is that the patient is comatose. At this hospital, the state of "being in a coma" was considered equivalent to being under a general anesthetic—that is, totally unconscious. The patient's condition and prospects were freely discussed in his presence. He was considered comatose when he did not respond to verbal or physical stimuli. The possibility that nonresponsiveness might mean an inability to respond rather than a general incapacity to hear what was said and understand what was taking place was not seriously entertained. Nevertheless, there were examples in which patients supposedly in a coma reported something of what was said or done in their presence.

The discovery of death—always an event of some social consequence—typically occurred in the course of ongoing ward activity of all kinds. The trained nurse's basic concern, with the exception of a few nurses of the alienated type, was to detect death as soon as possible after it occurred, so as to institute preparations to remove the body from the ward as soon as possible and to see that aides and orderlies did not neglect their responsibilities. In going about her work, the nurse periodically checked on the "dying patient." This check involved a long stare from the door to see if the patient was breathing.

To assume that a patient who has died is still alive leads to embarrassment. It is an emotionally disastrous experience, for example, for a young student nurse unwittingly to minister to a dead person; on

Dying in a Public Hospital [197

several occasions, this happened. In one case a student nurse was attending a man who had been severely burned and was almost totally wrapped in gauze, except for his eyes and small openings for nose and mouth. She spent several minutes trying to get him to drink some juice through a straw; having no success, she called on her instructor for help. "Well, honey, of course he won't respond, he's been dead for twenty minutes," the instructor said. The student explained that all she could see were his eyes and they had always been closed. Another student gave a patient an injection without noticing he was dead. Such occasions are not usually considered funny. Told that the patient was dead, this student cried nervously and trembled for several minutes; she was given a half-hour off to recover her composure.

Absence of a relative at the discovery of death, much desired in this institution, lent itself to the night nurse's common inclination to wait until quitting time to call the doctor in charge to inform him of deaths during the night. This in turn was a favor to her aides, because disposition of the body now passed on to the day shift. It would surprise the uninitiated how many patients died at or not long before 6:30 A.M., when the shifts changed. This forward displacement of death could not be carried too far without arousing suspicion, however, since it was obvious that all nighttime deaths would not occur within the same hour. The possibility that there would be several bodies to wrap, record, and remove was considered one of the disadvantages of being on the day shift.

Aides did not share the trained nurse's interest, borne of professional responsibility, in promptly detecting the presence of death (irrespective of when it was reported to the doctor). Aides typically made every effort to avoid discovering a patient was dead, partly because as soon as they informed the nurse it meant work for them. But aversion to the sight of death also was a factor. During the first several weeks that he was employed, one orderly refused to wander in and out of rooms, as an orderly must. He feared that he would not be able to control himself should he come upon a dead person.

The ritual of wrapping the body, mainly handled by Negro aides, and the further processing of a death are onerous chores which the personnel on the ward, if they could not escape them, preferred to undertake in easy stages. This required full recourse to all available knowledge of the impending time of death. One nurse on the male medical ward prided herself in her ability to predict what patients, if any, would die within the day. I made a short-term check, by asking for her predictions each morning and checking them against actual deaths; she was about 75 per cent accurate and in several cases predicted deaths of patients whom the doctors did not expect to die so soon. Aides, availing themselves of her forecasts, occasionally went into the room of such a patient, changed the bedsheets, inserted dentures, and in several cases of which I knew, put the post-mortem diaper on the still-living patient and also, as is routine, tied their feet together. Such initiative occurred mostly on the night shift when there was no danger of relatives coming on the scene.

Various other practices were devised to avoid workaday confrontations with death and its sequelae. A common one was the transfer of a patient from one ward to another. For example, the Emergency Ward might transfer a patient whose death was expected shortly to the Medical or Surgical Ward, on the ground that he was terminally ill and not properly a person for emergency care. One evening, a patient in quite critical condition was transferred from the Emergency Ward to the men's Medical Ward. The head nurse there refused to accept the obviously dying patient, and angrily complained that the Emergency Ward clerk sent him over to die on her property. She instructed the orderly to return the patient to the Emergency Ward with the message, "You tell Mrs. Smith to wrap her own bodies."

Death as a Self-Fulfilling Prophecy

Beyond the notion of a person being pre-wrapped for death lay the possibility that dying, under the circumstances described, took on the character of a self-fulfilling prophecy. The question is the relevance of a prognostication of death to the desirability of instituting or not instituting treatments to forestall death. Treatment without hope of cure or improvement falls under the general heading of palliative care, sometimes referred to as terminal care. This can be distinguished from euthanasia, typically conceived to be the purposeful termination of life through active intervention so as to shorten a painful period of dying. I saw no evidence of euthanasia, as such, in this county hospital. But palliative care, negatively defined by

Dying in a Public Hospital

admitted suspension of curative medical treatments and positively determined by admitted concern for treating pain only, was a commonplace. The progression from curative to palliative care was one of the practical consequences of regarding a patient as terminally ill. Insofar as the suspension of curative treatment, or care designed to prolong life, might have the effect of shortening life, then the declaration, "He is dying," could conceivably promote this result and thus to some extent operate as a self-fulfilling prophecy.

It is necessary at this point to file a disclaimer. The observations that I have made deal with one hospital of a particular type and in no respect can be interpreted as a generalization about all hospitals. As a matter of fact, my investigation, for purposes of comparison, of a voluntary general hospital, where private patients were cared for by private physicians, revealed an altogether different sense of responsibility and accountability. In this hospital, care of the critically ill patient was far more intensive, there was active resistance to the categorization of a patient as dying, and no organized effort to exclude relatives as witnesses of terminal illness. Whereas in the county hospital there was little time or occasion for interaction or interpersonal relationship between the patient's physician and the family, in the private hospital physicians were observed to show much consideration for relatives. It became apparent that this disparity of attitudes was conditioned by professional judgments about the social worth of the patient when it was recalled that persons of an upper-middle-class background brought to the county hospital for emergency care received more consideration and care than those of lower station. Indeed, in regard to the patient's condition on arrival at the hospital, it could be remarked that determinations of "dying" and being "dead" were partially a function of social class, and not simply in the usual sense of the wealthy getting better care. If one anticipates having a critical heart attack, it is best that he keep himself well-dressed and his breath clean if there is any likelihood of his being brought into the County Emergency Unit as a possible "Dead on Arrival." For the old, the poor, and the alcoholic bum, the inattention is such that the possibility could become an actuality without intervention.

I have used the term "social death" as a descriptive convenience, to vivify the ways in which an institution dealing with death may redefine the facts of death in terms of its own needs rather than those of the individual. Otherwise, I hold no brief for the entity and, of course, do not postulate a dichotomy between biological and social death, or propose that there is any real distinction between physical and social facts.

Impact of Organization on Dying

I should now like briefly to portray some organizational features of the particular hospital I studied, and show that some of the ways that the institution looked at death were conditioned by the ways that members of the institution looked at each other, rather than arising wholly from the way they regarded the human being known as the patient.

This 440-bed county hospital was of the short-term, general type devoted to care of acute illness; it was operated by the county mainly to meet the needs of the indigent. Its patients were, for the most part, in the active stage of a serious illness. Their average stay was six days, but the bulk of them came and went, dead or alive, in forty-eight hours. Only a few remained as ambulatory patients. Many were sent home. Those with chronic illnesses were referred to another facility. The physicians and nurses took it for granted that a routine question in their daily work with patients would be, "Will he make it?"

Although not affiliated with a medical school, the hospital was staffed—almost exclusively—by interns and residents taking part in an approved graduate training program. Supervision of the "educational program" was provided by private physicians from the community who served on a voluntary basis, in one-month tours of duty. Their influence and presence were more nominal and official than real. For all practical purposes, medical care was managed by the house staff, organized in the traditional hierarchy from chief resident down to junior intern. Quite seriously, the house doctors taught each other the practice of medicine with little help from more experienced practicing physicians.

The more prominent features of the organizational structure may be summarized as follows:

Dying in a Public Hospital

1. The hospital had no private patients, all being attended, whatever their source of referral, by the house staff during their stay. The hospital had an Emergency Unit which served the area in the care of accident victims and others with acute illnesses. Occasionally, a middle-class patient was admitted.

2. The system of patient management was traditional; the intern or resident was assigned to wards—medical, surgical, psychiatric, and so on—and rotated from one to another during his appointment. The assigned doctor took responsibility for all patients on a ward during the hours he was in charge. The Medical Wards had the highest death rate. Cases of diabetes, cancer, heart disease, kidney disease, liver disease, and the like were treated by all house doctors without regard to specialization.

3. Despite the lack of regular instruction, this was a so-called "teaching hospital" and the interns and residents so regarded it. These young doctors looked on the care of patients as the basis for a learning experience.

4. The patient population of the hospital was lower class. A large number of the patients were Negro. Much of the illness was related to alcoholism or the result of violence.

5. The hospital maintained a large nursing school. Nearly half of the nursing staff were students.

The effect of the teaching orientation upon decisions affecting terminal care are of particular interest. The method of case assignment, by wards, gave interns and residents not only a broad range of responsibility but also of freedom in the way they allocated their time and attention to patients in their care. This freedom was increased by the fact that these physicians had only minimal relations with members of the patients' families. This fact was the direct consequence of the rapid turnover, coupled with the rotation of three daily shifts of physicians through each ward. There was hardly time for formation of a doctor-patient relationship. The nature of the organization did not require assumption of any extended responsibility to particular patients and their families, as would normally be found in a private hospital, or daily accountability to a chief of service, as would be typically found in a medical school-affiliated hospital, where the house doctor works in regular consultation with a professor who is an established specialist in his field.

Focus on "Interesting Cases"

From the house doctor's standpoint, the locus of his involvement was "learning the ward" and what the cases present might teach him. While physicians in this hospital maintained an official adherence to the code that full attention must be devoted to the curative treatment of each patient, organizational pressures related to the teaching orientation operated to require an allocation of attention not strictly in line with this philosophy. In fact, the house officer's natural bent and unofficial guidelines coincided in the concentration of energies on the "more interesting cases." This selective interest was reinforced by the fact that the younger physicians, particularly the interns, were under continual strain to do good diagnostic discovery work. The discipline in this respect was of good quality.

As part of the periodic reviewing procedures, interns were under systematic surveillance of their ability to work up a case. Competition among junior staff members to achieve recognition for their medical diagnostic skills was often intense. Special consideration was available to those who achieved distinction. Rewards included assignment to relatively easy services and good shifts, access to more challenging cases, greater independence in decision-making, and good letters of recommendation for those seeking residencies elsewhere.

Not only for the interns but also for house staff at all levels, concentration on the unusual, perplexing, and diagnostically elusive situation was regarded as justifiable on pedagogic grounds, particularly for those who planned to specialize. The wide variety of case material provided a rich opportunity for a selective experience.

This emphasis on learning rather than service was of some consequence to patients known to have fatal illnesses and expected to die within their current admission to the hospital. The intern or resident on duty tended to write these patients off in the most routine manner, and, having done so, to lose interest in them. As indicated earlier, the care attitude changed from curative to palliative, with some exceptions to be described below. Subsequent care was modified partly by

Dying in a Public Hospital

the doctor's interest in the case, but also, it should be recognized, by the demands of other patients on his time.

In suggesting that institutional and professional considerations may affect the course of a fatal illness, I am not arguing that the judgment of a case as uninteresting necessarily led to improper care. Although in my judgment instances of this phenomenon—the operation of a self-fulfilling prophecy—were indeed common, I am not prepared to assert such a strong relationship as a general one. The often legitimate rebuttal of the staff physician would be that, no matter what care a patient defined as terminally ill had received, the patient would have died within a short period of time. This is the standard view of physicians in their exercise of discretion in such matters.

Whatever the relationship between principles of decision-making and their consequences, I simply wish to observe that in this hospital setting interest and time spent in the diagnosis and treatment of a case were influenced by the prediction of outcome. It is to be expected that, in this county hospital setting or in a private, upper-class institution, one can discover principles which guide decisions as to how and how much a fatally ill person is to be treated. Whatever the principles, they always will be formulated in medical circles as in the best interests of the patient.

Let me trace some of the ways in which interest in diagnostic experience operated; the relationship is by no means straightforward. One difficult problem involved a seriously ill patient, one expected to die shortly, who nevertheless presented "interesting symptoms" which challenged the young physician's knowledge and skills in differential diagnosis. But it was dangerous for him to deal with such a patient in a diagnostically enthusiastic way; if death should follow extensive attention to the case on his part, the competence of the physician to make a correct diagnosis might be subject to review. To avoid this danger, it was necessary for this physician, in view of his vulnerability, to obtain consensual validation that the patient would die. With such confirmation of his assessment, it was then safe for him to take a close interest in a case otherwise deemed, by common consent, hopeless. In general, it followed, it was in the attending physician's interest if his colleagues considered his patient's condition worse than it actually might be. If improvement occurred, his prestige rose; if it did not, collective opinion relieved him of personal responsibility for the negative turn in events.

A Medical Tightrope

On the other hand, there were counter-pressures against overly pessimistic prognoses, both in the form of administrative adherence to the doctrine that physicians do all they can to the very end and a concern that others might see pessimism as a rationalization for neglect when, in fact, the patient's outlook was simply not clear. This latter constraint operates to the extent that members of the family are heavily involved in the case, are articulate in their worries, and are vigilant in surveillance of the patient's care.

At best, the physician facing possible loss of a patient treads a thin line between an optimism that may prove unfounded and a pessimism that may be premature in relation to the actual time of death. The time of the physician's assessment that the patient has entered a terminal stage is best delayed with the family as an audience but is of less importance with only one's colleagues looking on.

Where there was uncertainty as to whether the patient would make it or not, it was of special importance to share this doubt with other physicians and nurses on the ward. In this way, the cost of failure to the young doctor could be lessened. In most cases of expected death, however, there was no basis for doubt. At this county hospital, most deaths involved patients who were deeply unconscious from the time of admission. The pronouncement, "dying," was perfectly straightforward in such instances, and validated the attending physician's allocation of attention to others who either had a chance of improving or who, while nonetheless fatally ill, offered an opportunity for a learning experience that, in its pursuit, would not reflect on the judgment of the physician.

We now come to cases in which there was neither hope for recovery nor loss of professional interest. Often, dying patients were subjected to treatments that had, as their essential aim, not the improvement of the patient's condition, but satisfaction of professional curiosity. Relatively radical procedures were undertaken as experiments or to gain experience. These included massive doses of antibiotics in excess of prescribed limits, massive surgical maneuvers, and the use of potent drugs in even more potent combinations. These were described as "last resort measures," but the fact that the patient was "terminal" was frankly regarded as providing the opportunity for scientific or educational experience.

The question of excusability in such instances is a delicate one. In each justification of procedures not calculated to benefit the patient on the basis, "He is going to die anyhow," it was strongly argued that there was no possibility of preventing death. My point in describing such practices is not to sit in judgment but simply to suggest that this is still another interest, in addition to diagnostic acumen, effective treatment, and staff accountability, that must be considered in an analysis of context for a prediction of death. Any more direct relationship between an action, such as semi-experimental surgery, and the outcome of the prediction that warrants the statement, "He is dying," is a subject for more careful investigation. Whatever direct relationship might be discovered, I have observed numerous cases where a negative prognosis was accepted as warranting procedures, particularly surgical, that were not expected to forestall death. Rather, they were termed important occasions for gaining experience in techniques that could not be attempted on healthier patients with similar problems.

One factor that influenced decisions made under some of the constraints discussed above was alcoholism, a common diagnosis in this hospital. A typical case was that of a middle-aged man who had been admitted to the hospital many times over a period of several years. Commonly, when admitted, he was in shock from loss of blood due to ulceration of the colon. He had undergone surgical repair of his ulcers several times, only to show up again a few months later with renewed bleeding. As compared to the symptomatology of, say, leukemia, stroke, heart disease, or diabetes, massive internal hemorrhage from ulcers induced or aggravated by alcohol offered little to interest an intern. Such a case might offer a surgeon a basis for dramatic repair work, but it did not require extensive laboratory testing and interpretation and simply did not challenge the imagination of a man in internal medicine.

To label a case of this sort (duplicated many times in my field notes) "terminal" is a relatively safe exercise of discretion. Assuming a relatively severe state of shock, sufficient indications of the extensiveness of the internal bleeding, and given the well-known social history of the patient, the doctors of this county hospital easily settled on a prediction of death when a critical juncture appeared. The consequences of such a decision were as follows: The patient was given blood transfusions, further surgical repair was not recommended, and a vigil over his vital signs was maintained. When the patient's strength deteriorated, administration of blood was terminated. The patient continued downhill to death.

The procedure was essentially routine with numerous patients who were familiar figures and had a history of repeated bouts with the same problem. Indeed, a large percentage of this hospital's seriously ill patients were admitted and discharged several times prior to their "fatal admission." In such cases the concern for consensual validation and ease in obtaining it were not unrelated to staff opinion of the moral character of patients. Not only were gravely ill alcoholic patients more readily assessed as terminal, but so were other classes of patients whose character and social background were regarded as less than desirable. Victims of violence from lower-class settings, prostitutes, suicidal cases, vagrants, narcotic addicts, and the like, when encountered in grave borderline illnesses, were normally accorded a more rapidly fatal fate. These patients were not only diagnostically less interesting but, from the viewpoint of the staff, less deserving.

A Question of Organizational Values

To bring these remarks into better focus, I should like to elaborate the contrast between the general organizational structure and practical experience orientation at this county hospital and some features observed at the middle-class hospital staffed by private physicians, mentioned earlier. Physicians in the private hospital were especially sensitive to the interpretation that might be made should they characterize the patient's condition as "terminal." They did not wish to be thought of as "giving up." The audience for the prediction of death, in contrast to that in the county hospital, was largely made up of members of the patient's family. To give up would mean endangering the doctor-patient relationship as it extended into the family.

The county hospital, on the other hand, was comparatively free from outside scrutiny; accountability was also entirely internal. Where the sensitivity of the charity hospital doctor to the question of

Dying in a Public Hospital [207

writing off a patient as "dying" was weak, I had to search much harder in the middle-class hospital to find patients whose condition would be acknowledged as terminal. Such judgments were carefully guarded and not matters of common ward knowledge.

These remarks suggest the importance of determining how the character of the organization may influence judgment on fatality. In this brief presentation, I have been able only to give a rough sketch of some of the components of these judgments, but it is hoped that a sense of organizational as differentiated from individual values has been conveyed. We could perfectly well imagine a hospital or society where notice was not taken of the fact that a person was dying, but our imagination would be naive. It would fail to note a whole set of interests—organization, career, family, work, nation, and so on—that operate to make the fact and rate of approaching death a matter of considerable importance to all involved.

For a physician the occurrence of death is a crucial matter. His timing of predictions must therefore be sensitive to the inferences available to those who bear witness to his successes and failures. We have observed that in one hospital the prediction of death was a signal for a sharpened sense of medical responsibility, whereas in another it could be taken as cause for virtual abandonment of the patient as an object for scientific and humane attention. The viewpoint in each instance was imposed by the organization's pattern of interests, by lines of responsibility or accountability, and by a social value system.

The social is in practice inseparable from the biological phenomenon of dying. Any discussion of terminal illness that treats "dying" as if one were dealing with a "disease" would, in my estimation, miss the essential character of the process as a socially situated, practically controlled, completely organizational concept.

Organizations Shape Morality

To suggest some broader implications of this organizational perspective, we may ask: What are the orders of consequences that may arise from such morally, as well as scientifically, significant issues as euthanasia, organ transplants, and related matters?

A first, general suggestion is that moral issues must be evaluated in terms of concrete consequences for, and effects upon, organized medical care. To state the matter bluntly, a danger exists in oversimplified formulations of the need for euthanasia, or in oversimplified justifications for the termination of one irreversibly deteriorating life for the sake of one that can possibly be improved.

The implementation of any particular moral attitude in medical care, no matter how justifiable theoretically, is always subject to the operation of an organization. The attitude will have to become part of a process, and this process includes the organization of the work load, selective allocation of work time, evaluations of moral character and social worth, sanctioned judgments on the value of a case for learning purposes, and probably more. To the extent that we might expect a new morality on "death care" to be applied on some large scale in the future, we inevitably would have to plan its application against a background of everyday work considerations.

Although no warrant currently exists for doubting the competence of medical personnel as prognosticators, and no strong basis exists for raising the possibility of error in such judgments as organ transplants involve, bureaucratically organized work routine will constitute the environment where any new practices are carried out. Currently, heart transplants are being made under closely controlled conditions, in facilities set apart from ordinary hospital ward management. We may, however, anticipate the day when such procedures, plus others, will become part of the daily treatment activities in our hospitals.

When that time comes, the decision-making processes concerning terminable life, likely death, and certain death as occasions for intervention will become progressively institutionalized and routinized within the daily hospital structure. The structure, it must be recognized, can affect the decision-making, as the decision-making can affect the structure. The analysis of the impact of the organizational milieu upon decision-making is perhaps one of social science's longest-standing interests.

The definition of the status or category known as "dying," it is my suggestion, is as much subject to analysis as the conceptual products of any organized decision-making activity. Unfortunately, the decision-making activities of medical practitioners have been only peripherally investigated. Decisions about matters of life and death would seem to be an especially important place to systematize such study.

PART THREE

Termination of Life—Social, Ethical, Legal, and Economic Questions

11

Dying as an Emerging Social Problem

Sol Levine and Norman A. Scotch

IT MAY APPEAR paradoxical to concern ourselves with death and dying in a society as advanced as our own, in which the value placed on human life is high and where the possibilities for warding off death are relatively good. Clearly, the United States and other highly developed societies have made major strides in decreasing various forms of morbidity and mortality.

Our secular society in recent years has emphasized death and dying only as something to be avoided. John Spiegel (1964:297) has explained this aversion to contemplation of death as a product of an American tendency to view death as a technical failure:

> In American culture the dying role is severely attenuated. The prospect of death does not fit well with the dominant values. Since there is little or no real belief in an afterlife, death represents the end of the line, the end of the story. In a culture that puts so much stress on the future, the prospect of not having any future at all becomes too dismal to face. That the dying role should turn out to be a transition to nothing, to extinction, robs it of some of its transitional properties. To make matters worse, the process of dying cannot even be treated as a tragedy since our Doing and Mastery-over-Nature values make it seem more like a technical failure. Tragedy, in our society, is something that should have been avoided rather than something to be appreciated. The implication is that someone slipped up or that research simply has not yet got around to solving this kind of thing. Thus dying is covered over with optimistic or reassuring statements and the dying person is scarcely given the opportunity to make the most of his position.

Why, it may be asked, have death and dying recently emerged as matters of concern if most secular societies prefer to repress rather than to examine these phenomena? It may seem that as a successful society we can engage in the luxury of focusing on dying—a luxury not enjoyed by the less developed societies where infectious diseases and hunger are rampant, where infant mortality is high, and where the life span is distressingly short.

It may also be argued that this recent interest is in part attributable to the inherently dramatic value of organ transplants and other heroic medical measures as exploited by the mass media. In addition, a relatively sophisticated public is focusing upon the medical profession and calling into question a range of ancient concerns: Whether and what the dying patient should be told? How long need he be kept alive? How should his psychological needs and those of his family be cared for? This sophistication dissipates the magical aura of the physician and makes the medical management of dying more difficult. Public scrutiny of the behavior of professionals has grown and the demand that they be accountable to the public is increasing in matters of dying as well as living.

The concern with dying is different from a concern about death. The process of dying and the eventual actual occurrence of death are so intertwined in our thinking that it is easy to blur them in our analysis and to treat them as a single phenomenon. In fact, however, death and dying differ significantly in the problems they pose for the patient, the family, the health professionals, and society. A true understanding of the problems requires that we unravel death and dying and attempt to ascertain their differential social impact.

While death remains a perennially tragic feature of man's fate, society has managed to develop relatively effective mechanisms to mitigate the disruptive aspects of death's impact. Certain features of man's contemporary plight may be dramatically mirrored and intensified in the death experience, but, in general, it appears that today death probably poses less of a problem for Western society than it has in the recent past.

The impetus behind the concern pervading this volume springs instead from the profound changes occurring in the character and duration of the dying experience. These changes are essentially at-

Dying as an Emerging Social Problem [213

tributable to the application of an impressive medical technology in the management of the dying patient. Although there is a burgeoning public concern about the dying patient, it is first and foremost a problem for medicine and health professionals. For, as we have suggested, it is not death per se but the question of how and to what extent the life of the dying patient should be prolonged that confronts medicine. The patient, once dead, quickly and abruptly moves outside the domain of medicine. It is precisely because the new medical technology has provided more options and alternatives and, at the same time, more conflicts and dilemmas for the physician in the management of the dying patient, that *dying* now as never before approaches the dimensions of a medical social problem. In managing the dying patient the physician, of course, is never a completely free and autonomous agent; he is subject to a system of social controls in which other actors and institutions set limits and play a part. Nevertheless, the task of managing the dying patient is primarily a doctor's dilemma.

Questions of Public Policy

The application of elaborate technology to extend the life of the dying patient also raises questions of fundamental social and public policy. As rising social expectations have kept pace with and indeed have outstripped the development, exploitation, and distribution of our national resources, it has become necessary to examine alternative measures in terms of their respective costs and benefits. The cost-benefit orientation given emphasis by the Department of Defense has been invoked in a wide number of social policy deliberations ranging from decisions involving foreign aid to the designing of domestic social welfare programs. In short, we have been compelled to pay attention to alternative ways of allocating resources. It is not surprising, then, that this orientation is beginning to manifest itself in the health field. What proportion of health resources should be deployed for kidney machines, or for heart transplants, and inevitably what magnitude of resources should be employed to keep the dying patient alive? Painful and repugnant as it may be, those who deploy resources in the health field must decide how much they wish to allocate for the prolongation of life as opposed to other types of investments in health. Research on chronic disease, expansion of existing health services, and the provision of health benefits to the poor all compete for resources with efforts to prolong the life of the dying patient.

While it may be contended that the dying patient is a relatively minor concern when compared with the more pressing problems of our time, we must appreciate that the problem may still be in its infancy. What may be an incipient problem largely confined to the medical profession and causing relatively mild stress to the social system may well assume much greater and serious proportions in the not too distant future. We live in an age in which technological innovations are rapidly occurring and unless we soon forge definite and effective policy guidelines with which to approach the dying patient, we will be ill prepared to meet the more massive accumulative problems that the technology will create tomorrow. The speed with which seemingly inconsequential irritants of concern to only a few soon grow into problems of primary import may be seen when we consider, for example, the rapid emergence of air pollution, population growth, and social congestion as salient concerns of our society.

We have suggested that the question of the dying patient is of serious concern to the medical profession, that it raises basic questions of how scarce resources are to be allocated, and that it is likely to mushroom in importance and increasingly command the attention of policy makers. Most of all, perhaps, we should not overlook the fundamental human dimensions of the problem—the anguish, the suffering, and the frustration of dying patients and their kin. Though their numbers are legion they are dispersed throughout the land. They are not an organized or visible public. Their agony is experienced quietly and privately. Society, in its wisdom, has developed efficient ways to shield itself from the daily tragedies of the dying so that it can go on with its tasks, unperturbed and uninterrupted. Hence, society is not confronted with the collective anguish or the outcry of the dying and their loved ones. As we gain systematic knowledge about the problems of the dying patient and as this knowledge begins to enter the public domain, however, the values of our society require that, to the extent possible, we formulate a more appropriate policy to abate the suffering and to meet the human needs of the actors in the drama.

Management of Death

Before we examine more intensively the problems of the dying patient and the strains they place upon different groups and institutions in our society, let us first consider briefly the problem of death itself. As we indicated earlier, in the present context death and dying are problems of a different order with respect to the strains they place upon other parts of the social system. A brief consideration of death will serve as a useful point of departure and a basis of comparison with the central subject under consideration—the prolongation of the dying patient's life.

Society, in fact, has developed effective means of managing death and of minimizing the impact of death on society. Hospitals have developed expeditious methods of classifying and routing dead patients; funeral parlors and morticians quickly and efficiently process and dispose of the dead body; funeral arrangements are formalized, conveniently sparing the family and friends of responsibilities and participation in the care for the dead. Even the mourning period is generally well handled by the society at large, allowing specific cultural groups to retain whatever psychological devices they have for handling the tragedy and bereavement accompanying death. Also, the long-term consequences of death have been attenuated. Life insurance has grown at a tremendous rate, and, together with the institutionalization of a social security system, tends to avert the traumatic and tragic disruption of the family historically associated with the death of a breadwinner.

Yet, the bureaucratization of death has negative consequences. It is often accompanied by despair, helplessness, and bewilderment, and reflects the alienation found in other areas of mass bureaucratized society. In many cases, as soon as death occurs in the hospital, the body is whisked away from the bereaved family often vainly attempting a final look at the departed. Crying relatives at the patient's empty bed, some having come without knowledge of his death, confirm their numbed realization that death has indeed taken place, and provide a tragic scene all too common to those familiar with hospital settings.

The routinization of events is evident as the body acquires an itinerary of its own and the family must muster its resources to keep pace with the events that are unfolding before it. Various hurdles must be surmounted. One is the first viewing of the body after it has been prepared by the mortician.

The grieving family is often compelled to make decisions quickly: Should the casket be opened? Where should the services and burial be performed? How should friends or relatives be contacted and assembled? Which clergyman should perform the ceremony? With each decision relatives strive to act in a manner consistent with the imagined wishes of the departed.

Although funeral parlors have demonstrated considerable ingenuity and success in maintaining dignified atmospheres, the volume of their enterprise and the bureaucratic need to process funerals quickly and expeditiously tend to violate the privacy and dignity that the survivors feel appropriate to the event. Some people may find themselves in the wrong section of the funeral parlor looking at the wrong casket. Others are unable to experience the unique quality of the occasion as they become aware of a similar ceremony next door. Furthermore, the clergyman who delivers the sermon often has had little contact with the deceased; he hurriedly acquires a few facts for his sermon and is compelled to speak on a platitudinal level. Bureaucratization prevents the family from immersing itself in and fully yielding itself to its grief. The mourners must adhere to the time scheduling requirements of the funeral parlor. Even the ride to the cemetery affords no relief:

> There is a newer road which now leads from the pleasant resorts of Eastern Long Island into the city; a highway eight lanes wide over which one speeds through the city's brutal outskirts in a hermetic trance, interrupted from time to time by streams of headlights, incongruously glowing in the daylight. These are cars of mourners following the hearses that come out of the city each morning to the immense new graveyards that ring New York, perhaps thirty or forty miles from the center. There is no time on this road for stately travel. The hearses race along, sometimes two or even three abreast, at the speed of other traffic or even faster, past the roaring trucks and lines of casual travelers. One watches and wonders how often, in this frightful race, a car of mourners, falling behind, becomes detached from the proper object of its grief and follows a stranger to his grave.

Dying as an Emerging Social Problem [217

Perhaps it doesn't matter. You die here as you live, more or less irrelevantly, and you grow accustomed to losing your way. (Epstein, 1966:15–16.)

Nevertheless, while some of the larger features and problems of American life such as bureaucracy and alienation are mirrored in death, American society, as we have seen, has developed institutionalized means for minimizing the social consequences of individual deaths. Aside from a recent growing concern with higher mortality rates among the poor, death is not viewed as an unusual problem except during times of war or where death occurs unexpectedly, as in children, or where death might have been prevented, as in disasters such as airplane crashes or mine cave-ins.

Management of Dying

But what of the process of dying? This has not been successfully bureaucratized and routinized. What was once a natural event is emerging as a social problem.

One of the underlying reasons why the management of the dying patient is emerging as a social issue is that there have been marked changes in the causes of death, primarily a shift from infectious to chronic diseases. This, in turn, has tended to lengthen life, reflected in a concentration of deaths in the later years. The nature of these deaths has shifted the place of death from home to hospital or nursing home, and there have been rapid and powerful technological developments so that hopelessly ill patients can be kept alive for long periods of time—but not forever.

Changing technology, then, has led to a significant enlargement of the process of dying, through changes in the causes of death and the development of treatment while dying. Duff and Hollingshead (1968) in a study of a small sample of terminal patients indicate that the median length of time between known onset of illness and death is twenty-nine months. "Terminal care" deals with this lengthened process of dying.

The key to understanding the social consequences and problems of dying lies in time—the hours, days, months, indeed years that it takes for the career of many terminal patients to unfold. To be sure, though

218] SOCIAL, ETHICAL, LEGAL, ECONOMIC QUESTIONS

death may be certain, dying, by virtue of added time, by virtue of a technology that often controls physicians rather than vice versa, adds powerful elements of uncertainty that produce strain for the entire social system involved.

Decisions are made affecting the quality of life in the final months and days of a terminal patient in a variety of ways. The question of basic human rights is often involved. The patient himself has little option as to what regimen, what therapy—or lack of therapy—may be administered on his behalf. As this book indicates in a number of places, patients are often treated in an evasive way, and are not permitted truly to know the circumstances or the conditions of their state.

Undeniably, there are many times when evasion or the lack of complete honesty may indeed be functional in filling the psychological needs of various patients. But there is little question that the will, the integrity, and the wishes of the patients are often not considered. The dying patient may be experiencing pain; he may need to resolve various legal matters, or to make final plans. In short, his essential right to have some decision-making power with regard to his own fate is violated. Even the fundamental question of whether his life is to be prolonged, at the cost of great pain and considerable financial outlay, is often not raised with the patient. Nor, incidentally, can a patient himself fully decide as to the disposal of his body. In many states the dying person cannot will his eyes or organs to others; only his next of kin have this prerogative.

It is clear then, that the dying patient is often defined as "irresponsible." It is tragic, that with so terribly little time left, that the very meaning of life—consciousness, self-control, decision-making—is taken away.

The uncertainties and problems of the dying process are evident when we consider the difficulties that the family may face. We will not attempt to deal with the psychological problems involved in the relationship between patient and family during the terminal period. It is worthwhile, though, to contrast types of problems that the family encounters when a member undergoes a prolonged terminal period with those problems that the family faces in his death. As we have seen, society has developed institutionalized means for handling the death experience, but society has not been nearly so ingenious in de-

Dying as an Emerging Social Problem

veloping devices to cope with the terminal period. The family, for example, may experience financial problems during this extended period that it would not face in connection with a quick death where life insurance would ameliorate such concerns. During this uncertain terminal period the family often is compelled to give up various plans and activities. Painful and traumatic as ultimate death is, it nonetheless offers clearly patterned devices or paths for the family to pursue. During the terminal period, however, there is a state of suspension, uncertainty, ambiguity, and nonresolution.

Like other actors in the total situation, the family cannot assume initiative in suggesting the termination of the patient's life. Because of the general moral imperatives of the situation, the family is in large part a victim of the overall situation. It has to witness and assent to a number of decisions that it does not understand and cannot control; to a range of new medical techniques offering little hope; to the introduction of new physicians, nurses, and attendants; to new sites where the patient is being sent or placed; and so on. Often the family is quite helpless to control its destiny or that of the patient during this period, no matter how hard it tries.

Clearly, the situation of the dying patient places a number of strains upon the smooth functioning and coping capacities of the family. Despite the fact that death is certain, it is difficult and often impossible for any legal machinery to begin to operate, for any probate process to be initiated, or for adequate financial assistance to be made available to the family.

There is also evidence that both the number and the unpredictability of dying patients are posing increasing problems for hospitals. For example, more and more patients die within hospitals. We know, too, that hospitals are compelled to devote considerable medical resources to the hopelessly dying patient and to render various services to their families. From the point of view of overall hospital operations and the appropriate deployment of personnel and other resources, the care of the dying patient represents a relatively ineffective and inefficient enterprise. Yet hospitals often must avoid relatively "rationalistic" and "efficient" alternatives because of pressure from the family to do everything possible on behalf of the patient. In many cases there is conflict between the hospital and the family, with the hospital attempting to

220] SOCIAL, ETHICAL, LEGAL, ECONOMIC QUESTIONS

encourage the dying patient to spend more of his days at home, while the family, feeling itself helpless to handle the emergency needs of the patient, insists on the staff maintaining the patient in the hospital.

In some cases, employers of the dying patient also experience their share of strain. They may be regarded as cruel and unfeeling if they abruptly terminate the dying patient's employment or, at any rate, income. It would be useful to learn whether the employer is often compelled to avoid filling the position of the dying patient in an effort to maintain the posture of expecting the patient to return to work. Does the employing organization have to postpone making various plans and decisions? It would be valuable to know more about the impact of the dying patient upon the organization where he works.

Role Conflict in Physicians

Let us briefly turn to some of the problems that plague the physician. Because of the extended and uncertain career of the terminal patient, the physician is frequently confronted with role ambiguity and role conflict. Trained to interact with the patient, he finds himself spending more time with the family; trained to deal with life, he must cope with death.

The physician is called on to devote valuable time, not in performing an instrumental role to which he is highly accustomed and for which he receives most of his rewards, emotional, financial, and otherwise, but in performing an expressive and nontechnical role when there is no opportunity for success. In short, much of the energy and time of the physician is dissipated in dealing with families, in listening to their suggestions of relatively hopeless remedies or alternatives, in being asked for assurance when no real assurance is possible, and in relating to the patient, when this is most difficult.

Although the attending physician bears the main responsibility for managing the dying patient, he is always subject to a larger system of social control. He must not only adjudicate the wishes and pressures of the family of the dying patient, but must also consider his colleague and peer group network and judge whether the action he is taking would meet professional approval. Thus, in one setting he may perceive his peers favoring a more conservative or traditional response; in another he may perceive his colleagues as favoring more heroic measures. Sudnow (1967) made this point vividly in contrasting a county hospital with a private hospital, both of which he studied.

Other factors that may impinge upon the physician's choice or decision are the size of the hospital and its types of activities and resources. The presence of a research team interested in new and experimental methods of treatment might influence the type of regimen he would be willing to prescribe for his patient. The availability of a cobalt radiation machine, dialysis machine, or heart transplant team might influence his decisions.

A number of institutions other than the health system itself circumscribe the behavior of the physician. The physician is always subject to the dominant norms and value orientations of religious institutions. The sacredness of life is fundamental and therefore in no case may the physician blatantly act to end the life of an individual, though we know physicians have developed informal norms and may refrain from excessive efforts in behalf of the hopelessly ill patient. The physician is bound not only by moral but by legal sanctions as well; the law takes a stern view of any act intended to shorten the life of the patient. The power of the new technology to maintain technical life considerably beyond the patient's capacity to function socially emphasizes the need to reexamine and reassess the application of religious and legal norms which govern the life-saving role of the physician.

Professional Agreement and Disagreement

The vexing problems posed by the dying patient have already stirred considerable discussion and deliberation within the medical profession. To be sure, much of the concern is narrow and pragmatic —for example, when is a person dead, and should dying patients be told. Close examination of the current literature indicates that within the profession there are cleavages surrounding issues such as the criteria for death and the allocation of new and scarce medical resources. The stances of different groups within medicine, such as internists and surgeons, often reflect the orientation and even the "self-interest" of each specialty.

The recent surgical "breakthroughs" associated with organ transplants have been accompanied by a landslide of medical editorials.

Some groups within medicine feel that transplants represent the medical frontier, and that the next major advances in medicine will be in transplantation, in organ storage, in synthetic organs, and the like. Other medical groups argue differently. They point out that dramatic and promising as many of these new technologies are, they may be raising more problems than they solve. They feel that by objective criteria—either in terms of the number of people served by the technology or the number of years added to the lives of those affected— virtuoso surgery as yet has accomplished little, especially when such surgery is adjudged successful on the basis of the "addition" of one or two years postoperative survival for the patient, and in many cases as little as two or three months. This position argues that scarce medical resources be used to reach more people, be oriented more toward prevention, and be used to improve the delivery of services.

Notwithstanding these differences that have appeared in the medical literature, some issues do not produce polarization within medicine. There is agreement at least that problems associated with dying exist and that solutions need to be found. With regard to the central question—that is, what kinds and quantities of medical technology should be brought to bear in behalf of the hopelessly dying patient— the physician is in need of help. He is trapped by competing values and social roles. On the one hand, it would appear that the physician has no alternative but to maintain his relentless efforts to prolong life. This mode of conduct is functionally related to the essential role of the physician, that of "being on the side of life." If the physician compromises this stance with the dying patient, it eventually may undermine the trust other patients are willing to put in him. On the other hand, it would also seem that the instrumental role of the physician may be distorted in his conduct with the dying patient; he is often compelled to act in a manner contrary to his medical training; this, too, may have negative consequences for the practice of medicine. It would appear that the medical profession is ill suited to solve this dilemma by itself and that it may have to turn to broader ,segments of the society to help forge appropriate policy regarding the prolongation of life of the dying patient.

There is the temptation, of course, to refuse to cope actively with this complex of problems and to rely instead upon the existing modes of managing the dying patient. Some even may argue that to focus directly on the problem of the dying raises more problems than can be solved—that it is actually better to rely upon the informal culture of physicians that has been handling a range of problems with some degree of efficacy than to open a Pandora's box with consequences that cannot be anticipated. Our stance, and the whole assumption of this book, is that our society is obliged to face and to solve problems directly, however painful and difficult this confrontation may be. Furthermore, to avoid facing the issues much longer may compound problems and further complicate or obscure solutions.

There is another important reason for our not being able to continue to rely upon existing methods of coping with the problem. We live in a period when the ideal values of equality are being asserted as never before and where departures from the ideal are subjected to the closest and most critical examination. In the health field, the continued discrepancy between reality and the ideal, the continued demonstration of inequality, may be greeted with vigorous protest. It is one thing to accept differential morbidity and mortality as stemming from variations in general modes of existence—though this view too will be increasingly challenged—but it is altogether another matter to observe a system of institutionalized inequality where life itself may appear to hang on a single decision—whether or not a person is eligible for artificial kidney service, for example, or for other new and potentially ingenious but nonetheless scarce devices for warding off death. Surely, the present procedures determining who gets what innovative health measure can no longer serve as a basis for public policy. No matter how judicious the decision makers try to be, their efforts within the present arrangements invite social ostracism. Public policy must be founded upon more fundamental values and more universally implemented procedures than the happenstance availability of technological resources.

At present, different elements of the health system are responding erratically, archaically, and even whimsically to the challenges entailed in the problem of the dying patient. The development of policy guidelines, however general they may have to be initially, offers hope of relieving needless and untold anxiety, tremendous cost, and wasted energy and effort. It is our belief that the development of some explicit policy guidelines, if formulated on the basis of solid empirical knowledge, can provide a desperately needed orientation for the participants in this drama: for patients, their families, physicians, and administrators.

REFERENCES

Duff, Raymond S., and August B. Hollingshead.
1968 Sickness and Society. New York: Harper.
Epstein, Jason.
1966 "Living in New York." New York Review of Books 5(January): 14–16.
Spiegel, John P.
1964 "Cultural variations in attitudes toward death and disease." In George H. Grosser, Henry Wechsler, and Milton Greenblatt (eds.), The Threat of Impending Disaster. Cambridge, Mass.: M.I.T. Press.
Sudnow, David.
1967 Passing On: The Social Organization of Dying. Englewood Cliffs, N.J.: Prentice-Hall.

12

Control of Medical Conduct

Osler L. Peterson

THE CONTEMPORARY PHYSICIAN who goes to a cocktail party is often showered with criticism: physicians are difficult to see, do not give their patients enough time, are opposed to Medicare, make too much money, and do not provide care in the ghetto. Such criticism contradicts objective evidence that Americans are getting more medical care than they ever had before. The modern, well-trained physician who is compared—it is scarcely necessary to add *unfavorably*—to an older doctor who made house calls in a Model-T Ford or even with a team of horses must feel that his problem is unique and the comparison unfair. The problems that provoke these criticisms are, no doubt, different from those of the past but criticism of physicians has been a characteristic of every age.

Physicians obviously long have held a special place in social organizations. Originally their status was presumably based on the character of the physician's responsibilities. In more recent history, one can see how it has been affected by higher education and more recently by the evident effectiveness of the care they give. The Hippocratic Oath must have had a very literal meaning to the Greeks:

> Into whatever houses I enter, I will go into them for the benefit of the sick and will abstain from every voluntary act of mischief and corruption and, further, from the seduction of females or males, bond or free.

From the specification we can assume that seduction was a cause for concern. Statistics on such mischief are seldom publicized but one can, from the published reports of disciplinary bodies, judge that it is now a numerically unimportant problem—though it has not disappeared and probably never will.

Henry VIII's charter to the Royal College of Physicians of London in 1518 described its functions as follows: "to curb the audacity of those wicked men who shall profess medicine more for the sake of their avarice than from the assurance of any good conscience; whereby very many inconveniences may ensue to the rude and credulous populace" (Stevens, 1966).

A recent lecturer on the history of medicine described his subject as follows:

> Social pressures, philosophical attitudes and scientific progress are some of the cultural factors which shape medicine. Medical history, particularly of the 17th century, shows how physicians and their doctrines respond to the revolutionary pressures that beset them, and reveals strong parallels to the present day medical tumult (King, 1968).

Social pressures upon physicians are constant, as the medical historian states, but the issues provoking these pressures change, as suggested by these two examples. We will deal briefly with this shift, particularly in the twentieth century, and will then examine the current effectiveness of professional self-government, with particular attention to pressing problems at this time.

Poorly Educated, Poorly Paid

As late as the last century many doctors were rustic characters in a society that was mainly rustic. Few physicians were well-educated men. Most were trained as apprentices by physicians who themselves had little education. It should be emphasized that the recent social prestige achieved by physicians of the United States (the profession enjoys more respect, we are told, than any other except justices of the Supreme Court) was a recent acquisition related to recent educational standards, excellent incomes, institutionalization of practice and, finally, real effectiveness in dealing with the problems of illness.

Meager medical incomes were once the mode in contrast to present affluence, and no doubt influenced physicians' behavior. Doctor Paget (1869), who studied the graduates of St. Bartholomew's Hospital, found that about 15 per cent had "failed utterly," meaning that they had been unable to make a living by doctoring.

George Bernard Shaw, in *The Doctor's Dilemma* (1913), spoke his opinions about medical men; they were, as usual, critical. Shaw contrasted Schutzmacher, a general practitioner from the Midlands whom he admired, and Blenkinsop, whom he made a pitiful figure. Schutzmacher was a shrewd man who explains to his scientist friend, Sir Colenso Ridgeon, the secret of his success. It was simple. He guaranteed the cure all patients hope for, and charged a sixpence. The sixpenny doctors were common enough in England's poorer districts and they often collected enough sixpences in a day to live comfortably or occasionally, like Schutzmacher, to become well-to-do. Doctor Blenkinsop, in contrast to Schutzmacher, was not a sixpenny doctor; he was desperately poor and his function in the play was to emphasize the poverty of many general practitioners.

Economic conditions in America for doctors at the beginning of the twentieth century were probably little better than in England. The number of doctors was large when compared with the present, and the demands for medical care were few. In 1930, United States physicians' mean income was low—somewhat lower than the modest incomes of lawyers and about 15 per cent above those of dentists, a situation that now has dramatically changed. The annual mean income of doctors in non-urban areas was then under $2,500 (Friedman and Kuznets, 1945). Physicians often spoke of their colleagues as "competition." It is unlikely that poorly educated physicians with small incomes would look kindly upon efforts at self-government in their profession. Severe competition between doctors no doubt fostered sharp practices. The general practitioner who said in 1930, "Your competitor always charges too much, prescribes excessively, and misbehaves with his office nurse," was caricaturing the intensity of competition in a less affluent society.

It is only since World War II that demands for medical care have intensified to a point where a medical degree almost guarantees a high income. Competition for patients is no longer important to the physician whose day is busy and whose appointment book is filled for weeks ahead. It is also during this same late period that we have seen the shift from empirical to scientific medicine.

Adequate training of physicians did not become common until

after World War II. The conversion of the medical profession from one universally engaged in general practice to one consisting mainly of coteries of well-trained specialists began between 1910 and 1920 and reached its peak after 1945. This transformation is particularly significant because most everyone in the profession now is well grounded and prepared for practice. The generally long residencies of physicians increase the likelihood that they will practice the quality of medicine learned in a Jesuit-like training process.

Lack of Government Regulation

The United States in some respects has been more poorly prepared than other industrialized countries for changes in a complicated institution such as medical care. In part, this may be related to the fact that our government was originally set up with checks and balances to assure the weakness of central government. The rather unusual organization of government with little of the party responsibility characteristic of parliamentary systems is, no doubt, related to the fact that, among the industrialized and wealthy nations of the world, ours is one of the last to deal with pressing social problems closely related to health and medical care, such as poverty, health insurance, and medical education.

In other countries, because of different governmental responsibility and some good luck, governments concerned themselves with medical care much earlier. In Germany, formation of the Krankenkasse in the last century established government's interest in the medical care field at an early date. In Sweden, the reorganization of government in 1862 gave counties responsibilities and taxing powers that soon were used to build hospitals staffed by full-time doctors (Engel, 1968). The remarkable Swedish system of county hospitals, many of which resemble American teaching hospitals with their hierarchical medical organization, training programs, and interest in clinical investigation and research, has eliminated some of the problems of medical control that are part and parcel of the North American system of open hospital staff organization.

In England, the early emergence of the Royal Colleges created two castes, consultants and general practitioners, providing a natural basis for the professional division between the important hospital doctor

Control of Medical Conduct   [229

and the humble general practitioner, finally formalized in the structure of the National Health Service in 1948 (Stevens, 1966). In Britain, where health insurance was legislated in 1911 and a Ministry of Health was established in 1929, there always has been deep governmental concern with medical care and the governance of medicine.

The United States, by contrast, did not establish its Secretary of Health until 1953, a generation or more after health ministries had become commonplace in other industrialized societies. The United States was also late in developing health insurance, voluntary or governmental, and this has had an important role in delaying government or other third-party interest in insurance payments.

Full-time hospital staffing does not eliminate problems of professional control but it has had a profound effect on their character. In most industrialized countries a salaried hospital medical service is the norm. Problems relating to quality of patient care or the influence of fees on hospital use are quite different under such organization. One example is the well-known tonsillectomy and adenoidectomy operations, accounting for about 5 per cent of short-stay, non-obstetric hospital admissions in New England. This routinely performed operation is no longer accepted as scientific in academic circles. In Sweden, with its hospital-based staff, it is performed infrequently. In the United States, "T. and A." operations are the leading cause for hospitalization of children. Presumably, the fact that they continue to be done in such large volume owes something to the fee received, to the far more mixed character of the physicians who use United States hospitals, and also to the type of professional government involved in American hospitals. The important problems of hospital standards and quality of care have a different character in a system with a hierarchical medical staff organization compared with the looser and more democratic staff organization in the United States.

The young European physician, like his counterpart in the United States, enters hospital training after graduation from medical school. Most of these young physicians probably hope to obtain the more prestigious and highly paid positions as hospital consultants. Many of the entrants will not achieve such appointments as they advance year by year from junior to senior assistants, to docent or deputy, professor, or chief; some of them will be selected for positions within the hospital or academic organization while others will be forced out. A doctor's conduct or the imposition of a standard of quality in such a system is seldom a problem. The rigorous selection of men who ultimately reach positions as chiefs of medical services or other services will not only favor good clinicians but will, for the most part, also select men who have scholarly credentials or have demonstrated administrative skills.

Salaried staffing of hospitals by specialists does not insure a medical millennium, as the experiences in different countries show. Quality of care obviously varies by country and by hospital in countries with full-time hospital staffing. The reasons for this are too complex and deeply rooted for discussion here.

American physicians work and practice in hospital environments that mostly have been extremely democratic. In these environments physicians have established systems of self-government partly because they are a responsible profession and also, it must be recognized, because to do otherwise might force the government to institute less congenial controls. Professional concern with cultism and quackery, important issues in the first half of this century, provides one example of self-government. The motivations were probably both selfish and more exalted, as the following examples show. Although this struggle was sometimes directed against external movements—faith healing is one example—it was often concerned with the splintering of medicine itself by movements such as homeopathy or osteopathy. The declining decades of empiricism were also characterized by frequent discoveries by allopathic or regular physicians of "cures" —often secret—for diseases such as tuberculosis and cancer. Maintenance of a mainstream in an empirical profession was no small problem and not invariably successful—as is shown by the continued separation of the medical and osteopathic professions at a time when their medical education and practice are nearly identical in content and form.

There was a time, as Doctor Geoffrey Freymann (1965) has reminded us, when the American medical profession spoke with a single voice—that of the American Medical Association. There is, he states:

> ... a tendency to ignore its work in maintaining high standards of education in medical schools and hospitals, in maintaining hospital

standards, in investigating drugs, in exposing quackery and in many other fields. This is probably because in an era of socioeconomic evolution, the chief image of the AMA in the minds of both physicians and laymen is as a political force.

Development of Self-Government

The AMA's preoccupation with achieving a sound system of medical education, culminating in the Flexner Report of 1910 and the enormous changes that followed, was an example of self-government at its best. Until those changes were achieved, distinguished medical school deans and professors often filled the presidency of the AMA. Examples cited by Freymann included Frank Billings, John H. Musser, and William H. Welch. The reform of medical education and the establishment of specialist societies, beginning with the founding of the American College of Surgeons in 1912, introduced a fractionalization of medicine into many different interests and voices. As Freymann observed, the medical educators, having achieved long-sought changes, retreated to their hospitals and laboratories. Colleges and academies increasingly claimed the time and interests of specialists.

The establishment of hospital accreditation, begun in 1918 by the College of Surgeons as a program of hospital standardization, marked an important date in medical self-government arising from the recognition that there was much unsatisfactory surgery. Early twentieth-century general practitioners often described themselves as "Physician and Surgeon"; they did not propose to give up surgery to a fledgling guild. The growing divergence of interests of general practitioners and surgeons is exemplified by the position long held by general practitioners that all doctors should be allowed to do whatever they felt competent to do without explaining how such competence was or could be determined. The College of Surgeons' accreditation program always was voluntary and more persuasive than demanding —the only possible approach when a majority of the medical profession was in general practice. This program set a pattern for a more general compliance with voluntary professional standards that has subsequently been adopted in many fields of medicine.

One example is the evolvement of the College of Surgeons' program into the Joint Commission for Hospital Accreditation in 1952 as a joint endeavor of the American Colleges of Surgeons, American

College of Physicians, the American Medical Association, and the American Hospital Association (American Hospital Association, 1964). Other examples are supplied by medical school accreditation and approval mechanisms for schools of medical technology, nursing, and the like. In many countries of the world such standards would have been accepted responsibilities of the government; they would have been approached through licensing arrangements, training requirements to determine eligibility for a post, and control of appointments. A philosophy of free enterprise and the absence of direct government involvement in medical care made voluntary compliance a logical and wise course for a responsible profession in the United States.

Four Areas of Self-Regulation

When we turn to the more specific problems of self-regulation of a profession, the problems and examples seem to fall into four somewhat different fields. The hospitals have been the focus of much attention and their problems, which are quite well known, will be considered first. Group practices present a special problem in which control by profession seems to have succeeded well. Their problems, in many ways similar to those of hospitals, will be taken up next and will be contrasted with other ambulatory care arrangements. A third major area deals with the application of disciplinary measures. The growing scientific basis for medicine has created some new problems. A final area will take up the questions of relationships between institutions and self-regulation on a basis transcending local institutions or by areas which are now receiving attention as part of medical care regionalization.

Hospitals For most doctors the hospital represents the point at which they come under the discipline of the medical profession. In contrast with most of the world, Canada and the United States have chosen to extend "hospital privileges" to all practitioners. The description of a physician's position in a hospital as a "privilege" presumably indicates the theoretical, if not the real, relationship. Although there are some physicians who do not have hospital appointments, this should not obscure the fact that most do. This has complicated self-government because the doctors vary in age, training, and the quality of patient care they give.

Control of Medical Conduct [233

The importance of self-regulation in the hospital arises from the fact that it is the site of the most important and critical episode of patient care—where the opportunities for good and the consequences of errors are great. We have already pointed out how much simpler the problem is under different hospital staff organizations where status and responsibilities are explicitly defined. Governance in United States hospitals is both more difficult and more complicated than is suggested by descriptions of self-government as democratic and voluntary. Voluntarism and democratic methods of governance of professional conduct are evident at all levels. Hospital approval by the Joint Commission on Hospital Accreditation, for example, does not depend upon prescribed procedures; its standards about rules governing desirable or required practices, services, organization, and the like are couched in broad and general terms.

In addition to its inherent weakness, professional self-government has to cope with serious structural problems. Hospital administrators during their training devote much thought to the fact that there is a separation between the legal responsibility for the hospital, which is invested in the trustees, and for the patient, which is vested in individual physicians. Although, in theory, the relation between a physician and his patient is a private and inviolable one, the efforts at self-government provide a continuing contest to define the boundaries of collective and individual professional responsibility. The hospital administrator, too, has great responsibility, limited powers and, naturally, many frustrations. The training of hospital administrators in recent years has given less emphasis to bookkeeping and other details of management and more to issues and philosophies relating to medical care. The administrator who is aware of the weaknesses of his institution and yet is unable to deal with them is a common phenomenon. While he may encourage more effective self-government, he must do so with consummate skill, for if he is too forceful or too active he may lose his point and his job.

In addition to a division of powers between trustees, administrators, and professional staff, there is the whole question of professionalism. It is sometimes said that most people are paid for their work, but professionals are paid so they can do their work. In a most extreme form, academicians insist that they are paid to do whatever interests them. This view of professional payments is not normally held with fee payments in mind but rather in consideration of what responsibilities and constraints should or should not be imposed upon persons with unusual skills. The view is utopian, and scarcely a realistic solution to professional self-government of an increasingly complex industry.

A question of major interest is: How well does this special status and self-government work out in practice? We have already pointed out that there are a number of conflicts within the medical profession related to self-government and changes in groupings within it. The half-century of conflict between surgeons and general practitioners about who should do surgery is one. The general practitioners' position that they should be allowed to do whatever they feel competent to do—including major surgery—has been slowly but increasingly limited by definition of a few of the common low-risk operations within their sphere. Two standards of surgical training have resulted.

Far more attention has been given to surgery than to other aspects of hospital practice for several reasons. The high incomes of surgeons may be one, because these pose temptations. Another reason is the manifest risk to the patient, both from the disease and from surgery. Another probably arises from the fact that the pathology examination of all surgically removed tissues has provided a better measure of diagnostic skill and outcome than is available in other fields. An appendix is either normal or diseased. In obstetrics, *per contra*, the caesarean section rate is given attention even though it is often difficult in the individual case to determine whether the decision was or was not a wise one.

The evidence about the quality of care given on the medical service of a hospital is less clear, and usually too laborious and costly to obtain.

The use of pathology examinations to provide an end result to measure quality is effective in some areas and less so in others. New England hospitals have lower appendectomy rates than hospitals in Sweden and England where study of the pathology of the appendix is uncommon (Pearson *et al.*, 1968). American surgeons who remove too many normal appendixes may be confronted by evidence that brooks no argument. In Britain or Sweden the lack of this evidence is a plausible explanation of the higher operating rates observed.

Control of Medical Conduct [235

In contrast to appendectomies, pelvic surgery rates in New England hospitals are high. For most of the common pelvic diseases the relationship between pathology and the need for surgery is much less clear. For example, myomas of the uterus, or fibroid tumors, which are often the basis for removal of the organ, are very common in the latter half of the childbearing period, often cause no symptoms, and regress in old age, whatever their size. Under these circumstances, the committee reviewing surgical records has an uncertain standard to apply in judging indications for hysterectomy. It may be that within the limits of knowledge judgments cannot be rigorous.

If we consider the circumstances in which the tissue committee does its work, it is easy to see the difficulties. In small hospitals doctors are likely to know each other well, they may cooperate in giving care, and refer patients to one another. When Doctor A joins the tissue committee he may find it difficult to be severe with Doctor X's performance both because of these personal relations and because next year their roles may be reversed.

Confronting the doctor with criticisms of his work is not pleasant. In larger hospitals with more departmentalization and specialist control of services, the problem of self-government and discipline apparently becomes somewhat easier and more effective. The relationships between staff members is less intimate and personal. As hospitals become larger, specialist staffing of services becomes the mode, so that agreement about practice standards is greater. In addition, administrators and trustees of hospitals are often more forceful and willing to give necessary backing to a review committee.

Although the duties of self-government in the hospital are often unpleasant, many physicians are willing to undertake them, not as a routine but as a serious challenge. Some are also very effective. One example is provided by the well-trained physician of a small hospital. As the chief of medicine, he was able to exercise some control over patient care on his service, but his efforts were directed mainly at the trustees, local factory owners and managers, many of whom were his patients. He first educated them about the institution's shortcomings and later forced them to take measures to improve practices in the hospital. In another hospital, a physician with remarkable personal skills dominated a large and heterogeneous staff and by force of personality enforced standards in all departments. In this hospital, for example, the young, well-trained surgeons operated under the supervision of experienced surgeons until everyone was satisfied that paper qualifications were matched by surgical judgment and skills.

Ambulatory Care In ambulatory private practice there are examples of both rigorous self-government and no self-government.

Most physicians are still in solo practice, small partnerships, or loose associations. In most smaller partnerships or solo practices, doctors are subject to little self-government other than that relating to ethics or the law. Physicians are, on the whole, a remarkably responsible group so that, for most, conduct that brings them into conflict with the law, licensing bodies, or ethics committees is an uncommon event.

Although serious breaches of law or ethics may call attention to themselves, other aspects of solo or small partnership practice receive little scrutiny. Whether a practice is conducted competently or incompetently is seldom known and often cannot be known. One physician, for example, was suspected of irregular practice by his colleagues because he attracted a certain type of patient from a wide area. The actual situation was otherwise. This physician, who had a rather strong personality, used a standard treatment for a group of patients in whom the psychosomatic component is believed to be important. The physician's personality and a wide experience with a single disease, rather than any hanky-panky, was the explanation for the success that had brought him under suspicion.

Group practice represents a quite different situation. The survival of a group often depends upon clear definition of clinical authority and acceptance by each doctor of his role, responsibility, and the group's standard of care. Jordan (1958) emphasized in his book that the purpose of the group practice should be "better medicine" and somewhat tangentially that the group's problems are much like those of a marriage. Joining a group should receive the same serious thought because acceptance of authority and responsibility are vital to achieving the practice goal.

The high quality of care given in some of the well-known group practices, while owing much to organization, also results from careful selection of new partners or members. Selection can be a very effective tool for obtaining men whose medical and general conduct will be appropriate. What little objective evidence there is supports the general impression that in group practices the quality of patient care is good (Peterson et al., 1956).

When we turn to the administration of self-government, it is found that the effectiveness of self-control by a profession is seriously hampered by the problems inherent in applying discipline to its members. The difficulties arise from the penalties that can be imposed upon doctors or other professional men; they are few and so severe that they are used reluctantly. The suspension of a doctor's license can be exceedingly damaging to a doctor's reputation, but most important, it removes his livelihood. It is a hard penalty to impose. Similarly, a doctor whose hospital conduct is unsatisfactory will be severely disadvantaged if he is removed from the staff. Under these circumstances, doctors are likely to be warned, reprimanded, or threatened with the loss of their hospital privileges or license repeatedly before such serious penalties are imposed.

Although attitudes are now changing rapidly, the abortionist has been an unwelcome problem to the medical profession. The operation is still illegal and contrary to medical ethics in most jurisdictions even though standards are now catching up with practice. Yet, laws have not prevented abortions and whether they have been curtailed in any important way can only be guessed. Even where the issue, as in this case, seems to be clear-cut, its control has seldom been effective or even seriously attempted. It appears that there has been a reluctance to interfere with a known abortionist if he is discreet. The lack of sympathy with the legal and ethical positions on abortion, the harshness of the available disciplinary measures, and reluctance to become involved in the unpleasant situations may explain this tolerance.

In England, when the National Health Service was formed and capitations were substituted for direct patient payments for care, it was deemed important to have milder disciplinary measures for physicians who failed to give proper care. A quasi-judicial system was set up to hear patients' complaints about shortcomings of care or treatment from general practitioners. Sufficiently grave misconduct charges, if proved, were punishable by a fine or by removal from the National Health Service. It may be a measure of the reluctance to apply a severe penalty, but it is more probably due to the responsible character of the general practitioners; at any rate, several years elapsed before one of the some twenty thousand general practitioners was forced out of the service for failing to give his patient necessary and appropriate care. The actual number of patient complaints has been small. Many have little substance; some are settled by discussion or an apology. A few doctors are fined but the numbers are small (Peterson, 1951).

Problems Related to Science Doctors have always made clinical observations and done studies but the establishment of clinical research institutes early in this century and the recent expansion of clinical research in all medical schools augmented the output without a corresponding increase in well-designed and controlled studies. For example, Simmons has recently pointed out that most studies of drug treatment of hypertension have been done without controls or have been inadequately controlled (Medical Research Council, 1962).

The drugs used to treat hypertensive patients are effective in lowering blood pressure but carry some risk—as do most medical treatments. As well-designed and controlled clinical studies have become more common, the risk of exposing patients to a drug, operation, or diagnostic procedure has increasingly preoccupied investigators. It is becoming generally accepted that patients should not be subjected to the risk of a poorly designed study that cannot settle a scientific question. Whether a physician should enroll his patient in a clinical trial is a related question. The Medical Research Council of Great Britain pointed out the ethical issue involved: "To obtain the consent of the patient to a proposed investigation is not in itself enough. Owing to the special relationship of trust which exists between a patient and his doctor, most patients will consent to any proposal that is made." Personal biases, which have to be eliminated in the conduct of an experiment, may also arise when a physician requests cooperation from his own patient. Sir Robert Platt (1963), in discussing informed consent, states that "It may become a kind of placebo to the experimenter's conscience." Standards of medical conduct are rising in science as well as in practice.

The Public Health Service has recently demanded that, when government funds are used for patient studies, there be institutional responsibility to ascertain that the interests of subjects of experiments are adequately safeguarded. University or hospital committees given responsibility for making these decisions must deal with awkward questions. Since there is little treatment of patients that does not carry some risk, the issues inevitably involve balancing the risk, large or small, against any expected benefit. Do preliminary animal experiments show enough promise to warrant trial of a treatment on a human being? Is the investigator competent? Is the design of the experiment such that it is likely to answer the question? These are questions which good investigators presumably have always asked themselves; now all scientists will have to face them when they apply their knowledge to human beings.

The outpouring of scientific results has produced other kinds of problems which are exemplified by recent technical developments. Physicians treating patients with end-stage kidney disease by renal dialysis early had to face the question of which patients should be or should not be treated, because facilities were insufficient to treat all. The answers in some instances involved medical questions, but in others included ethical issues and judgments that the physicians chose to solve by asking for help from the clergy and other nonmedical persons. It is probable that the physician is the best judge of what kind of person could cope with a life dependent upon a machine. Whether anyone can determine who should be selected or rejected for such treatment or whether life under such circumstances is worthwhile are questions for which there is little human experience to use as a guide. The important point is that physicians are now asking laymen to share in making important decisions whereas in the past the physicians' instincts have been the opposite—to reserve judgment for themselves.

The heart transplants have provided a different problem because there is a completely new element. The doctor who hitherto has accepted responsibility only for his patient now has his interest compromised because the treatment of one patient depends upon the death of another. The new and dramatic character of the dilemma posed for a physician has produced a quick response. Beecher and his associates (1968) have proposed a new definition of death which deals with the "brain death syndrome," or "irreversible coma," characterized by irrevocable loss of intellectual functions instead of "total stoppage of the circulation" and other vital functions diagnosed by a physician, the previous legal standard.

240] SOCIAL, ETHICAL, LEGAL, ECONOMIC QUESTIONS

The need for guidance in formulating solutions for some of the problems raised by heart transplants is evident in some of the comments made about this development. Heart transplants have been called "a grandstand play" and, more recently, a British physician described the "enthusiasm of doctors for the removal of vital organs as vulturelike" (*Manchester Guardian Weekly*, 1968). The Judicial Council of the American Medical Association (1968) has published ethical guidelines for organ transplantation containing some singular new features. In these they point out the physician's responsibility to his patient, the need to have independent confirmation of a donor's death, and the like. A most interesting recommendation is as follows:

Transplant procedures of body organs should be undertaken (a) only by physicians who possess special medical knowledge and technical competence developed through special training, study, and laboratory experience and practice, and (b) in medical institutions with facilities adequate to protect the health and well-being of the parties to the procedure.

This type of recommendation has been implicit in much of the medical profession's efforts to improve care; seldom has it been explicit.

While the ethical problems posed by dramatic new treatments have made us face and deal with them promptly, there are others, quite similar, which are not new and receive little attention. Senile dementia, a brain disease of aged persons in which there is progressive loss of intellectual functions ending in a vegetablelike state is one example. Formerly, it was not an important problem because there were fewer old people, and because senile dements soon died of "the old man's friend," pneumonia. It is not a reportable disease and is almost never a listed cause of death so it cannot be described quantitatively. Modern therapy has made it possible to treat successfully their pneumonias so many of these patients live on and on, requiring increasing amounts of care. Their care raises several questions: Should we not let these persons die when treatment is hopeless? Can we use resources for care of mindless, hopelessly ill patients, when there are children who would benefit from medical and dental care but receive inadequate or no care?

Another problem is presented by the terminal cancer patient. Fortunately, most cancer patients die with speed and in reasonable comfort, but there is a small number who linger on for long periods in great pain. The doctrine of the Catholic Church in this instance is clear. Undue effort need not be made to prolong life, but even more than this may be desirable. Every physician has known a cancer patient who would have preferred earlier death rather than continue to live in pain.

While there is much that we do not know about abortions, it seems probable that large numbers are done. The complications of criminal abortion—serious infection often resulting in sterility and occasionally in death—are seen with distressing frequency.

Abortions, it appears, are now obtained quite easily for the middle class and the wealthy but with more difficulty by the poor, who also seem to suffer the complications of criminal abortions more often. The arguments with respect to abortion are increasingly taking cognizance of this social-class difference and also of the implications of abortion for medical and social pathology. For example, illegitimacy is associated with high perinatal and infant mortality rates and with much severe social pathology. Out-of-wedlock pregnancies are one of the common reasons for abortion.

In this discussion we are much hampered by lack of information about the size of our problems. Senile dementia is probably increasing. The cancer patient who might wish to exercise the right to die, while not rare, is not common. But there are other patients who have good reasons for dying sooner rather than later. Abortions are, we believe, a frequent and serious problem.

The issues posed by these examples involve taking or shortening life. Some attempt to reduce the argument by redefining life. Some physicians insist that life cannot be regarded as human until there is a neural organization capable of supporting the intellectual functions characteristic of human beings and that abortion, which is done before such organization is reached, does not involve taking human life. This borders on casuistry; it would be better to face the situation honestly and accept the fact that the argument is about shortening life.

Both secular and theological positions on life have changed and can be expected to change more. Legal taking of life was once common but is now becoming rare. Though concern for life is increasing,

242] SOCIAL, ETHICAL, LEGAL, ECONOMIC QUESTIONS

it is not always consistent. The known high risk of mining is accepted because greater safety is too expensive. Unsafe cars and accidental deaths in epidemic numbers aroused little interest until Ralph Nader dramatically defined the problem as "unsafe at any speed." Clearly, if we want safer travel, something else must be given up. This is also true of medical care. Is it right to spend money on the extended care of senile patients and neglect children who are poor? Perhaps the difficulty is that such questions have never been raised forcibly enough to attract attention to themselves. In these circumstances the medical care industry goes on doing what it usually has done—care for the individual patient and hang the statistics.

Theologians do not speak with a single voice. While many hold to rigid positions, as for instance on abortion, others grant the validity of socially based arguments for change. Some certainly accept a patient's right to die. Similarly, some lawyers quote the law, but many others insist that laws must serve society and must be adapted to changed social needs.

When theologians and lawyers are willing to discuss these problems and to help the physicians establish new moral and legal positions more in tune with modern practice and need, what is the hangup? Physicians are as divided as theologians and lawyers on questions of abortion and the right to die. William Curran, Professor of Legal Medicine at the Harvard School of Public Health, states that liberalized abortion laws, strongly supported by some physicians, are applied very restrictively by other physicians and some hospitals. Thus, new laws may produce little change. In addition, medical ethics are not anyone's special business in the same sense as pediatrics or medical administration. Though many physicians must be concerned with medical ethics it is a casual preoccupation. There are no medical Naders.

Nevertheless, it does appear that we are beginning to face the problem of abortions. European countries that have developed a population policy have found a permissive approach to abortion, a logical next step. Although we have no explicit policy, there is increasing concern about quality of life and of population. In addition, what is probably freely available to the higher income groups can scarcely be denied to the poor who stand to benefit most from legal abortions.

Control of Medical Conduct [243

Laws have been changed in some states, the American Public Health Association has urged a liberal abortion policy, and New York clerics aid women to find abortions.

While abortion practices and laws are changing, the prospects for changes in the right to die and other awkward ethical issues of medical care are not good. But even here law and practice are diverging. Curran also points out that a physician or a family member who helps an incurably ill patient take his life is not normally punished by the law. Similarly, a patient who rejects a life-saving treatment cannot be forced to accept it and may exercise his right to die by calling a stop to treatment.

If physicians do something when the expected effect is shortening life, it is normally done with the conviction that the action is right. This is not a responsibility to be carried by a single physician. It should not be done covertly. Although there is no unanimity of opinion on these issues, it clearly is not healthy to tolerate increasing disparity between what is legal to what is done.

Regional Planning and Self-Government Hospitals, nursing homes, and convalescent care facilities are the responsibilities of states, cities, churches, community groups, individuals, and other groups. Hospitals built by religious, ethnic, or other groups undoubtedly satisfy their constituencies as well as providing professional opportunities for doctors, nurses, and other members of the group. This has created intense loyalties. Not surprisingly, expansion of a hospital or development of a new service is normally based on what each institution feels its needs may be. The evidence for the needs may be the opinion of the medical staff, demands of a constituency, the ambitions of a director, or occasionally the wishes of a donor. This institutional allegiance has produced a haphazard, occasionally inappropriate, and excessive array of facilities. Stone (1939), an authority on British hospitals, said that Britain had no system of hospitals, only a number of unrelated institutions; this is no less true of the United States in 1968.

Virtually all developed countries have accepted the idea of regional hospital and medical care planning since the last great war; a few, even before that. In the United States the recent enactment of legislation to support regional medical planning arose in part because of the recognition of the need for more systematic use of resources. The influences of the high cost incurred by Medicare may also have been a consideration in the timing of this legislation.

A medical-care industry that is built up institution by institution without consideration of the broader community and its total needs has created excessive local resources, left large areas untended, and also has adversely affected the quality of medical care. The popularity of cardiac surgery units, often described as hospital status symbols, has resulted in more units than are needed to meet current demands. It is generally accepted that an unnecessary risk is associated with a small heart surgery case load. The case loads of many units are very small (DeBakey, 1964). The situation of radiotherapy for cancer is similar. The Folsom Committee (1965) found that New York's facilities were far in excess of needs. Clearly, the wise course would be to have fewer centers, each with an adequate number of patients and presumably lower risk to each patient.

Superficially, regional planning may seem to have little to do with professional self-government. On deeper examination, however, it becomes clear that the general acceptance by physicians of responsibility for the quality and adequacy of medical care in a hospital and acceptance of responsibility for community or larger areas differ more in degree than in kind. Furthermore, any consideration of planning mechanisms inevitably leads to the conclusion that much planning must be local in nature. In other words, it represents only a transfer of responsibility from an institution to a community or service area. A few services demanding unusual personnel, equipment, or facilities can only be planned or supplied for a large population such as a state or region. Thus the major casualty of planning will be parochialism.

It is clear from regional medical program guidelines that serious planning is expected. The Surgeon General of the Public Health Service, for example, listed some of the steps involved, including setting of goals, analysis of problems, planning and selection of course of action, and restudy of the program to determine if the goals had been reached. If regional programs set out to determine whether goals have been reached, professional hospital personnel who are central in planning will be far more deeply involved in self-government than ever before. The hospital will become a goldfish bowl.

Regional planning presupposes not only new organizations and wider responsibilities but also new methods. A government program to improve patient care has two potential tools, coercion and encouragement, to accomplish its goal of improved care. The former is unlikely to be effective. The second, which is the chosen instrument, is represented by government funding, or earnest money, to encourage desired changes and developments. Theodore Marmor (1968) has concluded from his studies of medical politics that a government normally has to pay, and often has to pay dearly, for desirable changes in medical practice. Government funds to support changes is one major new element that is likely to make regional self-regulations effective where self-government within institutions often is not.

The creation of regional administrations with full-time personnel to aid with analysis of problems and formulate acceptable criteria for medical care developments and to undertake planning itself is the second new element. The provision of full-time professional staff to aid and encourage planning is likely to be an important element in making this new program more effective than previous efforts at self-government by part-time practitioners for obvious reasons. The part-time and occasional service given by a busy physician to the self-government of his hospital staff resembles the medical school faculties that were casualties of the reform set in motion by the Flexner Report. The regional medical program legislation stated that established practice patterns were not to be interfered with. This may have been tongue-in-cheek piety to make the bill swallowable because planning implies studied changes to effect improvement. The additional provision that planning be a cooperative process involving both providers and consumers of medical care indicated that decentralization and self-regulation were to be continued while the added provision of federal funds and an administration and planning staff would correct the major weaknesses of regional planning undertaken on a voluntary basis. These provisions are bringing medical care organization and government closer to the European model—as similar problems are prone to do in modern societies.

National Health Planning

Although regional planning may appear to some to be an exciting and somewhat daring experiment, it is probably not enough to meet the needs of a complicated modern state. The parochialism of hospital planning discussed above extends to other areas. When the regional programs were instituted as a means of improving the care of patients with cancer, heart disease, and stroke, some objections were raised. It was pointed out, for example, that money might more profitably be spent in trying to diminish infant mortality rates which are higher than they should be in the wealthiest country of the world (Burgess *et al.*, 1966).

The cancer, heart disease, and stroke program, which has been transmuted into regional medical programs, owed its impetus to a group of physicians and laymen who were interested in trying to reduce the large number of deaths caused by these "dread diseases." Alternative and more productive use of the allocated funds does not seem to have been considered. In other words, though there was a strategy, it was not broadly concerned with both health and medical care needs and opportunities. Why, otherwise, would one mount a large program to reduce deaths from diseases that occur mainly in old age and under circumstances where there is little evidence that good care can produce much improvement?

Scientific research policy has suffered from the same parochialism. Science is neither good nor bad but will go in directions charted by investigators' interests, opportunities, and by available funds. Scientists are no more or less wise or human than anyone else and are just as likely to serve their own interests.

The dietary treatment of babies with phenylketonuria, which some believe will allow these children to develop normally, has been introduced on a wide scale without asking whether the survival and distribution of the responsible gene in the population was an appropriate price to pay. Many biologists are deeply pessimistic about the possible consequences of a program preserving a disease-producing gene instead of allowing it to be eliminated by natural processes. This treatment was seized upon, not only by interested scientists, but also by health officers and legislators. Case-finding is now required by law in many states. Clearly, planning in this instance was too narrow, too much oriented toward a single rare form of mental deficiency, and did not consider the greater problem of the late results. It may also have been too hasty since the evidence does not clearly support the expected results of this now widespread preventive program.

The recent spate of heart transplants poses at least as many problems as it solves. Although my barber recently supposed that everybody would soon be getting a new heart, the fact that a majority of people now die of heart disease and the fact that there must be one donor for each transplant places boundaries on the operation—barring the use of hearts from lower mammals. The feasibility of organ transplants had been established before addition of the heart to the list, so this new surgery is more important technically than scientifically. The extraordinary cost of a heart transplant will undoubtedly be reduced with more experience but it is not likely to become cheap. The point is that advancements in technology are governed by possibilities and the interests of individual investigators. A successful development is likely to be applied and, once applied, demand rises. Policy questions are seldom raised.

While millions of Americans live in ghettoes without adequate medical care, no one has asked whether the enormous research and technical costs associated with heart transplants are appropriate or whether the money could better be spent on black children who, with decent medical and dental care, might grow into healthier adults. The surgeons who do heart transplants, like all physicians, feel that their responsibilities are to their individual patients and not to some impersonally defined group such as the poor, or the blacks, or the aged, and even less to some policy. Many physicians indeed would say that we can afford both heart transplants and medical care for the poor. The sentiment is admirable but, unfortunately, dead wrong. The creation of regional medical programs and of comprehensive planning bodies may serve as a counterbalance to the investigators who pursue a new field of patient care whatever the costs.

The fact, of course, is that we will never be able to meet all of our medical care needs. The superb care given to the late President Eisenhower during his series of myocardial infarctions under no circumstances could be extended to all persons in his age class. Clearly, planning for a region or a state is not enough. Medical policy formulation on a national basis is also necessary if both care and research are to be directed at problems where need is great, where there is reasonable expectation of favorable results, and where use of resources is not so prodigal that other efforts are penalized. This direction may also hold more promise of real improvement in health and longevity. Some untended health problems would have a very different cost-benefit ratio than heart or kidney transplants.

The Present Situation

One of the obvious conclusions of this examination is that modern physicians are, on the whole, a group whose conduct is both good and responsible. The present high standard of conduct has not always prevailed. Its achievement is related to many influences including a long professionalizing process, careful selection of students by medical schools, the tangible and intangible rewards given to physicians, the growing practice of medicine in institutions, and, finally, changes in the norms of society in which all professions participate.

The medical profession in America has developed a broader self-government than the medical profession of other countries. While self-government has not always been fully effective, and has occasionally been unable to cope with problems, it has achieved some important victories.

If the conduct of physicians is good and professional self-government is about as effective as the professional self-government can be, why is there so much apparent dissatisfaction and so many problems? Why is the doctor often treated like Doctor Scratch? Why is there general dissatisfaction with the availability of physicians when Americans are obtaining more medical care than ever before and, in addition, obtaining far more useful care?

The medical historian who emphasized the social pressures on physicians has, of course, anticipated the explanation. The establishment of research institutes in almost all medical schools since 1945 has given a hard push to the shift from empirical to scientific medicine. Medicine's increasing complexity has produced specialization and a division of labor that have made it complicated for patients to find needed care at comfortable prices. The medical profession does not have a sufficiently effective self-government so it can adapt its organization to what is now nearly a complete shift from general to specialty practice. Tensions have been aggravated by a revolution of expectations among the poor and not so poor who demand the good care that medical science has long given to the wealthy.

Control of Medical Conduct [249

Selection, income, and social position all incline the medical profession to be conservative. Its habitual stand in opposition to major social changes has aggravated relations between the profession and the public. It seeks for solutions but somehow the quiet and deliberate self-government that seemed to work in the past is inadequate. The size and complexity of problems is too great for solution by the profession. For example, the development of Blue Shield by the medical profession made available a good medical care insurance but it has remained to others to pioneer the more interesting and promising prepaid care plans, voluntary regional organization, and other experiments. A profession, in trying to meet problems, is hampered by its own attitudes but there are other more fundamental difficulties. The Blue Shield cannot provide protection for many persons—the unemployed, the elderly, the marginally employed, and the like—because it lacks both authority and funds. Certain activities such as the regional medical programs and comprehensive planning could be created only by government because only government can demand the planning that may involve the conflicting interests of different specialists and institutions and because only government can supply the funds to make planning effective. Major institutional innovations such as health insurance and regional medical organizations have been slow in developing in the United States. The fact that these sound medical measures were not legislated until a generation or more after they had been adopted by most other industrialized countries should not be attributed to the medical profession. They have been opposed by physicians in all countries. It is government that has acted or failed to act.

Although the last few years have seen a good deal of legislation relating to health and medical care services, we have not seen the end. There are planning needs in addition to those served by regional medical programs and comprehensive planning. Continued Federal support of categorical medical services for persons with certain diseases, of a certain age group, or of a specified social condition, the expenditure of larger sums for renal dialysis programs that benefit few persons, and the lack of adequate provision for persons who are too poor to purchase any care shows that we need a national health policy to ascertain that our funds are used wisely and effectively. In addition to wise use of resources for medical care, better informed choices of resources used in research is needed. It would be wise, for example, to determine the relation of positive cytology tests to cervical cancer so informed decisions could be made about screening programs—to cite an example of an expensive service based more on promise than on reliable data. Cytology testing programs were supported from Federal grants to state health departments until they became a casualty of recent reductions of government spending.

Complaint about the medical profession in the United States is unusual, for in most of the world physicians are popular. This may be because other governments have created institutions that can deal with the distribution of medical care nationally. In the United States, on the contrary, government policy—if it is policy—has been support of disease-centered research. The failure to assure that medical care is available to the population is blamed on the physician, but it is the government, with a single too narrow strategy, that has been neglectful.

REFERENCES

American Hospital Association.
    1964   Hospital Accreditation References. Chicago: AHA.
American Medical Association Judicial Council.
    1968   "Ethical guidelines for organ transplantation." Journal of the American Medical Association 205(August 5):89–90.
Beecher, H. K., et al. (Ad Hoc Committee of the Harvard Medical School).
    1968   "A definition of irreversible coma." Journal of the American Medical Association 205(August 5):85–88.
Burgess, A. M., Jr., T. Colton, and O. L. Peterson.
    1966   "Avoidable mortality." Arch. Environmental Health 13(December):794–798.
DeBakey, M. E. (chairman).
    1964   A National Program to Conquer Heart Disease, Cancer and Stroke. Vol. II. Washington, D.C.: The President's Commission on Heart Disease, Cancer and Stroke.
Editorial.
    1968   "The ethics of transplants." Manchester Guardian Weekly 99(September 19):1.
Engel, A. G. W.
    1968   "Planning and spontaneity in the development of the Swedish health system." The Michael M. Davis Lecture, Center for Health Administration Studies, Graduate School of Business, University of Chicago, Chicago, Ill.

Folsom Committee Report.
  1965 The Report of the Governor's Committee on Hospital Costs, State of New York.
Friedman, M., and S. Kuznets.
  1945 Income from Independent Professional Practice. New York: National Bureau of Economic Research.
Freymann, J. G.
  1965 "Whither the director of medical education?" New England Journal of Medicine 273(December 2):1253–1257.
Jordan, E. P.
  1958 The Physician and Group Processes. Chicago: The University of Chicago Press.
King, L. S.
  1968 1968–1969 Lectures on the History of Medicine, Countway Auditorium, Harvard Medical School, Boston, Mass.
Marmor, T.
  1968 "In transaction." Social Science and Modern Society 5(September):14–19.
Medical Research Council.
  1962 Paper #53/649, recirculated. London: Her Majesty's Stationery Office.
Paget, J.
  1869 "What becomes of medical students?" St. Bartholomew's Hospital Reports 5:238–242.
Pearson, R. J. C., et al.
  1968 "Hospital caseloads in Liverpool, New England, and Uppsala." Lancet 1(September 7):559–566.
Peterson, O. L.
  1951 A Study of the National Health Service of Great Britain. New York: Rockefeller Foundation.
Peterson, O. L., et al.
  1956 "An analytical study of North Carolina general practice." Journal of Medical Education 31(December):2.
Platt, R.
  1963 Doctor and Patient—Ethics, Morals, Government. The Rock Carling Fellowship; The Nuffield Provincial Hospitals Trust. London and Tonbridge: Whitefriars Press.
Romains, J.
  1924 Knock ou le Triomphe de la Médecine. Paris: Librairie Gallimard.
Shaw, G. B.
       The Doctor's Dilemma. New York: Penguin Books.
Shapiro, S., et al.
  1960 "Further observations on prematurity and perinatal mortality in general population and in population of prepaid group practice

medical care plan." American Journal of Public Health 50:1304–1317.

Stevens, S.
1966 Medical Practice in Modern England—The Impact of Specialization and State Medicine. New Haven and London: Yale University Press.

Stone, J. E.
1939 Hospital Organization and Management. London: Faber and Faber.

The Year Book Publishers, Inc.
1958 The Physician and Group Practice. Chicago: Year Book Publishers.

13

Legal and Policy Issues in the Allocation of Death

Bayless Manning

LAW IS THE MAJOR tool by which society translates its ethical value structure into action. In general correspondence to the value system currently prevailing within the society, a society's legal order allocates resources among its members, distributes powers, privileges, and immunities among them, and accommodates the competing claims of its members. Moreover, through its laws the society establishes the acceptable *procedures* by which disputes are to be resolved. The use of force as the determinant for resolving dispute is considered to be centered as a monopoly in the society's institutions of law enforcement. The more developed and sophisticated a legal order is, and the more widely its underlying value structure is shared, the greater its reach, and the greater its power to deny to members of the society resort to force as a method for resolving conflict. Where, as in the field of international relations, there is only a tenuous community of shared political and ethical values, the legal order is weak; participants in that environment can only resolve their conflicts by negotiation, where the issue is not considered to be of critical importance by the participants, or, where the issue is considered to be of critical importance, by violence.

Except in extremely limited circumstances, most animals display a deep instinctual inhibition against killing others of their own species. Man has little such reluctance. His powers of cerebration and imagination have enabled him to invent more reasons to kill his fellow, and more efficient ways to do it, than are available to his less gifted brothers of the animal kingdom. Thoroughly frightened of himself—and with good cause—man has long professed to the ethical injunction, "Thou shalt not kill." He has sought to enforce that injunction through social means—through law. Through law he has sought to contain the instinct to reach for the hand axe when frustrated, and also to provide alternative procedures for resolving conflict.

The legal order of organized society has achieved a degree of success in translating into action the ethical prescription against homicide. But that success must not be exaggerated. Even in the best-ordered and most homogeneous societies, violence of man against man remains a daily phenomenon. The law has also had to recognize, sometimes explicitly and sometimes tacitly, that the community is willing to accept some killings as permissible, the most obvious example being killing in self-defense. And in situations of mass violence, both law and ethics have had to give up entirely, explaining that the socially reprehensible practice of homicide becomes the socially laudable practice of war if the enterprise is adequately large-scale, well-organized, and expensive. Over the centuries, enormous investments of intellect and energy have been devoted to a delineation of the scope of the law's commitment to the prevention of homicide, to the pinpointing of exceptions, to the development of graduated series of sanctions to be applied depending upon the circumstances within which the killings took place, to the development of detection and enforcement institutions, and to the nurture of a generally anti-homicidal public attitude, at first in the family, then successively in the clan, the tribe, the province, the nation, and (dimly) the world.

It is, indeed, fair to say that the principal task to which the legal order has historically set itself has been to prevent or at least inhibit one man from taking the life of another.

This is the socio-legal backdrop against which one must view the problem of termination of medical care, and assess the explosive significance of emerging medical technology.

"Thou Shalt Not Kill"

A deep premise, or assumption, has always underlain the development of the ethical injunction, "Thou shalt not kill," and the corpus of

Legal and Policy Issues [255

legal principles based upon it. It has always been assumed that a man would die soon enough in any case, and that the problem therefore was to prevent other men from cutting his life short. Modern medicine, and the prospect of tomorrow's medicine, is slowly bringing into focus the possibility of a state of affairs that is wholly different from that premise. If science can extend a life indefinitely—or for a very long time past the Biblical three score years and ten—then, inevitably and inescapably, there will be, there must be, a social condition in which decisions will have to be made by human agencies as to who shall continue to live and who shall not, or, which is to say the same thing, how death shall be allocated, at least among the seriously ill, the badly injured, and the elderly. A legal order and ethical system based on "Thou shalt not kill" will be forced by the pressure of medical advance to move to a new plateau where the injunction will be "Thou shalt not kill, unless . . ." or, to put it less abrasively, "Thou shalt not kill, but thou may let die if . . ."

Analytically viewed, of course, the problem is not new. Doctors have always had to work with limited resources of time, medicines, and equipment and therefore have had to make choices among patients. They have always felt, and sometimes responded to, the pressures of patients *in extremis*, and their families, to whom death has seemed preferable to continuation of a life in agony. In the United States today, more than two-thirds of all deaths occur in hospitals or other institutions, and it is apparent that in a fraction of these cases it would have been medically possible for the doctors to extend the life span by a few hours, a few days, or a few weeks. Medical technology has not suddenly jumped, will not suddenly jump, from a level where it could do nothing to prolong life to a level where it can prolong life indefinitely.

But this observation, like many observations that are analytically valid and descriptively true, is not very important. Medical knowledge is undergoing, and will undergo, a dramatic quantum jump in the latter half of the twentieth century. The manifestations of that quantum jump have become headline news throughout the world. Geneticists and surgeons who are in the forefront of medical experimentation have become national and international figures whose faces and voices are familiar to television audiences worldwide. Practices that have been invisible are becoming visible. Problems that were thought to be individual will be seen to be recurrent and widely shared. Half-baked, semi-informed enthusiasts will see in the new medicine the arrival of the millennium; half-baked, semi-informed troglodytes will denounce each scientific advance as blasphemy. Tempers will rise, and denunciation will fill the air.

It can hardly be otherwise. The work of the doctors in the termination of care, in the allocation of death, will press hard not only upon man's resistance to change, but also upon his single most sensitive nerve—his instinct for self-preservation and his well-founded distrust of the homicidal proclivities of his fellow man.

Much of the debate and struggle that will swirl around termination of care will be cast in the vocabulary and rhetoric of the law—an invocation of allegedly existing law before the courts and proposals for new law before the legislatures. A useful way to survey some of the legal aspects of the topic is to break it into three parts: legal exposures of the doctor and hospital; legal consequences of life prolongation upon persons other than the doctor and hospital; and, from a broader social perspective, possible avenues of legal change in the short run and in the long run.

Liability Exposure of the Doctor and Hospital for Termination of Care

The situation that troubles the conscience and the security of the attending physician is easily described. The patient is very ill, or badly injured, or in great pain, or decerebrate, or some combination of these. As each day's dividend from the medical laboratories of the world, the attending physician is handed more drugs, more surgical techniques, more implements, and more therapies by which he can attack the patient's problem. Which of these should he draw upon, to what extent, and for how long, where—

—The effect of the treatment will be to prolong the circulatory and respiratory life of the patient, but will leave him permanently comatose.
—The effect of the treatment will be to preserve his "life" in the sense that the patient will be conscious and able to communicate, but will also permanently strip him of all physical mobility, forcing him to complete dependence upon full-time attendants for all his bodily wants.

Legal and Policy Issues

- The effect of the treatment will be to restore his bodily activity and his mental competence to communicate, but will completely destroy the existing personality structure.
- The effect of the treatment will be the economic obliteration of the patient and his entire family.
- The effect of the treatment will be to divert to the permanent monopoly use of this patient scarce equipment or resources, thus producing the certain death of other patients.
- The effect of the treatment will be to restore the patient to a state of life and health which he has already found intolerable and which he, and all members of his family, implore the doctor not to restore.

The variations are numberless. And, of course, the circumstances will often appear in combinations; the effect of a treatment (which itself may be uncertain) may simultaneously monopolize scarce resources, lead to decerebration or immobility, impose an insupportable economic burden on the family, and be contrary to the expressed wishes of the patient and his family.

If in such circumstances the doctor concludes not to reach into his kit of remedies, therapies, and surgical operations, or if he concludes that the time has come to switch off the respiratory machine, pull the plug on the circulator, or halt the ministration of life-sustaining drugs, what are the legal consequences?

Homicide—the Criminal Sanction   The doctor and his co-workers are as subject to the laws of homicide as other citizens, and the doctor's patient is as entitled to the protection of the homicide laws as any other victim. In fact, however, very few indictments have ever been brought against doctors for murdering patients, or even for manslaughter. Where such situations have arisen the circumstances have differed entirely from the topic at hand; the homicide charge might have arisen, for example, out of a love triangle, and the manslaughter charge out of the doctor's allegedly inept performance of his medical responsibilities. Occasionally one hears reports of doctors involved in "mercy killing," but so far at least criminal prosecutions on that theory have not found their way into the recorded cases.

What does the future hold in store on this point? One suspects that the heightened public perception of the physician's effective power to allocate death will tend to reduce the traditional unquestioning confidence in the physician's position, will tend to place the physician under greater scrutiny by his patient and his patient's family, and may, in time, lead some unshy prosecutor to file a homicide indictment against the physician. It is useless to speculate upon the outcome, for everything will depend upon the particular facts. Doctors will come to the support of their colleague. Lawyers will argue for directed verdicts, and the court may conclude that as a matter of "law" the prosecution has not made out a case. From the testimony of doctors and of others, the jury will learn for the first time (or say that they are learning for the first time) about the role of the medical profession in the allocation of death. If the court should let the matter go to the jury, it may be anticipated that the psychological state of the jury will be a complex thing. The juror may in part be horrified at the thought that his doctor may have actively helped Aunt Hettie over the threshold separating life and death. At the same time, the juror knows that further continuation of Aunt Hettie's life would have raised enormous problems, and, as a psychological matter, he is happy that it was not he who made the decision, but the doctor.

It is quite conceivable that no doctor will ever get tagged with a homicide conviction arising out of circumstances such as those listed above. The outcome will depend on the rate at which the public and the courts come to understand and accept the reality of the world that has been created by modern medicine—the inevitability that someone must be, will be, put into the position of allocating death through the withdrawal of supportive techniques. But it will probably be a close race, and if some doctor steps radically away from traditional termination practices—and if he attracts any significant newspaper attention, or publicly states that he pulled out the plug because he thought it more important that Aunt Hettie's family not be reduced to paupers than that Hettie's slender hold on life be continued for another six months—an indictment or two may come, and a jury or two may convict, especially in the communities where simplistic fundamentalism is more congenial than wrestling with hard problems of policy and fact.

If such an indictment should come, the doctor will not be significantly helped by the fact that the deceased patient had consented to, even desperately begged for, the termination of medical care. It is not

Legal and Policy Issues [259

a defense to a homicide charge that the defendant was helping the deceased to commit suicide. Consent by the next of kin to the termination of medical care is not likely to stand the doctor in any better stead in the event of indictment. The law may be pardoned for having developed a jaundiced estimate of the devotion that young heirs are likely to hold toward extending the life span of a testator.

Risk of Civil Liability

Where the doctor's decision to terminate care has led to the death of the patient, his risk of incurring civil liability, however small, is appreciably greater than his risk of incurring criminal liability. If for no other reason, this would be true because of the personal economic motivation of civil suit plaintiffs in contrast to the general public motivation of understaffed public prosecutors. But the risk of civil liability should not be exaggerated, and the number of actual winning lawsuits will likely not be great.

Where an action is brought, it will be under a so-called Wrongful Death Statute. Under some statutes, the plaintiff would be the executor or administrator of the estate, and the estate would be the beneficiary of any recovery obtained; under others, the next of kin may be the potential beneficiaries.* Some Wrongful Death Statutes still impose a fixed ceiling on the recovery. Unless the doctor has stepped radically out of line from existing practices, the plaintiff will not find it easy to hold him liable at all. The doctor will normally argue that his judgment was a practical one and that it would have been joined in, perhaps was joined in, by other doctors. On precisely that point, the court must make a critical decision of principle. To what extent should society, through its courts, adopt as its standard of not "wrongful death" that which the doctors do and think they should do? Only the doctors will have the range of relevant technical knowledge and a vision of the complexity of the problem with which they are dealing; on the other hand the ultimate decision contains a major ethical component that the doctors are no more equipped to make than are the court, the jury, or the society at large. For the time being at least, until public knowledge of the character of the life-death problem is far

---

* In these states, the consent of the next of kin to the care termination could well be useful to the doctor.

greater than it is today, it is highly desirable to contain the issue within as technical a framework as possible, to characterize it as being within the range of professional medical competence and do what can be done to equate the standard of wrongfulness under the Wrongful Death Statute with the standard of wrongful professional behavior as it is judged within the medical community. To the extent that that can be done, the doctor's decision on termination of care will not be an easy one, but at least his personal risks of being held liable will not be great. In the long run, as is suggested later in this chapter, the visibility of the process of life-death decision will become so great that it is unlikely that it can be left entirely to the doctors, but we will not be in a position to develop any alternatives until the level of public education in this field is much more advanced.

The Hippocratic Oath It would be of particular help to the development of the law in this area if the medical profession could bring itself into a relative unanimity in its interpretation of its own Hippocratic Oath. Although the lay interpretation of the oath assumes that it imposes upon the physician the obligation to preserve and continue the life of his patient, a more sophisticated reading is that the oath requires a doctor to do what he can to help his patient—a quite different proposition. No verbalized criteria are ever self-executing, or more than generally directive to the decision-maker caught up in a real situation. But if the doctors themselves could agree and make it clear that the Hippocratic Oath has limits, and does not bind the physician to the single unitary standard of a remorseless preservation of fractional life, regardless of other costs, the standard agreed upon by the doctor could have a substantial effect upon the court-declared law. And the reverse is also true; the doctor under fire will be in a precarious position if the profession should ever unanimously agree that its inexorable professional mandate is to extend the patient's life come what may.

Economic Consequences of Doctor's Decision It is possible to think of situations in which persons other than the estate of the deceased might seek to assert legal liability of some sort upon the doctor or hospital for an alleged premature termination of care. Under the terms of a will, for example, the termination of care of a patient might result in his predeceasing another person, thereby cutting out one series of

Legal and Policy Issues [261

beneficiaries of a will and installing others; long sustained preservation of a patient's "life" by extraordinary medical means could produce the opposite result. On the whole, however, it is not likely that the nephew who lost his inheritance would be able to persuade the court to hold the doctor liable, unless of course it could be shown that the doctor was aware of the terms of the will and was in some way working in cahoots with the beneficiaries who stood to gain by care termination.

The doctor is likely to find himself better off the less he knows about the peculiar economic consequences of his decision to terminate or not to terminate. But this principle is not an easy one to follow. Suppose, for example, that a member of the family of the patient implores the doctor to take whatever means necessary to keep the patient alive for just another seven days, for after that time a large property interest will vest irrevocably with the patient if he is still alive, and his estate and family will then be direct beneficiaries. Is that not a legitimate human consideration for the doctor to weigh? But then, suppose a property devolution will hinge upon which of two patients, each under the care of a separate doctor, shall predecease each other; should the doctors allow themselves to be drawn into a frenzied competition of temporary life-preserving therapeutic heroics?

Others of course may have an economic interest in the particular date of death of a patient—insurance companies, for example, or other persons in contractual relationships with the deceased. It is not easy, however, to imagine any significant likelihood that they could successfully bring claim against the doctor or hospital. The main concerns of the doctor and the hospital must be the risk of claim by the estate or next of kin of the deceased, and the related nonlegal risk that the confidence of patients in their doctors will over time suffer erosion.

In the interest of completeness it should be noted that wherever the distribution of significant economic interests depends in any way on the timing of death, there will be those who will be losers and who will be disappointed if the doctor extends himself to extraordinary lengths and manages to *preserve* the patient's life for an unusual period of time. Correspondingly, and more obviously, the extraordinary life-preserving efforts of the doctor can, and occasionally do, plunge the family into economic collapse. Does the family have any remedy against a doctor for an overzealous application of the Hippocratic Oath? Not at the present time. But if the oath comes to be given a multivariable interpretation, and if it comes to be generally accepted that doctors will make their final decisions about the allocation of death in a "reasonable manner" that takes many factors into consideration, there may come a time when precipitation of the family's bankruptcy through "undue" prolongation would be viewed as unreasonable behavior by the doctor.

Donor's Rights in Organ Transplantation Organ transplantations present a special set of problems in the field of continuation of care or termination of care. In the current excitement about the subject of organ transplantations, public attention is understandably focused upon the extraordinary technical achievement involved and the small chance of survival. But in time transplant results will have been stabilized and will join the arsenal of available medical procedures. The special characteristics of organ transplant as a therapy will then begin to become visible.

From the perspective of the organ donee, an organ transplantation is simply another life-preserving therapy. As the doctor considers whether to resort to this therapy in the case of a particular patient, he will encounter and have to weigh the kinds of considerations that attend any decision to terminate care or to go all out in an effort to preserve the patient's life. The doctor will find the decision no easier and no harder than in the case of any other available life-extending therapy.

But the peculiar and special circumstance about the organ transplant is that it also involves a donor. Put in the crassest legal terms, the donor, and his family and estate, represent for the doctor an additional and extensive source of potential plaintiffs—and potential plaintiffs who are psychologically motivated to sue.

The doctor's problem is quite acute enough where the organ involved in the transplantation is paired, as in the case of kidneys, and the donor survives the operation. More often than not, donors are likely to feel later that the donee has been insufficiently grateful for the sacrifice that has been made in his behalf. The donor is also likely to become hypochondriacal, and to attribute real and imagined discomforts to the loss of the organ. He is also apt to become persuaded

Legal and Policy Issues [263

that the doctor did not adequately inform him of the risks and consequences of the organ donation. Lawsuits come easily to one in this state of mind.

The donor's prior consent to the organ transplantation would of course be of great help to the doctor if sued. But it is important to recognize that such a consent does not and cannot provide an absolute bar against liability. To the extent that the plaintiff donor can persuade a judge and jury that the facts were not fully disclosed to him, he is likely to be able to pierce the consent. The donor plaintiff may also be able to overcome the effect of his earlier consent if he can demonstrate any real or implied environment of coercion, as where, for example, the donor was an employee of the doctor or the donee, or was a prison inmate, or a minor, or other dependent. On the whole, doctors have not been adequately sensitive to the difficulties of obtaining a valid and legally effective consent, and would be well advised to secure the best, most modern, socially sensitive legal counsel they can obtain to prepare consent forms for them and—far more important—to establish a careful interrogatory and disclosure procedure for using them.

Real as these problems are, the more serious difficulty comes in the case of an organ transplantation involving an unpaired organ—involving, in short, the possible survival of one of the participants in the operation and the sure doom of the other. We are not yet at a stage—and we may never be—where the society will consider organ donation as an acceptable justification for suicide or as an appropriate self-sacrifice for a loved one. The context of the transplantation problem is more narrow—and it corresponds exactly with the context of the more general issue of termination of care.

Vital organs deteriorate rapidly after blood circulation ceases. Although it is technologically possible to think of developing organ banks, and they are probably on their way, it is nonetheless essential that the organs be removed from their original human habitation as promptly as possible after "death." As the technology of transplantation stabilizes, the demand for organs will greatly exceed the supply. Every pressure will tend toward the development of an economic market in organs—whether overt and licit or underground and illicit. It may be expected that men with the economic resources to do so will seek to prolong their lives through contracts under which other parties will agree to make their organs available in certain situations. Doctors will be placed under enormous pressure to remove organs for transplants from patients who have just "died" in the hospital. And doctors will be subject to a powerful new incentive to terminate care, as they contemplate that the elderly or badly injured patient before them cannot survive more than a few weeks regardless of medical pyrotechnics while the organs removed from that patient could save the lives of three other patients in adjoining rooms. Where there is a prospect that over the next few weeks the organs themselves will become infected or otherwise useless, the pressure is obviously all the greater.

When Is the Donor Dead? There should be no mistake about the repercussive legal and political impact that transplantation of vital organs will bring to the subject of termination of care. In the past, we could live fairly comfortably with a vague subliminal awareness that the doctors were making crucial decisions on when to terminate care and when to continue it. We have no illusions that doctors are godlike in the wisdom with which they make the decisions, but they are at least as wise as any of the rest of us, and they have had the massive advantage of being personally disinterested in the outcome of the decision. The advent of organ transplantation changes that situation and it is just a matter of time until that change is felt and perceived. The technical possibility of organ transplantation introduces a possibility that the doctor might be tempted to terminate care of the donor patient earlier than he otherwise would. Especially is there room for that suspicion where the transfer of the organ to the donee is performed immediately after the "death" of the donor; the slower cycle of an organ bank into which organs are put in a routine way over time and are withdrawn in a routine way over time would appreciably mitigate the risk that a skeptical interpretation would be put upon the doctor's action in terminating care. It is not difficult to predict that the focus of public attention upon care termination where an organ transplantation is involved will have the by-product of bringing the entire subject of care termination under closer outside scrutiny. Interjection of transplantation techniques may therefore prove to be explosive, and have far-reaching consequences on more general practices of the medical profession in their administration of death.

As matters now stand, of course, it is assumed that no organs will be removed from a donor for an organ transplantation unless (1) he is "dead" and unless (2) the donation has been consented to. But both these conditions prove in practice to be much less manageable and predictable than appears on the surface. Some of the problems of consent have already been discussed in the context of the paired-organ transplantation. When one shifts to the context of a transplant of an unpaired organ, it is apparent that the burden of showing actual consent is much greater. Moreover, the issue of the donor's consent is most likely to be raised at a time when the potential donor is *in extremis* or perhaps unconscious. Who shall then be said to be able to give an effective consent?*

Then too there is a conditional consent: The patient on his way to the operating room agrees that his organs may be taken for transplantation if in the judgment of the attending physician the patient will not survive the operation, or has not survived the operation, or will survive the operation permanently decerebrate, or permanently immobilized, etc., etc. In that case again, the decision—a special instance of the decision to terminate care—will be vested totally in the physician, but in a context where a new motivation to terminate has been introduced. How well will such a conditional consent stand up as against a later suit by the estate of the donor against the doctor, claiming that he had not fulfilled his medical responsibility to preserve the life of the donor?

As for the other condition—that the donor be "dead"—the situation is not much clearer, while the emotional tensions involved could hardly be higher. To the mind of most, there is something distinctly macabre about the prospect—even the remote possibility—that the doctor might overeagerly turn off the respirator and immediately cut up the "dead" body in order to extract vital organs as rapidly as possible. As time goes by, and the point sinks in, the public will want clear assurance indeed that the donor was "really dead." But when does a person become "really dead"?

Classical theology has postulated, or simply asserted, that there is a

---

* The hair of at least one lawyer stood straight up to read in the newspaper account of the second South African heart transplant that the heart had been removed from the donor upon the consent of his *mother,* the donor himself having just died and his spouse being too overwrought to make the decision.

mystical instant when the soul flees the body and that at that point the person is dead. Regrettably, as inclines to be the way with the postulates or assertions of theologians, no one has yet observed that phenomenon take place. By contrast, the biologist finds elements of life within the human organism, and therefore no death, so long as any of the cells of the organism continue to be able to accept nourishment and re-create themselves; this cytological concept of death does not occur for several days after the respiratory and circulatory systems have stopped functioning. From the perspective of the psychologist or neurosurgeon, the key to death is the cessation of the capacity of the brain and nervous system to communicate, and to receive and respond to signals; an organism that had been physically decapitated would in this view be "dead" though the circulatory and respiratory system might still be functioning with the aid of supplementary machinery. On the other hand, the patient in a fully comatose state may produce a straight line on an electroencephalogram, while other physical functions of the body continue to be performed in normal fashion. A physician, and perhaps the usual layman, would likely point to the cessation of heartbeat and of breathing as the indicia of death. But it is now almost commonplace by massage and other therapy to restore palpitation to a heart that has fully stopped, and, with the aid of auxiliary respiratory and circulatory machinery, it is possible today to substitute fully for the pretermitted action of heart and lungs. In other words "death" is not an event but a process, is not unitary but is multiple, and is not absolute but a function of the perspective of the observer. And, most important for present purposes, the concept of death may be circular—the patient *would* be dead if certain medicological steps were not taken but would not, from some perspectives, be dead if those steps were taken. The question whether the donor of the organs was "dead" when they were taken, therefore, may resolve itself precisely into the question whether medical care was continued or terminated. The doctor who removes organs in such a case may well find himself accused of having brought about the "death" that was itself prerequisite to the removal.

Advantages of Alternative Research   It is a very real question—though a difficult one to raise seriously in the recent fever of excitement about organ transplantation—whether the medical profession

Legal and Policy Issues [267

might be much better advised today to pursue its research in other directions. A few years of concentrated work on the design and production of artificial hearts, or upon techniques for transplanting to humans the hearts of chimpanzees or other animals and upon the development of large-scale breeding of such animal resources, might be more promising and much less dangerous. Further support for that line of thought lies in the fact that it is inevitable that the demand for organs by prospective donees will always be far in excess of the numbers of vital organs that can be taken fresh from persons only recently dead. Artificial organs, once perfected, could be produced in any number, and organs taken from animals could be made available without limit. Organ removal from human donors will never produce more than a fraction of the supply needed and will be unavoidably accompanied by psychological tensions and liability risks of the kind just discussed.*

If organ transplantation is to continue, and particularly transplantation of vital unpaired organs, it is urgently desirable to develop a statutory framework under which doctors may operate. As things are now going, the new surgical procedure is bound to infringe upon anciently held legal propositions, some of them imbedded in statute. More important, the transplantation procedure points a scalpel directly at mankind's all-consuming concern with his own life and death and with his own body. What is needed is not a blanket authority for physicians to proceed with organ transplantations. Nor is it in any way useful to engage in definitional polemics about what is "death." The need is to establish procedures—procedures specifying what shall be and what shall not be a legally valid consent; procedures which, if followed, will give the doctor assurance that he will not be exposed to

---

* There are also other problems arising out of transplantation. Certain religious sects, for example, are opposed to any form of dismemberment or surgery upon a cadaver. At present, in most states, even post-mortem surgical exploration is forbidden except with the express consent of the next of kin or, in cases of mysterious death, a coroner or other public official. Typically, too, the cadaver is considered in law to be property of the estate, not of its former inhabitant, and, in the absence of special legislation, it is not clear that the consent to post-mortem surgery given by the deceased would be effective as against objection by the next of kin. In this connection, see the proposed Uniform Anatomical Gift Act. This model law, premising that an individual can decide the disposition of his body for scientific or humanitarian purposes, at this writing had been adopted in Kansas, Louisiana, and Maryland.

later liability; and—of particular importance to the medical profession and its relationships with its clients—procedures that will place the decision about the organ removal (and therefore the termination of care) in the hands of someone other than the physician who is eager to put the organs to use in behalf of another patient. If such a statutory scheme is not developed, and legislative bodies are not persuaded to adopt it, risks of doctor's liability will be substantial. More importantly, public unease about organ transplantations may well escalate to a more general unease about the way in which doctors are conducting their administration of death.

Legal Consequences of One's Life Prolongation for Others

So far, we have been considering liability risks to doctors and hospitals arising out of their administration of termination of care. It remains to be noted, however, that the spurt in medical technology, with its potentials for extending life or terminating it, will have other legal repercussions as well.

Already mentioned in the context of the physician's liability is the impact on significant property distributions of the doctor's decision to terminate or not to terminate. It is possible to imagine legal contests between other litigants that might depend upon a doctor's decision to continue or to terminate care. To put a simple case, suppose a husband and a wife are seriously injured in an automobile accident and the doctor decides to continue medical care in the case of one but terminate in the case of the other, with the result that one "dies" before the other. If under the terms of a will a devolution of property is determined by the sequence of the death, it is possible that in litigation involving interpretation of the will, one party might be arguing for recognition of the concept of "constructive death," or at least a constructive date of death—that date on which the injured person *would* have died had not the doctors intervened with massive medical technology. If that seems implausible, is it still implausible if the doctor removed vital organs from one spouse to maintain the life of the other? Is it implausible if care is terminated on one spouse, who dies at once, while intensive care is continued on the other, but it succeeds only in maintaining organic bodily functions and the patient

Legal and Policy Issues [269

never recovers consciousness or a capacity for communication; is it clear that for purposes of will interpretation one spouse should be considered to have died before the other?*

Perhaps these examples appear fanciful and perhaps they are fanciful. But at some point along the road of medical technological advance, when "life" can be sustained for long periods of time, there will arise real questions of the testator's intent when he provides in his will, for example, that on his (T's) death the income of his property should go to his elderly father until his death and thereupon to T's young son; is it a reasonable interpretation that T's entire estate should be devoted indefinitely to preserving the "life" of the elderly father until the age of 150 years while the son lives out a penniless life cycle and dies at age 70 without ever having received any part of the inheritance?

Possible Impact on Annuities It is interesting to speculate too upon the impact of the new technology on annuity premiums and other forms of insurance. The march of medical progress is apt to make life difficult indeed for actuaries and, one could even imagine, produce acute financial embarrassment for some annuity companies.

At root, the point is, of course, that many economic legal arrangements are built on silent assumptions about normal life expectations, based upon the history of man up to the latter half of the twentieth century. The advent of the new medical technology introduces an element of partial control over the time of death—either by termination of care or by application of radical new life-sustaining techniques—and in so doing can produce dramatic dislocations in those expectations.** Wherever, indeed, any legal event turns upon or is influenced by the time of the death of the person, the ability of the medical profession, however marginal, to determine the time of death will have significant legal repercussions and will contain at least the potential for a dispute as to when was the "true" time of death for the purpose of the legal matter at hand. As the life and death disposing power of the physician increases with the advance of medical technology, it

---
* Consider the application of the Uniform Simultaneous Death Act in this situation.
** Might an insurance company decline to pay a life insurance policy on the life of an organ donor on the grounds that he had in effect committed suicide?

may be anticipated that the courts will be periodically called upon to assess the impact of that new technology upon many of the inherited ways of the law.

Short- and Long-Term Approaches to Legal Problems of Terminating Life

Even at present levels of medical technology, it is apparent that a number of social-ethical-legal problems have come to surround the problem of termination of care and allocation of death.

The key problem of course is the one that has been discussed here at some length. Who should make the decision to terminate care for the patient? In what circumstances and by what standards? At present the topic as a whole is still subterranean, and decisions are predominantly being made by thousands of doctors in millions of different situations and by undefined, particularized, *ad hoc* criteria. It is arguable that, following appropriate data collection, an effort should be made to draw the attention of the public to this matter, to launch a general debate, and to try to work out a set of procedures and a body of principles that will gain legislative concurrence in the matter. But that proposal does not commend itself as a wise one. So great is the gap between the problem and the public's understanding of it, and so great are the psychological and theological tensions sparked by the subject, that it is most unlikely that the society can now be brought to a sensible overall long-term solution. The explosive rate of medical advance now being experienced and predicted for the balance of this century also warns against any effort to work out broad or definitive solutions at this time; we will not be able to do the job at all well (assuming we ever can) until we are much better apprised of the potentialities, limits, and shapes of the medical technology to which the society must adjust. The better course at this time would appear to be to address the topic in low key, to bring about gradual public education of the matter, and, for the time being, to leave to informal processes the slow development of commonly understood standards within the medical profession.

Doctors Proceeding at Own Risk As suggested earlier, a different route is called for in the matter of organ transplantations. The topic is already highly visible. The doctors are at present being forced to proceed largely at their own risk—an irrational and unjustifiable state of affairs. The traditional relationship of total and implicit confidence between patient and doctor is in potential jeopardy. And, unavoidably, basic policy decisions must now be made on where to invest available research funds—in the direction of more human organ transplantations or in the direction of developing substitutes, either by way of artificial organs or of animal organs. This issue is already upon us. Precisely because of its novelty, there is no inherited tradition or procedure. An intensive effort should be made to work out and install a procedural framework within which organ transplantations may proceed, and to bring public officials in responsible positions to focus clearly on the social implications of widespread use of transplantation techniques and upon the comparative advantages and disadvantages of alternative technological approaches.

The Longer Term Futuristic writing and forward social projection are currently enjoying a certain vogue. Most of the projections are grim. Man today does not face the future with a sense of ebullience and confidence. He has lost both his religious confidence that a beneficent God will take care of him and the rationalist confidence that mankind is a reasonable, reasoning creature who can be relied upon to solve his own problems. But fearful or no, we have no choice but to look into a farther term in the future and try to prepare ourselves for it. The only thing certain is that it will not be long before tomorrow is today.

What special issues may lie ahead relating to the issues of life continuation and life termination?

1. Somewhere along the way, consciously or unconsciously, explicitly or implicitly, society will have to make some basic decisions about the allocation of economic resources as between human beings of advanced years and those who are younger. The rate of medical advance will eventually force a decision. If a time comes—one is tempted to say when the time comes—when an array of therapies, drugs, supplemental machinery, and organ replacements will make it possible to extend the life, as somehow defined, of the individual, as somehow defined, to 150 or 200 years or more, it is quite clear that widespread application of that technology would produce a wholly different society. No aspect of economic or social life would stay as it

is today. At the same time, a massive fraction of society's total economic resources would have to be poured into the enterprise of life prolongation. The psychological capacity of the human being to operate as an integrated personality over a radically protracted life span is also a completely unknown quantity. We have only begun to recognize the existence of the field of study we call geriatrics. We have not begun at all to consider the violent social dislocations that would be brought about if a large fraction of the population were to be kept alive for significantly longer periods of time.

2. This paper, and the book of which it is a part, is addressed to no more than a small facet of the revolution that is taking place in the fields of health, biology, and human physiology. The truly dramatic explosions will not be in the fields of organ transplantation and other techniques for life prolongation, but in the work of the geneticist and the neurosurgeon. When the DNA code has been fully reduced to control, and we have gained an understanding of the aggregate surround of information about human development, man will himself be able to produce genetic structures on command, able to prescribe mutations, and able, in short, to control in advance the primary physical and intellectual characteristics of the newborn. Meanwhile, the brain surgeons will have learned how to effect radical changes in personality structure through intervention of surgery and drugs. Through these techniques, mankind will be presented with undreamed of powers of control over himself, over his successors—and over other men. How will he decide to use these new capacities; what kind of a world should he build with them; what kind of a world will he build with them?

3. When it is clear that man has the medicological power to sustain life for very long periods of time, to dictate its birth, and to shape its form, there will be no longer any escape from the necessity to make a direct assault upon the issues of termination of care that have just begun to become visible. In that future world, man will die either because he wants to die, or because someone else decides that it is time for him to die. One need not be much of a social philosopher to apprehend the seismic convulsions that will arise from the confrontation between the new technological state of affairs and the inherited ethical-legal injunction, "Thou shalt not kill." When technology has

brought us to that state, what kinds of procedures will man devise explicitly to allocate death and to supervise the allocation? Major spokesmen for some religious communities have not yet brought themselves to confront the reality of birth control. Abortion is just arriving at the stage where it is publicly discussable. If euthanasia is a term of shuddering horror and not at all mentionable, and attempted suicide remains a crime, how ready are we explicitly to address ourselves to the design of a systematic social procedure for the allocation of death?

4. When it becomes visible to the public that the continuation of life is discretionary, it will probably also become equally visible that the extension of life will, to considerable degree, depend upon the economic resources available to the patient. Of course it has always been true that the well-to-do have been able to command better medical attention than other men, and that their chances of health and long life are better. But so long as medical services are privately financed by the patient, rapid advances of medical technology will make it glaringly apparent that the rich can live longer but the poor must die. It is extremely questionable whether any society—at least any democratic society—will long tolerate a privately financed medical system in those circumstances. The American Medical Association may have successfully forestalled the efforts of social reformers to revamp patterns of medical service in the United States; the Association is less likely to be able to resist the long-term implications of expensive organ transplantations and other costly life-prolongation therapies.

5. The more exotic, sophisticated, and expensive new medical techniques become, the more pressure there will be to reallocate resources committed by the society to medicine, reducing the commitment to new research and discovery of new techniques, and augmenting the resources now being allocated to develop more efficient, widespread, and inexpensive delivery systems. The debate between those men in medicine who emphasize the need for further research and those who emphasize the need for wider distribution of knowledge already gained, is sharp, and is likely to grow sharper. Which way should the society lean on that issue and in what degree? And how shall the unavoidable risks and costs of medical experimentation be distributed as among patients, doctors, researchers, and the society at large?

Is all this simply a recitation of imagined crises? I doubt it. It is possible to argue about details of form and one can make different guesses about timing. But one needs only the single premise that the march of medical research and knowledge will continue to bring him eventually to the brink of these and similar awesome issues of social ethics and social organization. Because I am an optimist (and on no other empiric ground) I suspect that the twenty-first century will not in fact be a horror chamber of Brave New World tyranny or antisociety servitude. I suspect rather that our great-grandchildren, like our great-grandfathers and ourselves, will on the whole find some way to rock along in a social world that they correctly perceive to be chaotic, disordered, and functioning rather badly. New problems will have supplanted old ones, and their lives, like ours, will be caught up in the struggle to find consensus on the ways to cope with those new problems.

But it is certain that among the problems our children must face are those that have been the subject of this essay. Perhaps we could at this time take one step in the direction of making their lives somewhat more livable. Advances in medical technology, and the march of science in general, is shaking the underpinnings of society, and will do so to a greater degree in the future. Would it not be useful to bring into being now a major observation and study center devoted to the meteorology of scientific change? Such a center would be charged with the responsibility to detect scientific advances that bear the seeds of major social repercussions, to explore their potential and legal ramifications, to do what can be done to analyze the alternative social responses that are available, and to conduct a continuing program of education for intellectuals, legislators, judges, and the public in general so that society may at least be forewarned of the tidal waves that will next engulf it. We have come to view as indispensable the intelligence flow from our worldwide system of weather posts, of earthquake observatories, and of cosmic radiation stations. Does not mankind deserve at least equivalent advance notice of the social typhoons being generated in the world's laboratories?

14

Economic and Social Costs of Death

Richard M. Bailey

MEDICINE, AS A PROFESSION, has traditionally resisted efforts to relate death and conditions of illness to economic factors. Perhaps there have been good reasons for such a professional stance, since physicians typically have had more than enough to do caring for the ill without becoming embroiled in economic issues with which they had little familiarity.

Today, however, physicians are being forced to recognize the impact that our economic system has upon the organization, delivery, and allocation of health services. To force controversy to the surface, one need only raise the question of why we devote so many of society's scarce resources to the perpetuation of the lives of a few people —often with doubtful prospects of success—and, in this process, preempt the use of these resources for the prevention of premature death or disability of many others.

Such questioning of the present allocation of medical resources is not apt to be popular either with physicians or patients for, in essence, it shakes the foundations upon which the medical profession was conceived and upon which it has evolved in our society. Yet this question of resource allocation is a vital issue for our age, enraptured by the increasing possibilities of extending life through organ transplants, electronic heart pacemakers, and other technological devices.

Several issues subsidiary to the central theme of the paper must be discussed. We must (1) examine the factors responsible for the overall orientation of our health personnel and institutions to the production of high cost, curative services; (2) question the current relevance of many traditions perpetuated by practicing physicians and by our medical schools; (3) specify how economists should attempt to measure the economic costs of death and, the other side of the coin, the economic value of life, and (4) consider how government (and others) may effect a reallocation of health resources using criteria that emphasize the most good health for the most people.

All of these issues are here framed in the analytical viewpoint of the economist; this creates a problem in itself both because of the assumptions that must be used and because of the distinct distrust many physicians and other social scientists feel for the ability of the economist to speak to such social issues. Despite this burden of credibility, we will proceed, not, we hope, as a fool walking where angels fear to tread, but as a concerned observer who is distressed by the reluctance of so many to raise the gut issues surrounding the topics of death and dying. We recognize that not all of the issues are economic and, hence, cannot be resolved by economic analysis alone. But many issues can only be examined in their total perspective by introducing a number of economic concepts and measures.

The Economist's Value Measurement Dilemma

There are at least two issues that must be faced squarely when an economist becomes embroiled in discussions of the economic costs of death. The first issue revolves around the question: What economic value does an individual place on his own life? The second issue concerns the value that society may place on the lives of its members either directly—in the sense of making expenditures to prevent premature death of specific individuals—or collectively—in the sense of financing projects or programs reducing the statistical probabilities of death for groups of persons but in ways not aimed at saving the lives of particular individuals (Chase, 1968:15).

A favorite tenet of economists is that man is rational. Given a high degree of freedom to make personal choices in a capitalist economy such as the United States, the individual can choose among many alternative goods, services, occupations, and leisure time activities that

Economic and Social Costs of Death [277

differ greatly in the degree of risk to the purchaser or participant. Some persons may express a preference for "risk-taking"; others for "risk-avoidance" (Friedman and Savage, 1962:297–298).

When we observe the many ways that individuals evaluate their own lives, we are struck with a wide spectrum of behavior. Some truly seem to be risk-takers. Individuals purchase and use many dangerous products: LSD, cigarets, lead-based paints, guns. At one time or another, many of us engage in dangerous activities—football, automobile or motorcycle racing, skiing, hunting. In these, the consumer or participant is generally aware of potential danger. Yet he perseveres. In doing so, he exhibits clearly that self-preservation is not the ultimate aim of his life. After all, life is to be lived, not sheltered. Hence, we all accept trade-offs between danger and longevity just as we continually make decisions between current versus future pleasure. But some are more willing to incur risks than others.

It is clear that the value that any person places on his own life cannot be adequately reflected by his purchases of life insurance; there is no possible way the purchaser can benefit from the proceeds of the policy. What the person loses at death is impossible to define, but there is abundant evidence to indicate that the loss may be considerable by virtue of the effort and personal expenditure one is willing to make to avoid it. As Schelling (1968:132) has noted: "If we ask, who is willing to make an economic sacrifice to prevent a death, in most societies there is at least one unequivocal answer: the person who is to die."

When we consider death in this personal context, there are good reasons for classifying those expenditures made by an individual to avoid death as purely consumptive in nature. If one believes in the principle of consumer sovereignty, expenditures that individuals make to purchase a reduced probability of death may serve as a first approximation of the value they place on their lives. Of course, it may be difficult for the individual to make such decisions because the information that he might require to be rational in such matters is unavailable—or at least so costly to obtain that for all intents and purposes it is unavailable.

The expenditures that individuals make to avoid death can be of many types. Some economists have preferred to restrict the expenditures largely to the purchase of medical care services. By so doing, they are able to argue that government has little reason to think of medical care services as being different from other goods and services; hence, there is no need for national health insurance systems or compulsory national health insurance (Lees, 1961). But it is also obvious that even in the setting of strictly private market transactions, individual purchases of seat belts for automobiles and construction of storm cellars in the tornado belt or retaining walls in landslide areas can be viewed as decisions explicitly or implicitly including an element of reduced probability of premature death. If freedom of consumer choice is valued as an end in itself, we should be willing to concede that these options for purchase decisions should be preserved as a province of individual consumer action.

Opinions vary widely on the degree to which individuals must fully bear the costs of risks that they knowingly incur or the extent to which society, in some sense, has the responsibility of sharing such costs. If a "risk-taker" becomes involved in a situation where expensive medical services may be required in order to prevent death, these questions must be faced:

1. Why should society (government) bear all or share part of these costs?
2. Why should those persons who contribute to private insurance funds share these costs? Why shouldn't "risk-takers" be required to pay above-normal insurance premiums because they are admittedly in a high-risk group? (An analogy may be found in the automobile insurance field where accident-prone drivers are considered insurable but must pay very high premiums reflecting their poor driving experience.) Why shouldn't sound principles of insurance be applied in the health field as in other areas of life where people desire to insure themselves against risk?
3. What is so sacrosanct about health services that makes us, as a nation, feel that premiums for insurance against expensive hospital treatment should be computed on a community basis (Blue Cross) rather than on a risk-group basis (the typical commercial health insurer)?

Economic and Social Costs of Death [279

Another significant issue for those concerned with how society allocates its scarce resources is: How does society place a value on the lives of its members? This issue has been part of a larger debate raging among welfare economists for several years; when we talk about how society places a value on a life, we come terribly close to implying that there exists a commonly accepted social welfare function.

Arrow (1951), in a classic work discussing the derivation of a social welfare function, has concluded that this is almost impossible to construct. The problem, simply stated, is that society is perpetually torn by conflicting objectives. On the one hand, we value individual decision-making highly and typically conceive of the market mechanism as being the means by which individual choices can be most adequately expressed. But, for society to exist, it is also necessary that some decisions be made collectively. It is at this point that problems multiply rapidly because we do not have a political marketplace that is sufficiently sensitive either in timing or in response to the "votes" (choices) of the public-at-large to enable us to determine a socially optimum decision (Downs, 1957 and 1962). Quoting Arrow (1951: 462), "We must look at the entire system of values, including values about values, in seeking for a truly general theory of social welfare." Since the market mechanism is able only to measure the economic value that individuals place on specific goods and services, economists are at a real disadvantage in their efforts to discuss the aim of society as it relates, say, to valuing human life.

Measurement of Individual's Value to Society

These caveats notwithstanding, many man-years of economists' thinking have been devoted to the theoretical development and measurement of this elusive social welfare function. The use of a social welfare function is frequently described as society's attempt to maximize the utility derived from the use of its resources, subject to whatever constraints environment may impose upon the society. Thus, we find many economic analyses directed to consideration of alternative expenditure decisions (implying use of resources) with the objective of finding *the* alternative that maximizes society's well being. The general conclusion is: (a) as regards purely private goods and services, social welfare is maximized by unlimited free choice by individuals subject to the income distribution that exists; but, (b) when we consider goods that are in a sense "public" and may require collective consumption, social welfare is maximized by obtaining the greatest benefit for a given level of expenditure.

How do we measure this benefit? Usually in the measure of value that economists are accustomed to: the dollar. In essence, dollar values have to be placed on the goods or services purchased and, as you can see, we have come full circle to Arrow's conclusion. We are back to saying that someone first has to place a value (other than but including economic value) on something in order for it to be measured. But when someone does this, we are not able to say that his values reflect the values of society at large. There is no way to determine society's values! Joan Robinson (1964:14) states this issue succinctly when she says, "It is not possible to describe a *system* without moral judgments creeping in. For to look at a system from the outside implies that it is not the only possible system; in describing it we compare it (openly or tacitly) with other actual or imagined systems. Differences imply choices, and choices imply judgment. We cannot escape from making judgments and the judgments that we make arise from the ethical preconceptions that have soaked into our view of life and are somehow imprinted on our brains."

Only if one assumes that there is an objective social good defined independently of individuals (by God, a dictator, or the like) can one state that there is *a* social welfare function. Regrettably, most economists like to sidestep this issue and don their hats as technicians setting forth to determine empirically the most efficient way to allocate resources. But the problem does not disappear that easily, for, as Oskar Morgenstern (1963) has titled one of his insightful articles, *Qui Numerare Incipit Errare Incipit* (He who begins to count, begins to err). Measuring without being extremely sensitive to the limitations on measurement lends an impression of precision to economics that more thoughtful economists eschew.

An underlying complication in the effort to measure the value of the lives of others to society is that economists deal in values that are determined in the marketplace—where goods and services are exchanged. But human life is no longer traded in the marketplace, so economists have no direct way to value life. Attempts to impute a value to life indirectly through marginal analysis of decisions which may affect life (the purchase of seat belts, storm cellars, or the like) are open to serious questions of validity because people are not buying and selling their own lives in these decisions. At best, they are attempting to reduce the statistical probability of premature death. Purchases of food, shelter, and other items needed to sustain life also would have to be included as proxy expenditures that reflect one's value of life, but efforts to allocate properly the portion of these expenditures that are "needed" as contrasted to "pleasureful" strain the imagination.

The most commonly accepted measure of the value that society can place on the lives of its members requires that economists consider persons in their roles as producers. In this way, economists can discuss the economic consequences of the curtailment or prolongation of life. Human life can be viewed as an investment: production by the person that exceeds total investment yields a net contribution to society while anything short of the investment becomes a drain. To the economist qua economist (perhaps I should say, the laissez-faire economist), human life has economic value only as a function of its ability to produce goods and services that are demanded by others. The reasoning underlying this arbitrary measure is applied to material goods as well. It is based on a fundamental proposition of economics that credits the marketplace with the ability adequately to reflect the relative value that people place on various goods and services. Thus, the price that a consumer is willing to pay for a particular good or service is viewed as a proxy measure of its value to him: If the price were to rise, he might refuse to buy it because it is not "worth that much"; if the price were lowered, he might buy more of it—or he might buy the same quantity and use the dollars saved to buy something else.

Just as the consumer is deemed sovereign in the marketplace, economic theory views the price that the producer will pay for labor or material goods as a proper reflection of their value. Thus, the price of labor services appears to be directly determined by the producer— Marx even went so far as to describe labor as a commodity to be bought and sold by capitalist owners. But, on deeper examination, one finds that the price of labor services is ultimately determined by consumers in the marketplace. If the final product or service offered for sale is in great demand, the price may rise and the various factors of production (both human and physical) may demand and receive higher payments for their inputs. Conversely, if the final product is not demanded by consumers at the going market price, the producer will find it impossible to pay as much as in the past to either labor or other resources—their value falls.

Although this discussion is elementary, it is important to emphasize these economic theories. They are basic to everything that follows. Children have economic value only as future producers. Society makes an investment in children with the expectation of future payoff. (Payoff is defined as production in excess of consumption: netting a return on the investment.) Thus, in an advanced economy like ours, the economist supports many private and public expenditure programs that not only feed and maintain the health of children so that they will reach adult ages, but also large educational programs that will raise their level of skill and hence their future value as producers.

At the other end of the age spectrum, we have the elderly. Both in terms of law and physiological status, most people in our society are viewed as unemployable after 65 years of age. Their value as producers drops to zero. In perspective, we interpret the life cycle as:

1. Youth, a period in which consumption exceeds production and society makes an investment in the child with the expectation that not only will he become self-supporting in the future but will return to society some surplus of production—a form of payoff justifying the investment made in him during childhood.
2. The adult years—21 to 65—during which the person is actively engaged in one or more forms of productive work. During this period, the individual usually produces considerably more than is required to maintain his own well-being: He produces (earns, if you will, for this is how his value is measured) in excess of his own needs and the residual is used to support others (his family, directly; others in society, indirectly, through the payment of taxes, part of which are used, in turn, to support those incapable of earning their own living).
3. The elderly, who again return to the status of the child where consumption continues but production ceases.

Economic and Social Costs of Death [283

But there is a crucial difference between the elderly and the child: With the elderly there is no prospect of being able to produce in the future; no way of justifying economically the investment of resources in humans whose present and expected future economic value is zero (or negative). Just as physical capital is viewed as having a limited life and is destined for the scrap heap when its value in production becomes zero, so also does human capital depreciate to the point where it can no longer be supported on economic grounds. Here, the economist must give way to a value system that looks at life with different criteria.

Several important points must be considered when we speak of death, particularly in relation to age and economic and social position. Age, alone, is especially significant; a person dying in his 20's, 30's, or 40's has embodied within him a substantial amount of capital investment made by his family and society. Economic valuations of such persons tend, therefore, to be high and expenditures made on their behalf either by the individual or society to reduce the probability of premature death are likely to have a high payoff (Weisbrod, 1961). In many respects, society acts quite rationally in providing health services for this age group through company-paid fringe benefits. Of course, society also exhibits just the contrary behavior in its willingness freely to expend the lives of its young men in wars.

It is also apparent that there is a difference in the magnitude of the loss that society bears in the deaths of specific individuals. Consider, for example, the relative loss to society through the death of a 35-year-old unemployed coal miner versus the death of a 35-year-old president of an expanding electronics firm. The issue raised here is one of externalities: What are the relative losses to the community that result from each of these deaths? The medical profession has been faced with this problem increasingly in the last few years, especially in terms of assigning patients to renal dialysis machines (Haviland, 1965).

Demand and Supply in the Health Services Industry

For a variety of reasons, economists long have neglected analyses of the health services industry. One of the major reasons has been the belief that the industry is organized largely around nonprofit institutions and, as a result, is not readily susceptible to economic analysis. This is not true. Many branches and components of the health services industry are profit-motivated. Further, as more mechanisms and procedures are established in our society to enable greater numbers of people to obtain health services—and to subsidize through public funds certain types of medical care—the profit incentive is being used increasingly as a means of inducing change and new productive efforts. For example, within the last decade the availability of more public and private funds to pay for hospital care has resulted in a rapid growth in numbers of hospital-based medical specialists and a sharp increase in the use of hospitals. As the health care industry becomes increasingly like other industries in response to market demand, it should be expected that economic incentives and profit-making institutions will assume an even larger role in the production of health services.

Although physicians have been reluctant to look at their professional activities in purely economic terms, a good case can be made for this approach. When one considers medical services in this light, he observes that the behavior of the health services industry is not too different from the behavior of industry in general.

First, the industry has been much more demand-oriented than need-oriented. In other words, the purchase of medical services has been oriented along the traditional lines of a market economy where the producers play a largely passive role of waiting for the consumers to present themselves (to express effective demand) and then they begin to organize the inputs needed to conduct proper treatment. The kind of demand expressed has been predominantly for curative services. Even more significantly, those services that have been accorded the highest priority are naturally the ones to prevent death or severe, permanent disability.

Second, because the medical profession has maintained a posture of strongly believing in a free enterprise approach as regards the production of medical services, the majority of all health professionals, care institutions, educational institutions, and insurance companies are oriented *only* to the production of curative services—treatment of the individual patient in a highly individualistic manner! The profession has accepted as its objectives the fulfillment of those demands that are expressed in the marketplace, nothing more.

My personal preference for analyzing consumer demands for medical services is to divide these demands into three types: (1) the immediate demand for services to prevent death or serious disability (life-or-death situations); (2) the demand for services to alleviate pain where the problem may be relatively minor (caused either by accident, short-term acute illness, or a chronic condition), and (3) the demand for health services in the absence of symptoms of illness (Bailey, 1969). The first two types of services are of a curative nature; the third, preventive. Since physicians are educated not only in the basic sciences and techniques of diagnosing and treating illness but also, presumably, in an epidemiological approach to disease, it seems strange to the casual observer that medical practice is so inclined to the production of care services that often fall in a "too little and too late" category. In essence, this means that medical services directed to forestalling or detecting and resolving health problems at early stages of development have been neglected—health services that might, in the long run, preclude the need for expensive curative services later in the individual's life.

Since the medical profession has held rigorously to its position that the free enterprise practice of medicine can solve all problems of meeting health care needs, we find that high-cost, curative medicine is the norm—it is *the* American system of health care. As a result, hospitals are equipped with expensive equipment that is used infrequently; medical centers teach future physicians more about the diagnosis and treatment of complex, unusual diseases than how to produce those services most frequently required on an efficient, low-cost basis; organ transplants and other heroic ventures to save the lives of a few are heralded far more than efforts to insure that medical services are distributed fairly equitably in geographic terms.

The health care system is designed to provide many services for the "really sick" individual, but pays little attention to the basic health problems of society. Often, no costs are spared to prevent the death of one person (in part this occurs because our financial mechanisms for subsidizing such treatment are biased in this direction). Conversely, few funds are available for attacking the problem of how best to prevent diseases from becoming far advanced. This subject appears to be one which physicians have avoided traditionally other than on a disease-by-disease basis. One noteworthy study dealing with the overall issue of planning for health has recently been completed (Blum, 1968). A strong case can be (and has been) made to support the proposition that the production of medical services should remain in the private sector in order to achieve the benefits of production efficiency and variety of service offerings that should be available to consumers in an economy such as ours. Medical resources, like all resources, are limited both as to quality and quantity. To expect that everyone can have equal access to all the medical services that he might wish to consume at no cost is a dream. But it is one thing to argue about how the production of medical services will be organized and where economic incentives will be used to encourage production; it is another matter to ask the question if the "right" medical services are even being produced, given such heavy reliance on the marketplace.

Thoughts about what might be possible if medical services were produced somewhat differently are more likely to be frightening than challenging to physicians. Their economic self-interest and continuous focus upon *individual* human beings makes it comfortable for them to conceive only of doing more of what is presently being done. Physicians rarely raise the big question of how the health of mankind might be better served, disregarding any constraints of how medicine has been or should be practiced. (Witness the debate on health care for the aged.)

Health Services as an Investment

It is apparent that the normal workings of the medical marketplace have carried the inference that medical services are basically consumption goods. Lees (1961:19–21) has probably presented the most cogent case for this view. But I submit that his view is extremely narrow, and should like to expand upon this point.

First, it is probably quite true that many of the *curative* medical services purchased directly by individuals or provided by various governmental or philanthropic organizations can be classified as consumption goods. When such is the case, there are legitimate grounds for questioning whether society should "promote" the use of more medical services. In a sense, we may agree with conservative medical spokesmen who fall back upon the rationing apparatus of the market and the philosophy that only he who is willing to pay should get these medical services.

But there is another side to this story that also deserves telling. It is based on a section of the theory of welfare economics arguing that government may quite properly inject itself into so-called provinces of the private sector under at least three conditions:

1. To produce a good or service where the market cannot be expected to perform adequately. Such goods or services are referred to as "pure public goods" and include such activities as national defense and atomic energy development, police and fire protection, or the like. The reasoning behind public production of these services is that if each individual had to buy them, many individuals would attempt to avoid paying their fair share of the cost while at the same time receiving benefits paid for by others. (Those side benefits made available to others are called "externalities.") Moreover, even if each person willingly paid for his share of the expense, market demand could hardly be expected to lead producers to produce a balanced mixture of goods and services—everyone might want to have their dollars go for the purchase of machine guns; no one might like to see his dollars buy poisonous gases for use in chemical warfare. Thus, government acts for the public as a whole buying or producing what is deemed necessary because the market is inadequate to carry out its normal allocative functions.

2. To purchase certain goods and services where it is believed that the market could work but probably inadequately or only part of the time. These goods are often called quasi-public goods. Examples are education, highways, postal service, research, and so on, where a variety of different governmental policies exist. In some cases, government runs systems—education, for example—that are competitive with private enterprise; in other cases, government purchases goods or services from the private sector but owns and operates them—for example, highways and some research activities; in other cases, the government produces the services even though they might be produced under contract by private parties—postal service and some research activities to name two. In all of these examples, there is the presence of externalities—if the goods or services were sold only in the marketplace an underconsumption or underinvestment in the areas might occur (research) or someone would be getting benefits without paying part of the cost (education).

3. To correct some of the grossest inequalities of income distribu-

tion. It was mentioned earlier that people in our economy reap economic rewards largely as the result of producing goods or services that are valued by others. (Some of these rewards are the result of good fortune; some arise from hard work; others come from finding and exploiting a monopoly situation.) If consumers value a product highly—even something as simple as an electric knife—huge profits may be made by the owner-producer. Other services, which may appear to have great intrinsic or long-run value, may not be treated well in the marketplace—school teachers, for example. By and large, we accept these differences in income as being normal. But society is increasingly aware of the fact that some people are exploited in the marketplace, and, strive as they will, they cannot earn enough for a decent living. Others, because of illness or old age, are also frequently unable to earn a bare subsistence. Government intervenes in these circumstances and through use of taxes and subsidies redistributes income from the more well-to-do to the poor.

With passage of the 1965 Amendments to the Social Security Act, government announced that access to medical services is a right and not a privilege. Placing such an objective in an economic context gives one an appreciation of how fundamental a change is occurring. In the past, access to medical care services has been a privilege: Those who could afford to purchase the services and valued them above other goods and services mainly were the ones to receive the services. Treating medical care as a privilege was quite compatible with allowing market transactions to determine the proper balance between supply and demand in this industry.

Once one states that medical care is now a right—a term meaning that care should be available even if one cannot pay for it—the whole structure and operation of the health care industry becomes subject to scrutiny. Can the industry really deliver the services that may be demanded by those previously unserved? Is the existing mixture of services produced in response to free market demand the same services that may be rational under this new objective?

Will government as a consumer be willing to pay for services devoid of preventive measures and replete with frills irrelevant to mass health? Can an industry that has many monopolistic elements meet the new demands that are expected to be generated without further

Economic and Social Costs of Death [289

governmental regulation and control; for example, may we not have to treat the health care industry as a giant public utility and regulate prices to be charged, quantity of output to be produced, and so on. Will government have to take over much or all of the production of health services because the market cannot respond adequately? In summary, stating that medical care is a right, not a privilege, implies that we are not just moving from the eighth into the ninth inning; we have an entirely new ball game!

Government, having made the promise that all people should have a right to medical services, has had to consider how it can accomplish the task. By analyzing the demand characteristics for medical services, government has correctly concluded that making all services free would probably create more problems than it would solve. After all, the words "access" and "right" do not necessarily mean free—at least, not free to everyone. On the other hand, the word "right" implies that even the poorest person should have opportunity for medical care of good quality and should have some choice as to where and from whom he will seek care.

Cost-Benefit Analysis in Health Resource Allocation

In spite of the difficulties mentioned earlier in finding a social welfare function that can adequately represent society's values, it is now time to mention just what economists have been trying to do in the way of applying these concepts in a limited manner in the health field. The term generally applied to such activities is cost-benefit analysis.

There have been relatively few cost-benefit studies conducted in the health field encompassing all of the points that an economic theorist would expect from such analyses. Since a number of recent analyses are purported to be of the cost-benefit type but have not approached this ideal, let us consider some of the essential ingredients of cost-benefit studies so that we may differentiate them from other similar but not-so-comprehensive analytical efforts.

Before we define explicitly what should be measured, a word must be said about two important issues in any cost-benefit study. These are the issues of efficiency and equity. Efficiency, used in the context of welfare economics, is concerned with obtaining the maximum value of output given the use of one or more inputs. Specifically, optimizing efficiency in the economy means that resources are used in their most highly valued way—letting the market price of goods and services serve largely as a proxy for value. Most of the time, economists focus only on the issue of efficiency—how to get the greatest output with the least input. But the other issue that needs to be raised is that of equity—the issue of who receives the benefits and who pays the costs. As you may guess, advocates of efficiency are often in conflict with advocates of equity.

Attempts to measure costs and benefits must include efforts to estimate all of the relevant effects of a given action. These economic costs are described as direct costs and benefits and indirect costs and benefits. Direct costs and direct benefits are usually labeled as explicit and can be traced quite easily. Indirect costs and benefits are called implicit—they include effects that are felt by the person involved, other persons, and involve some consideration of the incidence or distribution of costs or benefits among various groups. In many instances, problems arise in differentiating costs from benefits. In the health field, future costs avoided are often regarded as benefits. We will generally follow this pattern of distinction in this paper.

In the case of health services purchased to avoid death we would classify costs and benefits as follows:

1. Direct costs—those expenditures made to purchase health services.
2. Indirect costs:
   (a) The loss of earnings of those who die prematurely.
   (To calculate these earnings, we generally assume that the economy is functioning at full employment. We also estimate the average length of working life of the persons, their earning capacity, etc.) (This could be the same figure as in 3 below.)
   (b) Subsidized care—cost paid by others over and above payments made by the individual and which may not show up in direct expenditures.
3. Direct benefits—earnings of the individual made possible by avoiding premature death. (This figure could be the same as in 2(a) above.)
4. Indirect benefits—the increased production of co-workers made possible because of the avoidance of death of the ill person.

Economic and Social Costs of Death

The Direct Costs of Death As cited earlier, it will be best to consider the direct costs of death in two ways: the cost to the individual and the cost to society. Burial costs are not considered as a direct cost of death in our analysis—they are bound to occur to everyone, sometime. Our focus is on the costs of medical care preceding death. In direct costs of death to the individual, the economist includes those payments for medical care associated with a terminal illness or accident as separate from costs of care incurred in connection with medical problems that do not result in death. Accordingly, if through an accident, heart attack, suicide, or the like, instantaneous death occurs, we would say that there has been no direct economic cost to the individual (or to his survivors). From an economist's point of view, death that comes quickly is preferred over a lingering terminal illness because direct costs are reduced.

In contrast to the relatively few cases of instantaneous death, we see many instances in which death is preceded by a lingering illness or a period of hospitalization following an accident or severe, short-term illness. In these cases, various medical resources may be employed to treat the acutely ill person, frequently at high cost to the individual. Emergency medical services received often are very expensive because they include twenty-four-hour observation by trained nurses, ambulance services, the use of intricate equipment and facilities, and the services of highly specialized physicians.

For a moment, let us examine why these medical resources are necessarily expensive. One of the underlying reasons for the high cost of short-term emergency medical services is related to timing. For instance, it is commonly accepted that the large supermarket can sell many of its items at a lower-per-unit price than the small corner "mom-and-pop" delicatessen because of higher sales volume. What is not often recognized is that the higher volume/lower-per-unit price also is made possible because the sales are spread over a considerably shorter period of time. After all, time is valuable. If a productive factor can be employed full-time (at capacity), it can usually produce its output at a lower-per-unit cost than if it occurs intermittently.

If the productive factor has economic value, it will have a going price. The ambulance driver expects to earn $120 per week regardless of how many trips to and from the hospital he makes. The nurse, the laboratory technician, even the neurosurgeon, have similar expectations of a satisfactory income. The analogy applies also to material factors of production. In a similar vein, the hospital administrator has an expectation of the revenue to be earned from use of the ambulance, the operating room, and the intensive care ward. All of these productive factors have costs; the prices attached to their use is accordingly a function of how frequently they are used and how long they may reasonably be expected to yield valued services before wearing out.

Indirect Costs of Death Before we consider indirect costs (sometimes classified as benefits), some assumptions and ground rules need to be stated. The first assumption is that society desires to make the best possible use of its resources. This means that the return on society's investment in resources allocated to health should exceed, or at least be equal to, the return received on investments in other sectors. From the viewpoint of society, there are trade-offs between the use of resources to produce health services and the use of these same resources to produce other goods and services. Faced with the alternative of using scarce resources to produce a medical product or some nonmedical product, the benefits from both alternatives must be weighed.

Second, it is assumed that all resources can be given a dollar value. This assumption is always challenged by non-economists as being unrealistic, inhuman, and the like. The counter agreement is that this is a reasonable assumption because: (1) All resources are limited (we are even beginning to recognize that air, always previously considered as a free good in abundant supply, is now frequently viewed as a scarce good both in certain cities and throughout the world). (2) The use of a resource in one way (for example, air combined with gasoline in the carburetor of an automobile) deprives us from using the resource in other ways. (3) In our economy, the more highly valued use of the resource generally holds sway; for example, we continue to use the air to make our private automobiles operate because there still seems to be enough oxygen content to support human life and thus we place a high value on the use of air to support combustion. But, when we reach the point when our choice is narrowed to the option of air to help power automobiles or to sustain life, there is good reason to believe that we will recognize life as being the more valued of the two.

Economic and Social Costs of Death

Some may contend that placing a dollar value on human life is unthinkable—especially when doing so creates a bias against an entire age group: those 65 and over. But it bears repeating that society often seems to value life more than do the individuals whose lives are at stake. Conversely, at times society appears to treat individual lives quite callously and it then remains for the individual to declare his opposition to such circumstances (as in the case of the current anti-Vietnam conscientious objectors). It is also clear that neither society nor the individual always values life above other things. For example, we do not insist that every product offered for sale be absolutely safe: food poisoning still occurs, brakes and other safety devices on automobiles are often defective, and so on.

Just as we do not insist that all commercial products be safe, we find that few "public goods" have an overriding concern with the value of life. Practically every community has its deadly highway intersection, yet it is not eliminated. Government regulates many forms of transportation but overtly ignores hazardous conditions in the control of air space and detailed inspection of equipment used by all carriers.

The point is: Society does place a dollar value on life in a multitude of ways each and every day! True, many such decisions are subconscious and hence permit us to avoid the issue. In economic terms, we can say that the marginal cost of *complete* safety is excessive. Insistence on applying such a criterion would drive the cost of most goods and services beyond the point of feasible economic use. Hence, we accept a trade-off. We hope that drivers will approach the dangerous intersection more carefully if we place signs nearby letting them know how many have died there previously. Such risks are incurred because of the high cost of safety.

It is evident that society has considerable concern for the future. In fact, the time horizon of society is generally longer than that of the individual for obvious reasons of relative perpetuity. Thus, we find society making investments in its members as a means of achieving its long-run ends. In the process, it often uses a social rate of discount considerably below the private rate of discount—another indication that society values the long-run more than the private sector. Though most of these ends of society are continually in the process of being redefined, one underlying goal seems to be the attainment of a more prosperous, comfortable, growing economy. Taking this goal as a reasonable end, we can understand why valuing lives as investments may be seen as contributing to this long-run economic growth goal. Finally, since our concern is with national objectives, both direct and indirect cost and benefits must be calculated. Inasmuch as we are using dollars as acceptable for the purposes of determining the relative value of different resource allocations, the data base for making calculations should be the national income accounting system.

Costs and Benefits Not Usually Measured There are a number of costs or benefits that typically are not measured in a formal cost-benefit analysis. The explanation for such omissions is based on two points: (1) the objective is to focus on the efficient use of society's resources with an overall view; hence we cannot include all of the details that might be relevant to someone who had a different analytical objective in mind; and, (2) there is no method yet existing to measure such intrinsic values as the quality of the healthy life. So, we have the following types of costs or benefits that are not usually measured in a cost-benefit study:

1. Direct costs:
   (a) Borne by the institutions involved in providing care.
   (b) The numbers and types of personnel involved in providing health services and their cost and period of involvement.
   (c) The institutional use of facilities and timing of use.
   (d) The burden placed upon the family in times of stress, reduced consumption, etc.

2. Indirect costs:
   (a) Time devoted by family and others (free) to assist the ill person.
   (b) Possible need for children to quit school and go to work to support the family resulting in a reduction in the opportunity for the child to achieve his potential.

3. Direct benefits:
   (a) Increase in overall production (both that at work and at home) resulting from avoidance of death or prolonged illness.
   (b) Number of years added to life (working and total).

(c) Opportunity to reach one's capacity as a worker and an individual.
(d) Effect upon the quality of life of the individual and his family.

4. Indirect benefits:
   (a) Better level of living that a worker can provide his family because of being employed than would be the case if forced to be on welfare due to illness.
   (b) Avoidance of the social stigma of "being on welfare."
   (c) Effect upon the community of better outlook of the individual and his family toward life.

Implications of Using Only Those Costs and Benefits That Are Typically Measured Since certain costs and benefits are excluded from measurement—and since the conceptual base of our national income accounting system is used as a determinant of dollar values to be assigned in various cases—a number of biases are likely to be present in any cost-benefit study. These biases should be explicitly recognized not for the purpose of criticizing the entire analytical concept but for noting where strengths and weaknesses exist. In other words, cost-benefit analyses have limitations that are based in part on the way data are gathered and used. By understanding the problems involved, some changes may be introduced in future analyses and/or we may be given the incentive to develop better analytical tools. These are some of the data constraints and resulting implications that follow from their use in the typical cost-benefit analysis:

1. We are forced to count as output a number of factors that often are referred to as inputs by health personnel, for example:
   (a) Expenditures for hospital care are considered to be representative of the dollar value of the output of hospital services even though these services might also be thought of as an input to the patient which, combined with other things, enables him to recover from his illness.
   (b) Physician's services are represented by measures of gross expenditures (payments) to physicians—if the physician is not

paid, no value is inferred; if he receives high pay, the implication is that the services have high value.

2. Given the conceptual base of the national income accounts, the following measures are adopted:
   (a) The value of housewives' services are counted as zero (services are assigned values based upon what they are "worth" in the marketplace. Since housewives fulfill a number of roles (more than domestic servants), there is no generally accepted way to value their services. (Sometimes housewives are imputed to be worth the wages of domestic servants—with apologies.)
   (b) Working women are valued less than working men because their earnings are lower.
   (c) The elderly (past 65) have no implied economic value because they are beyond their productive years by definition.
   (d) Youngsters contracting serious illnesses might have negative economic value if their long-run consumption costs exceed their future potential value as producers.
   (e) The poorly educated would be valued less than others; so also would Negroes and other minority groups whose lifetime earnings are typically below average.

3. The logical outcome of applying these criteria strictly in a cost-benefit analysis would be:
   (a) To direct even more health resources to the care of those who are best able to pay for the services—for example, those who have higher earnings currently or whose potential earnings are high.
   (b) To reduce the quantity of government health services made available to the elderly, minority groups, incapacitated youngsters, etc., because their economic value is less than others.
   (c) In essence, there would be an emphasis upon shifting further from the poor to the affluent the already recognized maldistribution of health resources. Values assigned by market forces would have to be accepted as final; those persons that value health highly and can pay for health services would get

them; those who either do not value health highly or cannot pay for health services would be denied access.

(d) Using pure cost-benefit analyses, future allocations of public funds would probably be altered to: favor the young over the old; favor services provided in the short-run over research which is so difficult to justify on terms of payoff because there is so much uncertainty about its effectiveness; favor the educated over the uneducated; favor the rich over the poor; encourage treatment of acute illness and downgrade concern over chronic illness; stress preventive care for some age groups, disregard it for others; provide more funds for high income states and local areas, deny funds to the less affluent; encourage more private health outlays, reduce the share of total health expenditures made by government.

It is obvious that a literal application of cost-benefit analyses to various health programs would lead to their complete demise. Perhaps that would be good. But it should also be made clear that wholesale application of the cost-benefit tool to all health problems is patently wrong. If one does this, he is implying that the economic value system is paramount to all other values.

Probably what we need to recognize is that some public expenditures for health services may be justified on the basis of economic criteria (externalities, and so on), whereas others can only be supported on grounds of income redistribution—from the more wealthy to the poor. Medicare is an obvious example of the latter case. Nevertheless, at some point the question must be asked as to how far we can go in providing health services as a means of redistributing income in contrast to making long-run investments in younger people. For this reason and also because of the opportunity costs of using health resources in this fashion, we must return to the relevance of the cost-benefit tool in the health field. At the very least, using this tool raises some serious questions about the relative merit of certain approaches to health problems. Likewise, even if we decided that we would keep certain programs on humanitarian grounds, we would have some idea of how high an economic value we are placing on being humanitarians. The point is, let us not be afraid to conduct such analyses for fear that they may tell us something we do not want to hear. We need to be informed if we are to make wise decisions. Holding to criteria and analyses that emphasize economic efficiency is one way to develop insights into problems that should not be overlooked.

Recent HEW Disease Condition Studies

Some of the earliest analytical efforts of the Office of Program Analysis in the Department of Health, Education, and Welfare have resulted in several important studies that have been published within the last two or three years. It is hard to classify these studies as being of a true cost-benefit analysis type but they approximate it closely. Probably the most significant of these studies—because it developed the methodological and data framework upon which all later efforts have been built—was done by Dorothy Rice (1966). In her *Estimating the Cost of Illness,* a wealth of information is brought together on the annual cost to the nation associated with many major diseases and accidents. The costs that are measured are both direct (expenditures made for the purchase of health services) and indirect (earnings lost because of premature death or disability and lost production). Through such estimates of the total (direct plus indirect) cost of major illnesses, we are given a picture of the relative significance of different types of illness as they affect our economic well-being.

Following this study, several analyses of specific disease conditions were undertaken (cancer, heart, kidney, automobile accidents) to consider the costs of alternative approaches to treating the disease. However, it was soon recognized that the only alternative is not to consider various forms of treatment—it may be cheaper to prevent some disease or accidents than it is to effect a cure or partial rehabilitation. To be relevant, we are finding that a cost-benefit analysis of a disease must be based upon the prior careful work of the epidemiologist. The cost-benefit analyst then builds upon this information by assigning costs to the various interventions that are possible, estimates the dollar benefits to be gained (or costs saved) of each intervention, considers the sequence of timing of costs and benefits, and provides one with a set of data that may be evaluated in terms of relative medical and economic effectiveness.

As government has looked for a way to achieve adequate medical

Economic and Social Costs of Death [299

care as a human right, these analyses of the costs of illness and specific diseases are resulting in a broadening of focus for all parties concerned. The view that government has quite properly adopted is that too frequently we have regarded expenditures for medical services as being consumption goods exclusively; that is to say, medical services have primarily redounded to the benefit of the individual alone. But if one looks at people as being one of the most valuable resources of the nation, health services that result in a prolongation of productive life take on more and more of the characteristics of an investment good. Moreover, when government considers how it must meet the medical needs of the poor, it cannot help but become interested in the entire health care delivery system and how various interventions may or may not yield a payoff in terms of adding to the present or future productive capacity of our people. As the relative advantages or disadvantages of particular interventions become better specified, this knowledge will increasingly become the basis for planning and expenditure decisions.

The disease condition analyses mentioned above have been framed in the context of decision-making for an optional allocation of society's resources in the health field. Rather than calculate the dollar value of man-years saved by a certain medical procedure by specifically estimating the incomes of all the different persons involved, the average income for all persons of a specific age group is used. Thus, an argument often expressed by health professionals to the point that we should not try to value certain lives more highly than others is countered by the fact that we are only using average figures. If we were to use actual figures, the man with a low income would be valued less than the man with a high income. If one is really humanitarian, he should opt for using average income estimates in making analyses of the costs of illness. Using any other figure will create the same kind of bias in decision-making that we presently find all about us.

We are all too familiar with the growing level of expenditures for medical services. Annual outlays for the treatment of heart disease, cancer, mental disorders, and injuries run into billions of dollars. But when we look at expenditure data alone, we often miss the most significant costs—those of premature death or disability. In 1963, quoting from *Estimating the Cost of Illness* (Rice, 1966), morbidity losses caused by mental illness were twice as large as direct expenditures; premature mortality costs (lost years of working life) caused by heart disease were more than six times as large as costs of care; and morbidity and mortality losses associated with injuries were more than five times as great as direct medical expenditures for care and treatment.

As a nation, public expenditure decisions in the past have often been based upon the relative importance of problems as indicated by annual costs of direct care. Losses to the nation caused by morbidity and mortality have rarely been considered. Yet it is in these very areas of neglected measurement that cost-benefit analysis spotlights the problems because it includes *all* costs. In another context, these analyses may focus on new points of intervention in a given disease or accident area by indicating where trade-offs among research, prevention, and treatment may occur. As these analyses are completed and examined for accuracy and completeness, it is inevitable that priorities of public expenditures will be reoriented to the most important issues as seen from a societal point of view.

The analyses will undoubtedly also call into question many current treatment practices that are expensive (and whose cost must be covered by private insurance or public aid) but where the payoff in terms of numbers of lives saved per dollar expended are small. After all, we are making decisions each day that indirectly are leading to the death of others. When Blue Cross spends $28,000 to cover the cost of a single heart transplant operation—and the patient still dies—there is $28,000 less in their insurance fund to pay benefits to young women who need surgery for cancer or for children who need to have their tonsils removed. "There is no such thing as a free lunch" is an old saying; there is no such thing as using vast quantities of either public or private insurance funds to pay for very expensive treatment for a few patients without depleting the available resources that might be used for assisting many others to recover their health. But can we avoid placing a dollar value on life? No. And it is far better to do so explicitly than implicitly because when we follow the latter course, we may not even be aware of what we are doing.

As more of these disease condition analyses are accomplished and government uses this information to restructure interventions in the health care delivery system, it is to be expected that more private parties will become interested in the findings. It should not be anticipated that government actions alone will bring about the major changes in the orientation of physicians and health institutions that are contemplated. Rather, government actions in this field may be compared with government actions in the area of fiscal and monetary policy where they influence marginal changes and create a leverage effect which induces others to follow suit. In the process, it is expected that a new rationalization of the entire health care system will result.

REFERENCES

Arrow, Kenneth J.
  1951   Social Choice and Individual Values. New York: Wiley.
Bailey, Richard M.
  1969   "An economist's view of the health services industry." Inquiry (March):3–18.
Blum, Henrik L., and associates.
  1968   Notes on Comprehensive Planning for Health. San Francisco: Western Regional Office, American Public Health Association.
Chase, Samuel B., Jr.
  1968   Introduction and Summary in Problems in Public Expenditure Analysis. Washington, D.C.: The Brookings Institution.
Downs, Anthony.
  1957   An Economic Theory of Democracy. New York: Harper.
  1962   "An economic theory of political action in a democracy." In Landmarks in Political Economy, Vol. II. Chicago: Phoenix Books.
Friedman, Milton, and L. J. Savage.
  1962   "The utility analysis of choice involving risk." In Landmarks in Political Economy, Vol. II. Chicago: Phoenix Books.
Haviland, James W.
  1965   "Next step in meeting the nation's health goals." Bulletin of the New York Academy of Medicine (December):1255–1267.
Lees, D. S.
  1961   Health Through Choice. Hobart Paper #14. London: Institute of Economic Affairs.
Morgenstern, Oskar.
  1963   "Qui numerare incipit errare incipit." Fortune (October):142–181.
Rice, Dorothy P.
  1966   Estimating the Cost of Illness. Publication #947-6. Washington, D.C.: U.S. Public Health Service.
Robinson, Joan.
  1964   Economic Philosophy. Garden City, N.Y.: Anchor Books.

Schelling, T. C.
 1968 "The life you save may be your own." In Problems in Public Expenditure Analysis. Washington, D.C.: The Brookings Institution.
U.S. Department of Health, Education, and Welfare, Public Health Service.
 1966 Estimating the Cost of Illness. Health Economic Series #6. Washington, D.C.: Government Printing Office.
Weisbrod, Burton.
 1961 Economics of Public Health. Philadelphia: University of Pennsylvania Press.

CONCLUSION

Dying and Its Dilemmas as a Field of Research

Diana Crane

THERE SEEMS to be general agreement among the authors of this volume that the nature of dying has changed qualitatively in recent years because of advances in medical knowledge and technology. A shift in the statistical frequencies of deaths toward chronic disease has taken place. This, in conjunction with increases in the sophistication of treatments capable of prolonging life, has had the effect of lengthening the average amount of time that elapses between the onset of a fatal illness and the termination of life. As a result, problems of dying that always have existed have multiplied. This contrasts with the fact that American society in many ways has contained the impact of death by releasing the aged from active participation in occupational roles and in family roles before their deaths occur. Even deaths of young persons are not highly disruptive in a society such as ours, since, for the most part, occupational and even marital roles are interchangeable. Continual adjustment of social roles is expected and accepted in an era of geographical and social mobility. The dilemmas surrounding dying, however, are more difficult to resolve. As a result, dying frequently disrupts social relationships more severely than death.

The authors of this volume have been concerned with a number of issues related to the process of dying. They are aware of the steady improvement in medical technology for prolonging life and they are worried that at times lives are needlessly prolonged. Are bodies that are no longer sentient or, if sentient and racked by pain, kept alive too long? Some authors are concerned that, in the haste to obtain organs for transplants, lives will be terminated prematurely. Other authors point out that measures that could prolong life are frequently not used, either because the doctor is unable to diagnose his patient's illness correctly or because he sees other goals as being more important. Thus, while some authors are concerned about the consequences of decisions to prolong or terminate lives, others are interested in the process of decision-making itself: the difficulties involved in making such decisions and the ways in which nonmedical issues influence them.

Several authors point to the problems involved in interacting with dying patients. What should the doctor tell the patient? Why is it so difficult for doctors and relatives alike to speak frankly with dying patients? How does the dying patient himself respond to his situation? Finally, one or two authors allude to the fact that bereavement is a threat to life. Is the aftermath of a lengthy process of dying so stressful that the survivors are sometimes unable to make a satisfactory adjustment?

It appears, then, that in dying as a social process there are three sources of conflicts and dilemmas, each of a kind difficult to resolve: (1) decisions regarding the prolongation or termination of life; (2) interpersonal relationships involving dying persons; (3) adjustment to bereavement. The following pages discuss the difficulties involved in designing research related to these problems and review previous relevant research.

Decisions to Prolong or Terminate Life

The authors have asked whether decisions to prolong or terminate life are being made wisely. Such decisions are difficult to study systematically because they are extremely complex. First, it is difficult to isolate such decisions from many closely related decisions. Such decisions actually have several parts; these will be described shortly. Second, there are several sets of norms and values that can be used in making such decisions. Third, such decisions are made in various organizational contexts presumably affecting them in various ways. Finally, a variety of actors participate in making such decisions. Doctors

Dying and Its Dilemmas as Field of Research [305

and other medical personnel probably have the most influence but relatives and dying persons themselves are frequently involved.

Although the prolongation or termination of life is certainly a problem in medical care, it is essential to place it in the perspective of medical treatment generally. It is clear that this problem arises under rather special circumstances. In the deaths of many persons, the issue is never recognized. Decisions to prolong or terminate life must be seen as part of a process which involves at least two sets of stages: (1a) the perception that an individual's life is threatened; (1b) a decision to mobilize medical resources to withstand the threat; (2a) the perception that death is inevitable for a particular patient; (2b) a decision to attempt to prolong or to terminate life. These pairs may occur consecutively or separately.

It is obvious that many deaths occur before a threat to an individual's life has been perceived. They are accidental, sudden, and completely unexpected. Where a threat to life is perceived, it seems likely that the nature of the disease affects the character of the prognosis. For example, a patient suffering from heart disease may appear to require intensive care to save his life while the death of a cancer patient may seem inevitable. One patient is defined as dying, the other is not; yet both may die.

Whether medical resources are mobilized when a threat to life has been perceived probably depends upon the availability of such resources and the patient's ability to pay for them, by being sufficiently interesting from a medical point of view to influence the doctor's decision in his favor, or by having some special characteristic or combination of characteristics which endow him with social value. When death is perceived as inevitable, the patient has lost his social value (for reasons to be discussed later), but, under certain circumstances, attempts may be made to prolong his life. Here different qualities of the patient play a role such as his degree of sentience, his age (appropriateness of death for that person), and the extent to which social value can be restored to him through participation in a medical experiment.

Thus, the first part of each set is essentially a problem of prognosis. The questions require rephrasing. Given certain types of diseases, what types of prognoses tend to be made? How often is there disagreement among doctors regarding the prognosis and the appropriate treatment? How frequently do doctors fail to assess accurately the likelihood of death? (Duff and Hollingshead, 1968). What is the role of the following factors in such failures: (a) characteristics of different types of illnesses, (b) the organizational environment of the hospital, (c) the social background of the patient?

The second part of each set involves the allocation of medical resources. The pertinent questions are: How are medical resources allocated to patients whose lives are perceived as being endangered? How are resources allocated to patients for whom death is believed to be inevitable? How are decisions made to withdraw resources entirely? In the case of a patient with an illness extending over months or even years, attempts may be made to prolong life until the symptoms become very severe, at which point efforts to make the patient comfortable are likely to take precedence (Glaser and Strauss, 1965: 194–203). Efforts of the latter type include measures as drastic as surgery and may at times be interpreted by nurses and families as attempts to prolong life. If the patient deteriorates but continues to live although suffering considerably, the doctor may decide upon measures to terminate his life.

The issue of termination is cloudy. The prohibition against actively terminating a patient's life means that a doctor who believes that a patient's life should not be prolonged may wait for some event such as pneumonia to hasten the process of dying. Some doctors resort to "invisible acts" in which patients' lives are deliberately shortened by manipulating dosages of pain-killing drugs (Glaser and Strauss, 1965: 198). A similar effect can frequently be brought about by discontinuing measures that have been sustaining life by supplementing or replacing essential bodily functions. Obviously the legal sanctions against termination of life make it difficult to study it empirically.

Medical innovations should be examined separately. Are they allocated differently from routine medical resources? How explicit are the procedures used by hospitals for selecting recipients for innovational treatments? What are the social characteristics of patients who receive innovational treatments (a) under conditions of high risk and (b) under conditions of scarcity? The heart transplant operation is a high-risk innovational treatment. Kidney dialysis is a low-risk, high-cost treatment. In cases of innovational treatments requiring donors, how are donors selected when (a) donors have to be dead to contribute; (b) when living donors can contribute organs? These and other issues are discussed in reviews of particular types of innovations by Simmons and Simmons (1970) and Swazey and Fox (1970).

Norms and Values Concerning Treatment of the Dying

American culture contains various norms and values influencing the conduct of both medical personnel and laymen in their decisions regarding dying persons. While American culture has a fairly consistent attitude toward death, it does not have a unified viewpoint toward dying. The individual is faced not with a single set of normative prescriptions regarding the prolongation of life but with a number of inconsistent and contradictory orientations.

All of these views are found in Western culture but two of them are strongly linked to medical institutions. They are part of the medical ethos and describe ideal behavior, behavior doctors like to think is typical. The first involves *the sanctity of life*. It is often assumed that medical personnel attempt to prolong life as long as is medically possible. This norm is based on the belief in the sanctity of life which is strong in Western culture (Shils, 1967). This ideal has its source in Christian religion at least in part and stems from the belief that man's survival is part of God's design. Those who are irreversibly comatose or who have suffered severe brain damage are frequently exempted (Glaser and Strauss, 1968:105). The normative basis for these exceptions is probably to be found in the fact that only human life is considered sacred. We do not hesitate to destroy other forms of life if it suits our needs. When life continues after its peculiarly human qualities have been lost, it frequently but not always loses its sanctity.

The second norm stresses *humanitarianism*. Humanitarian norms prescribe the alleviation and prevention of suffering. Although both are part of the medical ethos, it is only recently that temporary and permanent relief of illness have begun to contradict each other in specific cases since life can now frequently be prolonged even though it entails unbearable suffering. The conflict is intensified by the fact that humanitarianism seems to have become steadily stronger in Western culture. As our experience of personal suffering decreases, our sensitivity to its occurrence in others appears to increase.

Neither of the medical norms are applied in all situations. A number of general social norms frequently take precedence over the two medical norms. The first is *social differentiation*. In all human societies, members are ranked according to certain characteristics. Certain classes of individuals are considered more important or valuable than others. A specific example can be observed in our attitude toward the appropriateness of death in particular types of cases. One of the clearest statements of norms regarding the appropriateness of death is that of Parsons and Lidz (1967). They point out that attitudes toward dying in our society differ depending upon whether the process occurs at the end or as a break in the life cycle. The first type of event is considered normal; the second is the object of vigorous intervention. Efforts to minimize this type of death are highly valued. Thus we react to a threat to the life of an individual with apathy or activism depending upon our assessment of the appropriateness of death for him.

The requirement of differential ranking of individuals interacts with that of *utilitarianism* in the allocation of scarce resources. There is a strong emphasis in our culture on a cost-benefit basis for such allocations. This norm is also applied to medical resources. To the extent that medical resources are scarce, those whom health professionals perceive as contributing more to the society are more likely to be the objects of heroic life-saving efforts. Attempts to prolong their lives sometimes may be continued beyond the point of effectiveness. Concomitantly, those who are perceived as deviant or marginal, such as drug addicts, chronic alcoholics, or prostitutes, are likely not to receive even the minimal attention that could prolong their lives (Sudnow, 1967). The same utilitarian approach prescribes the withholding of scarce medical resources from those whose lives are defined as beyond hope. In many cases, such resources are considered better spent on those whose lives can be saved.

American society places a high value on the advancement of scientific knowledge. Medical personnel sometimes make extraordinary efforts to prolong life not with the goal of actually saving lives but with the intention of learning something. Science is anti-humanitarian in the sense that scientists treat human beings not as individuals but as research subjects. It provides a context for decisions to prolong or terminate life not in accordance with the welfare of the patient but to suit the demands of a research design or to make it possible to try out

Dying and Its Dilemmas as Field of Research [309

a new medical technique. Glaser and Strauss (1968) describe cases of dying patients who were kept alive because they were subjects of research studies. If such patients are in pain, humanitarian values can conflict with the motivation of the doctor-scientist to complete his project.

Finally, personal goals can also influence decisions in this area. Sudnow (1967) has shown how residents' desires to advance their careers affect their decisions to prolong lives. The absence of third parties, such as relatives, facilitates such distortions of interest. When families are present, their emotional reactions to the dying process determine the amount of pressure that they exert in either direction. Desire to protect their emotional well-being can influence them to try to shorten the dying process while a sense of guilt toward the dying person may have the opposite effect.

The various sets of norms can be classified into two categories, those which are altruistic and those which are instrumental. Norms prescribing prolongation because life is sacred and those prescribing humanitarianism are altruistic in the sense that the welfare of the patient is the primary consideration. Utilitarian and scientific norms, and those requiring social differentiation, tend to be instrumental since the goals of an organization, institution (science), or society as a whole are placed ahead of the welfare of the individual patient. This distinction has been made in other settings (Blau, 1955; Caudhill, 1958). Behavior conforming to medical ethics tends to follow the altruistic rather than the instrumental norms. Which set of norms is actually followed in any particular case depends upon many factors: (1) characteristics of the patient (his age, social value, degree of consciousness, amount of suffering); (2) the presence or absence of family members and their ability to influence medical personnel, in turn often depending upon their social class background, on the one hand, and their emotional toughness under stress on the other; (3) the personal values of the physician; and (4) the organizational setting. This last is most likely to be the hospital or the family. Previous studies of the influence of organizational settings upon the development of and conformity to norms suggest that the setting is an extremely important factor in affecting this type of behavior (Carlin, 1966; Coleman, 1961). For example, Carlin showed that conformity to legal ethics was lower in less prestigious law firms. Is conformity to medical ethics lower in less prestigious hospitals?

Hospital Settings and Treatment of Dying Persons

It is likely that each hospital (or specialized units within large hospitals) has and fairly consistently follows a value system regarding the treatment of dying persons. The characteristics of the norms may vary depending upon the type of hospital, public or private, academic or nonacademic, religious or nonreligious. Private hospitals may be more likely to have norms favoring the prolongation of life due in part to the economic status of their patients, who can afford to pay for expensive treatment. The low economic status of patients of public hospitals favors the opposite type of norm in that setting. Hospitals affiliated with universities are likely to have a strong orientation toward medical research. Duff and Hollingshead (1968) have shown in their study of an academic hospital that patient care was secondary to the research interests of the staff. Glaser and Strauss (1965:201) found that greater efforts were made to prolong life in Jewish hospitals than in Catholic hospitals.

It would be of interest to examine the ways in which such norms develop and are reinforced in hospital settings. How much influence do directors of medical departments have in this respect? Does their tendency to recruit doctors who share similar values produce considerable consistency in the behavior of a hospital unit in this respect? To what extent do doctors influence each others' decisions by their comments and implied criticism? Glaser and Strauss indicate that such decisions were frequently the subject of considerable controversy in the hospitals studied. This implies that variations in the behavior of staff members occur It is possible that controversy develops when the behavior of one or a few doctors is contrary to the normative orientation of the group as a whole.

The Dying Patient and Decisions to Prolong or Terminate Life

The role of the patient in deciding to prolong or terminate his life is exceedingly constricted. One of the implications of the belief in the sanctity of life is the proscription against taking life (except in war), either one's own or that of another person. This denies the individual the right to exercise rational control over his own demise. However, sanctions against suicide, formerly extremely severe (Parsons and Lidz, 1967:162), are becoming milder. Attempted suicide is no longer a crime in England (Hinton, 1967:32–33). In the United States, it remains a crime in only a few states (Shneidman, 1963:41). A social movement has been trying unsuccessfully for decades to give the individual legal control over his own demise.

There is some evidence that people would prefer to control their mode of dying. When asked where and how and under what conditions they would prefer to die, people respond that they would prefer to die quickly, painlessly, and with as little fuss or inconvenience as possible (Fulton, 1965:81). This suggests that they would like to be able to maintain as much control as possible over their deaths. An additional finding that people say they would prefer to die in their own homes (Fulton, 1965:92) can also be interpreted in this manner.

Glaser and Strauss found some evidence that patients who realized that they were going to die wanted to get it over with quickly and tidily. While obviously a period of suffering is not desirable, an underlying motive is probably their response to their perceptions of their own loss of social value. It seems likely that the dying person does not feel he has the right to be a burden to others.

Cappon (1962), who questioned dying patients, other patients, psychiatric patients, and nonpatients, found that the majority of each group favored euthanasia. It was most favored by the dying patients. On the other hand the complexity of the problem is indicated by the fact that in the same study dying patients were less likely than healthy patients to want to be told whether they were going to die from their present condition (an illness or injury imagined by those who were well but real for the patients).

Attitudes toward suicide among the terminally ill reveal the normative conflicts in this area. Glaser and Strauss (1968:104) indicate that, while measures are usually taken to prevent such suicides, the patient's attitude toward his death sometimes influences the amount of effort the staff will make to save him. Shneidman (1963:35) found that although suicide by terminal cancer patients is often considered as justified and reasonable, when such suicides actually occur both family and hospital staff express guilt, surprise, and embarrassment.

These contradictory types of behavior reflect a norm in the process of changing. The proportion of suicides among terminal cancer patients is believed to be small (Shneidman, 1963), suggesting that taboos against it are still strong. Since many such suicides are carefully concealed, however, the phenomenon is difficult to measure. A careful inquiry might reveal that the proportion is higher than is generally realized. Stewart (1960) examined all suicides occurring in a town in England during a seven-year period. He found that only one-third had no organic disease; the remaining two-thirds had either severe hypertension or a wide variety of "painful, disabling, or fear-engendering diseases." The relationship between physical illness and suicide deserves further study. Can potential suicides among the physically ill be identified and, if so, could they be helped to make a satisfactory adjustment to their condition?*

There is also some evidence that the dying have more control over the timing of their natural deaths than is generally realized. Phillips, in an interesting study (1969), has shown that mortality rates decline prior to important social events, such as presidential elections, the Day of Atonement, and one's own birthday. A number of explanations for this effect have been suggested but Phillips has shown that the data are inconsistent with all interpretations except the one stating that the dying appear to be able to delay their deaths in order to experience important social occasions. Weisman and Hackett (1961) have described patients who correctly predicted their own deaths when medical personnel did not anticipate them. Beigler (1957) suggests that a patient's anxiety increases prior to death and that this is an indication that he is consciously or unconsciously aware of his impending death.

Summary There is a need for systematic information regarding decisions to prolong or terminate lives in various types of cases. To obtain this information, it is necessary to examine (1) the types of prognoses that tend to be made in connection with various types of diseases and the degree of ambiguity and controversy surrounding such prognoses; (2) decisions to allocate medical resources when

---

* Studies by Farberow *et al.* (1962) and Farberow and McEvoy (1966) represent a beginning in this direction.

there is a chance that a life can be saved; (3) decisions to allocate or withdraw medical resources when there is no possibility of averting death. Several sets of norms relevant to these decisions have been identified. Research is needed to find out how the characteristics of organizational settings and of participants affect the type of behavior chosen.

Relationships with Dying Patients

While there are several sets of normative prescriptions to which one can refer in deciding whether or not to prolong life, there do not seem to be norms regarding appropriate behavior toward a person whose death is considered inevitable. Without exception, studies indicate that communication between dying patients and both staff and relatives is poor. To some extent, this can be explained by the fact that interaction with persons who have no future is frustrating in our culture. Such individuals suffer a sharp loss in social value.* Attitudes toward these patients are very different from attitudes toward patients for whom some hope remains. The latter are socially rewarding because they can be made the objects of heroic life-saving efforts. Those for whom death is inevitable do not provide such satisfaction. Until recently, when belief in an afterlife was common, the dead were perceived as having a future in the next world. They retained their social value until death occurred, as is seen by the fact that their deathbed pronouncements were taken seriously (Gorer, 1965). If dying patients were still perceived as having social value, it seems probable that medical personnel and relatives would wish to interact with them and that norms regarding appropriate behavior in such situations could be located. Such norms still exist in other cultures. For example, as Glaser and Strauss (1965) point out, it is the custom in some cultures for relatives to gather around the patient a day or two in advance of the expected death and to remain until death occurs.

The absence of norms is not only due to the fact that such interaction is perceived as unrewarding, however. There is also strong emotional resistance to such interaction by relatives and medical

---

* The use of dying patients in medical experiments represents an attempt to restore their social value, at least temporarily.

staff alike.* The resistance is so strong that it prevents the development of appropriate modes of behavior. The reasons for this resistance require further exploration. It is possible that the literature on attitudes toward death is misleading. The literature suggests that the fear of death is not strong in American society and that death is seldom a subject of concern (for a review of this literature, see Lester, 1967; for some recent data, see Riley, Chapter 2 in this volume). However, such questions probably evoke an evaluation of the respondent's attitude toward death coming at the end of his life cycle. The prospect of death coming as a break in the life cycle may actually be terrifying in a society where death for most people is not a preface to an afterlife. Since death in the middle of the life cycle is a relatively unlikely possibility for most people, such a fate is ordinarily not the subject of more than passing concern. Interaction with dying patients may bring such fears to the surface and make such interaction intolerable. Discussions with dying persons in which the truth is mutually accepted have been described as extremely trying (Quint, 1964; Glaser and Strauss, 1965). Feifel's suggestion (1959) that doctors exhibit more fear of death than the average person may simply reflect their greater exposure to the incidence of death as a break in the life cycle. Their greater awareness of this type of death has made them more conscious of the fearful aspects of death.

The dying patient's role tends to be defined negatively rather than positively. He is expected not to be difficult, not to complain. There are no clear prescriptions regarding behavior considered appropriate in bringing one's life to a close. It seems likely that the lack of norms concerning the expected behavior of the dying person increases his mental suffering. The dying person is a special kind of marginal man.

---

* Some interesting evidence of this was provided by Lawrence LeShan who computed the length of time it took hospital nurses to respond to call-lights for terminal cases compared to the time for non-terminal cases. The nurses were startled to learn how much they delayed answering the ring of the dying (Bowers et al., 1964). Using a modification of the Bogardus social distance scale with a sample of college students, Kalish compared the extent to which interaction with dying persons in various types of hypothetical situations was avoided with the amount of avoidance elicited by 14 other ethnic and non-ethnic groups. In hypothetical situations which involved frequent face-to-face encounters, the dying person was avoided by more than half the sample (Kalish, 1966).

Increasing alienation is an almost inevitable aspect of his condition. This process has been brilliantly documented by Ross (1969).

Thus relationships with dying persons are of an unusual type; there are few normative guidelines for behavior and a high degree of negative affect on both sides. In order to study such relationships, it is necessary to consider the following aspects: (1) Who is interacting with the dying person—medical personnel, relatives, friends? (2) What is the content of the interaction—information or emotional support? (3) What are the conditions under which the interaction is taking place? The conditions are the awareness contexts described by Glaser and Strauss (1965), the extent to which a patient knows he is dying, and the extent to which staff and relatives are willing to admit their knowledge of this condition to him. (4) How has the dying person adjusted to his condition? What is his intellectual position and emotional response toward his situation?

Medical Personnel and Dying Persons

Medical personnel prefer to treat dying persons as if they were expected to live (Duff and Hollingshead, 1968). The motive, conscious or unconscious, may be that of maintaining their control over the doctor-patient relationship. The dying patient who is aware of his fate is more difficult to handle. Oken (1961) found that not only did 88 per cent of the 219 physicians whom he studied prefer not to tell cancer patients their unfavorable prognoses but their commitment to this policy appeared to be largely based upon emotional reactions rather than upon a rational assessment of the situation. Their resistance to change in this area was such that a significant proportion indicated that their approach was not likely to be changed by the results of research.

Effective emotional support of dying persons by medical personnel apparently occurs relatively infrequently (Duff and Hollingshead, 1968). In this volume, Glaser and Strauss argue that medical personnel need to be systematically educated in the appropriate ways of handling dying patients. While such training would undoubtedly be useful, it seems unlikely that this would provide a complete solution to the problem. As Glaser and Strauss have themselves pointed out, there are no rewards in the hospital for the quality of a staff member's interaction with dying patients. Effective interaction with dying patients is an exacting and delicate task. Such efforts are unlikely to be forthcoming unless there is a major change in the allocation of rewards by hospitals.

In the meantime, evaluation would be useful of the effectiveness of professionals such as clergy and psychiatrists who do perceive this task as within their domain. Cappon (1959) indicates that the prevalence of psychiatric illness among the dying is high, so that psychiatrists could be expected to be particularly useful. Hiring psychiatric social workers to perform as their primary task the role of helping dying patients cope with the reality of their situation would also seem promising. Such interaction is resisted to such an extent that only as a kind of specialty is it likely to be satisfactorily and dependably handled.

Studies of attitudes toward dying persons and of the fear they arouse in those who interact with them would be useful. Perceptions of death may influence behavior toward and by dying persons. For example, Chandler (1965) differentiated between three different perspectives of death: (1) perception of the existence of death in a general sense without a feeling that it is of vital concern to the individual; (2) perception of the presence of death in terms of the existence of an incurable, terminal disease; (3) the presentiment of death or the recognition that death can occur at any moment in a patient although he might also live for a longer time than is expected. The last is the most threatening. Staff interaction with patients whose deaths were imminent was characterized by negativism and withdrawal. Chandler compared these relationships to the "double-bind" process, "a situation in which no matter what a person does he can't win."

Kastenbaum (1965) suggests in a different type of study that doctors prefer to perceive their patients as having a longer life expectancy than mortality rates would indicate was likely. He hypothesizes that doctors may need to deny the possibility of death in the near future in order to maintain an interest in caring for their patients. Concomitantly, one might infer that, when death as an immediate possibility can no longer be denied, the quality of medical care declines because of lack of motivation upon the part of the physician.

Relatives and Dying Persons

Relatives also prefer to deny the reality of the situation or to withdraw from interaction altogether. Weisman and Hackett (1961) refer to the "bereavement of dying" and suggest that the dying patient may suffer more from abrupt emotional isolation and deprivation than from his illness. Quint (1964) has described how women who had had mastectomies were unable to discuss their fears about dying with their families. We have already suggested that dying persons may react to this type of behavior by losing their desire to prolong their lives further.

It would be useful to know more about the types of persons who, as relatives, react in various ways to dying persons. Do relatives who are unwilling to face their fears realistically prefer to interact with a dying person as if he did have a future, that is, by denying the fact of his imminent death? Do relatives who are more sensitive to the loss of social value by the dying person prefer to withdraw from the situation altogether?

It is known that marital relationships vary considerably in the amount and characteristics of the communication occurring between spouses (Blood and Wolfe, 1960). Middle-class spouses have more communication with each other about a wider range of topics and share more interests with one another than lower-class spouses. With increasing age, however, the amount and range of communication between spouses declines in both social groups. This suggests that middle-class spouses would be better able to support dying patients than lower-class spouses and to resolve the normative conflicts which develop more satisfactorily. One would also expect that for similar reasons younger spouses would perform this role more effectively than older spouses.

The Adjustment of the Dying Person

Medical personnel and relatives have been criticized in the literature for their failure to provide frank information to dying persons and for their ineptness in providing emotional support (Glaser and Strauss, 1965, 1968; Duff and Hollingshead, 1968; Quint, 1965).

However, it is likely that the dying person himself affects both the kinds of information he is given and the amount of emotional support he receives.

People who are healthy tend to say they would want to be told that they were going to die. Those who are actually dying are less certain (Cappon, 1962). Since the implications of this knowledge are so horrendous, it is likely that patients vary in their responses to such information and in their abilities to adjust to it. Uncertainty about a person's ability to adjust to the knowledge that he is dying affects the decision about whether or not to tell him the truth.

We know many of the ways in which individuals respond to the information that they are dying but there is not much indication as to the frequency of different types of reactions. Glaser and Strauss state that among geriatric patients the end is often welcomed. Among younger patients, responses range from positive to negative. A positive response entails an attempt by the patient to make appropriate arrangements for his exit both in terms of business matters and in terms of his relationships with relatives. Negative responses reflect mental disorganization. The individual is unable to organize his business affairs or to interact meaningfully with anyone. Kalish (1968) has defined "social death" as the individual's perception that he is "as good as dead," that his social role has ceased. This type of perception appears to represent a form of anomie, the feeling of isolation and meaninglessness which the individual tends to experience when he is not a member of any cohesive group (Durkheim, 1951). The most acute form of this reaction may induce death sooner than it would otherwise occur. There is some indication that sudden, unexplained deaths occur in both men and in animals when they face situations in which they perceive themselves to be in danger and to have absolutely no defense against it (Richter, 1957). The physiological processes that lead to death in these situations are not understood.

Between these two poles are a variety of responses in which denial and acceptance are mixed. These have been well documented by Glaser and Strauss. Suicide may actually result from either a positive or negative reaction. An individual who foresees that the end of his life will be unpleasant for himself and for others may try to shorten his existence. An individual who is overwhelmed by the knowledge of

Dying and Its Dilemmas as Field of Research [319

his impending death may resort to suicide rather than attempt to adjust to it.

Obviously the nature of these responses to the knowledge of terminality will affect the efforts of medical personnel and relatives to interact with patients. Suspected terminality can also have psychological consequences for the patient which can impede effective interaction with others.

There is also some indication that, particularly among older patients, mental changes occur prior to death which affect the individual's ability to interact with others. These changes are indicative of "diminished competence, control, perception, and performance" (Weisman and Kastenbaum, 1968:28). Lieberman (1966) has found that learning capacity diminished, mental organization became simpler, and efficiency declined in the same degree as the subject's proximity to death. Cappon (1959) has also found some evidence of a relationship between mental illness and certain types of physical illness. Anxiety and depression seem to be connected to heart disease and schizoid and schizophrenic reactions to cancer.

These findings suggest that, if communication with dying patients is to be meaningful, skilled assessment of their psychiatric status will be necessary. It may be that in certain types of cases only a psychiatrist can interact with any degree of effectiveness. Unfortunately, psychiatrists apparently prefer not to work with dying patients.

Summary Investigation of the factors affecting the "quality" of dying is needed. What are the conditions which enable the dying person to accept and to adjust to his situation? How can his relationships with others in his environment be improved? Can the generally low level of communication between relatives and dying patients be attributed as much to the mental state of the patient as to the inability of his relatives and medical personnel to interact with him in a realistic manner? Can the effect of the disclosure of terminality upon different types of patients be assessed in quantitative terms?

Dying and Bereavement

After death occurs, one would expect that the bereavement period would be affected by the normative conflicts that have preceded it. Adjustment to the death of a family member may be more difficult if relatives are uncertain that their decisions regarding that person while he was dying were appropriate.

The literature on responses to death by relatives suggests that pathological reactions to bereavement occur fairly frequently. Gorer (1965), in his study of English persons who had lost a relative, characterized the grieving as "unlimited" in over one-third of his sample. Many of these people were unable to adjust to their loss. Lindemann's study of bereavement (1944) also revealed intense reactions to death on the part of relatives. A number of studies have shown that the incidence of death among the recently widowed is higher than among married persons of similar age (Hinton, 1967:174; Rees and Lutkins, 1967). Another study has also shown an increase in physical ailments and psychiatric symptoms among the recently widowed (Parke, 1964).

On the other hand, accounts of the interaction between dying persons and family members tend to emphasize the inability of relatives to respond meaningfully to the fact of death before it occurs. Systematic examination of the relationship between events which took place while a relative was dying and the nature of the subsequent grief reaction have not been made. Gorer alludes to the fact that "the whole relationship between the dying and their partners or close relatives is falsified and distorted in a particularly degrading and painful fashion" (p. 17). He does not, however, attempt to relate the mourners' doubts about their own behavior while their relatives were dying to the characteristics of their grief reactions.

It seems likely that deaths of family members create acute anxiety since individuals typically have few dependable ties outside the family. Prior to the deaths of such persons, the individual desires to deny the possibility of death while at the same time withdrawing his emotional involvement from the relationship in preparation for its complete severance. After the death has occurred, however, the extent to which he has perceived normative conflicts concerning the treatment of the dying person may affect his adjustment to bereavement. One study reported hostility by relatives toward doctors after death had occurred (Hinton, 1967:169). It is possible that some of this hostility may be due to resentment over the ways in which the normative conflicts surrounding the dying process were resolved. For example, adjustment to bereavement may be more difficult if the relative feels that decisions regarding the prolongation or termination of life were made upon an instrumental basis rather than upon an altruistic basis. Decisions are probably more likely to be made on an instrumental basis in hospitals than in patients' homes. Rees and Lutkins (1967) found that the risk of close relatives dying during the first year of bereavement was doubled when the primary death causing the bereavement occurred in a hospital compared with at home. The hospital is apparently more stressful for relatives than the home. Concern over these problems may be lessened if relatives have many family members and friends in the community to provide emotional support.

Conclusion

Our argument here has centered upon normative ambiguities as the source of current social dilemmas surrounding the process of dying. We have shown that these ambiguities affect decisions to prolong or terminate lives. The absence of norms regarding appropriate behavior toward dying persons creates another type of ambiguity, a situation where none of the actors knows exactly what to do. As a result, the reality tends to be denied or to be discounted in advance, producing a kind of social death for the dying individuals concerned. Similarly, there is no behavior generally expected from the dying person. Not only is he not permitted control over his own demise but there are no appropriate rituals for bringing his life to a close. It seems likely that these dilemmas surrounding the process of dying affect adjustment to bereavement.

What are the prospects for this type of research? A number of factors have inhibited its development in the past. One is lack of awareness of the problem. The dying are not a vocal constituency. Their relatives do not realize that their problems are shared with many others. Among medical personnel who care for the dying, it is mainly psychiatrists who have concerned themselves with the behavioral aspects of the prolongation of life. The majority of doctors, as laboratory scientists or clinical practitioners, have not been sensitive to these issues.

For different reasons, social scientists have also not paid much attention to these questions. Other social problems have seemed more urgent, because the solutions would benefit particular groups, such as juvenile delinquents or the unemployed, whose effective participation in society could be thereby increased for considerable periods of time. Improvement in the environment of the dying seems, from this point of view, a luxury item in social science. It can benefit a relatively small class of people who in turn do not contribute anything to the rest of society.

This interpretation, however, is incomplete. Some of those who are needlessly defined as dying could be restored to useful roles in society. Not only have the numbers of people for whom the process of dying is an extended one increased but concomitantly the complexity of the issues involved in their care has become more serious. Aside from the altruistic goal of improving the "quality" of dying, those who must make decisions concerning the allocation of medical resources to the dying, relatives and medical personnel alike, are increasingly in need of the information social scientists can provide. The problem also has ramifications extending beyond these groups. As the government becomes more involved in paying for medical care, policy makers on that level could benefit from more information about these problems. The resolution of legal questions concerning the dying could also be improved by studies of the kind being suggested here. In short, these problems have ceased to be the concern solely of doctors and their clients. Members of other institutions are involved in the decision-making process. New knowledge could help to ascertain that these decisions will be made wisely. No solutions are likely to be entirely satisfactory, however. In the last analysis, death is the one human problem that can never be completely resolved.

REFERENCES

Beigler, J. S.
    1957   "Anxiety as an aid in the prognostication of impending death." Archives of Neurology and Psychiatry 77(February):171–177.
Blau, P. M.
    1955   The Dynamics of Bureaucracy. Chicago: University of Chicago Press.
Blood, R. O., and D. M. Wolfe.
    1960   Husbands and Wives. New York: Free Press.
Bowers, M. *et al.*
    1964   Counseling the Dying. New York: Thomas Nelson.

Cappon, D.
　1959　"The dying." Psychiatric Quarterly 33:468–489.
　1962　"Attitudes of and toward the dying." Canadian Medical Association Journal 87 (September):693–700.
Carlin, J. E.
　1966　Lawyers' Ethics: A Survey of the New York City Bar. New York: Russell Sage Foundation.
Caudhill, W.
　1958　The Psychiatric Hospital as a Small Society. Cambridge, Mass.: Harvard University Press.
Chandler, K. A.
　1965　"Three processes of dying and their behavioral effects." Journal of Consulting Psychology 29 (August):296–301.
Coleman, J.
　1961　The Adolescent Society. New York: Free Press.
Duff, R. S., and A. B. Hollingshead.
　1968　Sickness and Society. New York: Harper & Row.
Durkheim, E.
　1951　Suicide. Trans. by J. A. Spaulding and G. Simpson. New York: Free Press.
Farberow, N. L., E. S. Shneidman, and Calista V. Leonard.
　1963　"Suicide among general medical and surgical patients with malignant neoplasms." VA Medical Bulletin (February).
Farberow, N. L., and T. L. McEvoy.
　1966　"Suicide among patients with diagnosis of anxiety reaction or depressive reaction in general medical and surgical hospitals." Journal of Abnormal Psychology 71:289–299.
Feifel, H. (ed.).
　1959　The Meaning of Death. New York: McGraw-Hill.
Fulton, R., and G. Geis.
　1965　Death and Identity. New York: Wiley.
Glaser, B. G., and A. L. Strauss.
　1965　Awareness of Dying. Chicago: Aldine.
　1968　Time for Dying. Chicago: Aldine.
Gorer, G.
　1965　"The pornography of death." In Death, Grief and Mourning. London: Cresset.
Hinton, J.
　1963　"The physical and mental distress of the dying." Quarterly Journal of Medicine, New Series 32 (January):1–21.
　1967　Dying. Baltimore: Penguin Books.
Kalish, R. A.
　1966　"Social distance and the dying." Community Mental Health Journal 2 (Summer):152–155.

1968 "Life and death: dividing the indivisible." Social Science and Medicine 2:249–259.

Kastenbaum, R.
1965 "The realm of death: an emerging area in psychological research." Journal of Human Relations 13:538–552.

Lester, D.
1967 "Experimental and correlational studies of the fear of death." Psychological Bulletin 67:27–36.

Lieberman, M.
1966 "Vulnerability to stress and the processes of dying." Proceedings of the 7th International Congress on Gerontology, 8, 513–519.

Lindemann, E.
1944 "Symptomatology and management of acute grief." American Journal of Psychiatry 101 (September): 141–148.

Oken, D.
1961 "What to tell cancer patients: a study of medical attitudes." Journal of the American Medical Association 175 (April):1120–1128.

Parke, C. M.
1964 "Effects of bereavement on physical and mental health—a study of the medical records of widows." British Medical Journal 2(August):274–279.

Parsons, T., and V. Lidz.
1967 "Death in American society." Pp. 133–170 in Edwin Shneidman (ed.), Essays in Self-Destruction. New York: Science House.

Phillips, D.
1969 Dying as a Form of Social Behavior. Unpublished doctoral dissertation, Princeton University.

Quint, J. C.
1964 "Mastectomy—symbol of cure or warning sign?" General Practice (March):119–124.
1965 "Institutionalized practices of information control." Psychiatry 28(May):119–132.

Rees, W. D., and S. G. Lutkins.
1967 "Mortality of bereavement." British Medical Journal 4(October): 13–16.

Richter, K.
1957 "On the phenomenon of sudden death in animals and men." Psychosomatic Medicine 11(May–June):626–633.

Ross, E. K.
1969 On Death and Dying. New York: Macmillan.

Shils, E.
1967 "The sanctity of life." Encounter, 39–49.

Shneidman, E. S.
1963 "Suicide." Pp. 33–43 in Norman L. Farberow (ed.), Taboo Topics, New York: Atherton.

Simmons, R. G., and Simmons, R. L.
 1970 "Sociological and psychological aspects of transplantation: kidney transplantation and dialysis as a special case." In J. Nazarian and R. G. Simmons (eds.), Transplantation. Philadelphia: Lea and Febiger (forthcoming).
Stewart, I.
 1960 "Suicide: The influence of organic disease." Lancet 2(October): 919–920.
Sudnow, D.
 1967 Passing On. Englewood Cliffs, N.J.: Prentice-Hall.
Swazey, J. P., and Fox, R. C.
 1970 "The clinical moratorium: a case study of mitral valve surgery." In Ethical Aspects of Experimentation with Human Subjects. New York: George Braziller (forthcoming).
Weisman, A. D., and T. P. Hackett.
 1961 "Predilection to death." Psychosomatic Medicine 23(May–June): 232–256.
Weisman, A. D., and R. Kastenbaum.
 1968 The Psychological Autopsy: A Study of the Terminal Phase of Life. Community Mental Health Journal Monograph, No. 4.

Death and Dying

A BRIEFLY ANNOTATED BIBLIOGRAPHY

Richard A. Kalish

A NOTE FROM THE COMPILER. This bibliography is drawn from a more comprehensive effort which began in 1963, emerged in mimeographed form in 1964, and was augmented by a supplement produced in 1965. Initial funding came from Equitable Life Assurance Society through the efforts of John W. Riley, Jr. Additional funds were obtained from the Department of Psychology, California State College at Los Angeles, and from the School of Public Health, UCLA.

The bibliography is not completely coordinated with articles in the book. Rather, a separate set of criteria for including references was used. In compiling these materials, I have tried to be as thorough as possible in covering the literature of psychology, sociology, and psychiatry; also included are items from nursing, general medicine, pastoral counseling, theology, hospital administration, and anthropology. I have limited items to those published in English and to those available in libraries (i.e., no dissertations, mimeographed materials, speeches, etc.). With a very few exceptions, I have also omitted articles on mourning and grief, suicide, abortion, cryonics, birth control, and homicide. An excellent bibliography covering historical and philosophic materials, and not limited to the English language, may be found in *Modern Man and Mortality* by Jacques Choron (New York: The Macmillan Company, 1964).

The present bibliography forms the basis for a more extensive collection to be published in a self-contained volume. Nevertheless, I welcomed the opportunity offered by the editors of this book to make the literature known, and I eagerly accepted their suggestion that this material become part of their volume. If that goal is achieved, the work involved will have been well rewarded.

A

ABRAM, HARRY S.

1965 "Adaptation to open heart surgery: a psychiatric study of response to the threat of death." American Journal of Psychiatry 122(December):659–667.

A clinical study of 23 patients undergoing open heart surgery revealed the operation presents a symbolic and realistic threat to life. Anxiety and the use of denial are described.

ABRAMS, RUTH D.

1966 "The patient with cancer—his changing pattern of communication." New England Medical Journal 274(February):317–322.

Unique problems appear for the physician with respect to patients in whom cancer is considered irreversible. Fears of death, dying, and abandonment must be attended to at a time of decreasing overt communication and increasing depression.

ABRAMS, RUTH D., GERTRUDE JAMESON, MARY POEHLMAN, AND SYLVIA SNYDER.

1945 "Terminal care in cancer." New England Medical Journal 232 (June):719–724.

The discussion centers about the following topics: elements involved in providing adequate terminal care, including medical and nursing needs; family acceptance of the medical situation; family ability to care for the patient at home; patient's wishes with respect to care at home; and existing conditions.

ACKERKNECHT, ERWIN H.

1968 "Death in the history of medicine." Bulletin of the History of Medicine 42(January–February):19–23.

This theoretical article surveys medical involvement with death which historically has addressed itself to three points: prediction of death, fixation of moment of death, distinction between actual death and apparent death.

AITKEN-SWAN, JEAN.

1959 "Nursing the late cancer patient at home." Practitioner 183 (July):64–69.

The article reports results of an investigation into the attitudes and opinions of relatives concerning the treatment of late cancer patients at home.

AITKEN-SWAN, JEAN, AND E. C. EASSON.

1959 "Reactions of cancer patients on being told their diagnosis." British Medical Journal 1 (March):779–783.

In an interview study of 231 selected cancer patients who were told of their diagnosis, results were tabulated for approval, disapproval, denial, and delayed reactions. Only 7% of the subjects disapproved of being told.

ALDRICH, C. KNIGHT.

1963 "The dying patient's grief." Journal of the American Medical Association 184 (April–May):329–331.

Criticizing the traditional determinants of a person's ability to accept his own death, the psychology of the dying patient is explained from the perspective that loss of personal interrelations is more important than fear of dying.

ALDRICH, C. KNIGHT, AND ETHEL MENDKOFF.

1963 "Relocation of the aged and disabled: a mortality study." Journal of the American Geriatrics Society 11 (March):185–194.

The opportunity to study relocation effects without family or health factors was provided when a home for incurables was closed for administrative reasons and patients were moved to other nursing homes.

ALEXANDER, IRVING E., AND ARTHUR M. ADLERSTEIN.

1958 "Affective responses to the concept of death in a population of children and early adolescents." Journal of Genetic Psychology 93 (December):167–177.

Affective responses to death words were measured in a population of males from 5 to 16. The population as a whole showed increased emotional involvement with death words on both response measures. All subgroups showed significant increases in response time to the death words.

1959 "Death and religion." Pp. 271–283 in Herman Feifel (ed.), The Meaning of Death. New York: McGraw-Hill.

Religious college students believe that death does not bring extinction, while irreligious students accept death as the end. Either position reduces anxiety.

1960 "Studies in the psychology of death." Pp. 65–92 in H. P. David and J. C. Brenglemann (eds.), Perspectives in Personality Research. New York: Springer.

This article looks at man's reactions to death and cites the results of empirical studies. Generally, results showed that there is a direct relation between magnitude of affect and age, asymptoting at about college age. The studies did not uphold the notion that religiousity decreases anxiety about death.

ALEXANDER, IRVING E., RANDOLPH S. COLLEY, AND ARTHUR M. ADLERSTEIN.
1957 "Is death a matter of indifference?" Journal of Psychology 43 (April):277–283.
Thirty-one male college students responded with greater emotional intensity to words logically related to the concept of death than to words equivalent in frequency of usage, length, etc., but not logically related to death.

ALVAREZ, WALTER C.
1952 "Care of the dying." Journal of the American Medical Association 150(September):86–91.
A physician relates from his own experience techniques in dealing with the dying patient and the family.

ANONYMOUS.
1969 "Death: the way of life." Harvest Years 9(April):19–34.
An article directed at the older person himself, touching on many aspects of death and dying, and without the usual euphemisms and pollyanna approach.

ANTHONY, SYLVIA.
1940 The Child's Discovery of Death: A Study in Child Psychology. New York: Harcourt, Brace.
This is the study of death in children through the expression of their conscious thought and phantasy, expressions in which conscious and unconscious elements are interwoven. The author treats death as an isolated external reality, knowledge of which has to be acquired by the child as an intellectual process.

ARONSON, GERALD J.
1959 "Treatment of the dying person." Pp. 251–258 in Herman Feifel (ed.), The Meaning of Death. New York: McGraw-Hill.
A psychiatrist states that care of the terminal patient should (a) enable him to continue as a human being, (b) enable him to maintain his roles and identity, and (c) keep him from becoming depressed.

B

BACK, KURT W., AND HANS W. BAADE.
1966 "The social meaning of death and the law." Pp. 302–329 in John C. McKinney and Frank T. de Vyver (eds.), Aging and Social Policy. New York: Appleton-Century-Crofts.

A Briefly Annotated Bibliography

Sociological forces tend to isolate the dying and the dead person from American society, but the law (through such devices as wills and trusts) permits the dying and the dead more power.

BAILEY, MARGARET.

1959 "Survey of the social needs of patients with incurable lung cancer." Almoner 11(January):379–391.

One hundred fifty-five patients with incurable lung cancer were surveyed for their needs, and for the problems stemming from the nature of their disease.

BARBER, THEODORE XENOPHON.

1961 "Death by suggestion: A critical note." Psychosomatic Medicine 23(March–April):153–155.

Voodoo death is neither mystical nor the outcome of environmentally initiated biochemical changes. Rather, it results from self-starvation or dehydration based on refusal to take liquids or a similar behavior change.

BARCKLEY, VIRGINIA.

1964 "Enough time for good nursing." Nursing Outlook 12(April): 44–48.

Survey of training program supporting an ambitious effort to provide enough nursing time for over 100 terminal cancer patients, where half the patients are in critical condition every day, and where professional registered nurses are unavailable.

BEATTY, DONALD C.

1955 "Shall we talk about death?" Pastoral Psychology 6(February): 11–14.

Apropos of the fact that we avoid talking or even thinking about death, doctors and nurses in hospitals keep patients from knowing that they are dying.

BECKER, ARTHUR H., AND AVERY D. WEISMAN.

1967 "The patient with a fatal illness—to tell or not to tell." Journal of the American Medical Association 201(August):646–648.

The pros and cons of informing patients of fatal diagnoses, including the views of a clergyman and a physician.

BECKER, HOWARD, AND DAVID K. BRUNER.

1931 "Attitude toward death and the dead and some possible causes of ghost fear." Mental Hygiene 15(October):828–837.

The authors trace various possible explanations of attitudes toward the individual's own death, the dead, ambivalence in human relations, and fear of ghosts.

BEECHER, HENRY K.

1962 "Nonspecific forces surrounding disease and the treatment of disease." Journal of the American Medical Association 179(February):437–440.

This article offers evidence for the tenet that fear can kill.

BEIGLER, JEROME S.

1957 "Anxiety as an aid in the prognostication of impending death." Archives of Neurology and Psychiatry 77(February):171–177.

A somatic illness can sometimes be detected for the first time by its psychiatric manifestations, such as dreams, by the course of psychotherapy or psychoanalysis, by hysterical symptoms, and by euphoria.

BENDER, LAURETTA.

1934 "Psychiatric mechanisms in child murderers." Journal of Nervous and Mental Diseases 80(July):32–47.

The author concludes that child murder by parents represents suicide via identification processes.

1953 Pp. 40–65 in Aggression, Hostility and Anxiety in Children. Springfield, Ill.: Charles C Thomas.

Previous studies have shown that people are unconsciously more concerned with death than they realize. Generally, children have a realistic appreciation of death which is thought of as occurring through violence. Death for the child signifies deprivation.

BERMAN, MERRILL I.

1966 "The Todeserwartung syndrome." Geriatrics 21(May):187–192.

The feeling of uselessness and idleness and the loss of an effective, satisfying environment set the stage for the Todeserwartung syndrome of "waiting to die" communicated by residents of old-age homes.

BIORCK, GUNNAR.

1968 "Thoughts on life and death." Perspectives in Biology and Medicine 2(Summer):527–543.

Reflections on the enigmas of life and death, including a discussion of transplants and the law and euthanasia.

BLAUNER, ROBERT.

1966 "Death and the social structure." Psychiatry 29(November): 378–394.

Explores the social and cultural consequences of modern society's organization of death. Social arrangements designed to contain the impact of death are emphasized, including their relation to the demographic characteristics of a society.

BLUESTONE, HARVEY, AND CARL L. MCGAHEE.

1962 "Reaction to extreme stress: impending death by execution." American Journal of Psychiatry 119(November):393–396.

Death row inmates were examined for defense mechanisms used to avoid reactions to their overwhelming stress. Denial, projection, and preoccupation were encountered in various combinations.

BORKENAU, FRANZ.

1955 "The concept of death." The Twentieth Century 157(April): 313–329.

This article advances the thesis that the self-contradictory experience of death is a basic element in shaping the course of human history; that changes in the popular attitude toward death mark great epochs of historical evolution, etc.

BOWERS, MARGARETTA, EDGAR JACKSON, JAMES KNIGHT, AND LAWRENCE LE SHAN.

1964 Counseling the Dying. New York: Thomas Nelson.

The authors feel that people who work with the dying should encourage a more effective communication with the patient, and that it is important to try to develop a different climate in the professional and general community in regard to death and dying.

BOZEMAN, MARY F., CHARLES E. ORBACH, AND ARTHUR M. SUTHERLAND.

1955 "Psychological impact of cancer and its treatment, Part III: the adaptation of mothers to the threatened loss of their children through leukemia: Part I." Cancer 8(January):1–19.

A study was conducted to determine adaptation of mothers to threatened loss of their children from acute leukemia. All mothers tried to integrate this injurious experience, mostly by extending relationships and asking for emotional and physical support.

BRAUER, PAUL H.

1960 "Should the patient be told the truth?" Nursing Outlook 8(December):672–676.

The author asks the question, "What is the truth?" All words have different meanings for different people. Each case should be handled individually.

BRODSKY, BERNARD.

1959 "The self-representation, anality and the fear of dying." Journal of the American Psychoanalytic Association 7(January):95–108.

Fragments of 3 case studies of psychoanalytic patients were discussed in support of the postulate that during the anal stage, the fear of death becomes the fear of turning into feces due to the conceptual equation of dead bodies and feces.

1959 "Liebestod fantasies in a patient faced with a fatal illness." International Journal of Psychoanalysis 40 (January):13–16.
The psychiatric case history of a young woman who has a fatal illness is presented.

BROMBERG, WALTER, AND PAUL SCHILDER.

1936 "The attitude of psychoneurotics towards death." Psychoanalytic Review 23 (January):1–25.
Early experiences determine death attitudes of an individual and these may be expressed through neurotic manifestations.

1933 "Death and dying: a comparative study of the attitudes and mental reactions toward death and dying." Psychoanalytic Review 20 (April):133–185.
This article discusses empirical data contrasting attitudes toward death in normal and neurotic individuals.

BROWN, NORMAN O.

1959 Life Against Death. Middletown, Conn.: Wesleyan University Press.
This book deals with the psychoanalytic meaning of history. It examines Freudian and psychoanalytic theories and applies them to the state of man and the world.

BULGER, ROGER J.

1963 "Doctors and dying." Archives of Internal Medicine 112 (September):327–332.
Physicians, who through training have become experts on life, have a responsibility to become experts about death. Article gives examples of how death has been met in the works of some well-known authors.

C

CAIN, ALBERT C., AND BARBARA S. CAIN.

1964 "On replacing a child." Journal of the American Academy of Child Psychiatry 3 (July):443–456.
Several cases of moderately or severely disturbed children who were conceived shortly after the death of another child are discussed. These were all substitute children.

CANNON, WALTER B.

1942 "Voodoo death." American Anthropologist 44 (April–June):169–181.

Objects of voodoo hexes have ominous and persistent fears which cause intense action of the sympatico-adrenal system and a disastrous fall of blood pressure, resulting in death.

CAPPON, DANIEL.

1959 "The dying." Psychiatric Quarterly 33 (July):466–489.

Bedside interviews were conducted with dying and nondying hospital patients; a special effort was made to obtain fantasy material at sleep and waking levels of awareness.

1961 "The psychology of dying." Pastoral Psychology 12 (February):35–44.

Article discusses a study of 20 dying patients; there was a positive correlation between acceptance of death and religiosity.

1962 "Attitudes of and towards the dying." Canadian Medical Association Journal 87 (September):693–700.

This paper discusses a study by the author regarding conscious, public attitudes toward death and dying.

CAPRIO, FRANK S.

1946 "Ethnological attitudes toward death: a psychoanalytic evaluation." Journal of Clinical Psychotherapy 7 (April):737–752.

Death plays an important part in our lives at the unconscious level as evidenced by early preoccupations of various peoples with problems of death and the fact that many ancient death customs have survived in modern culture.

1950 "A study of some psychological reactions during prepubescence to the idea of death." Psychiatric Quarterly 24 (July):495–505.

One hundred unclassified adults selected randomly were asked to recall and relate by the free association method their mental reactions toward death during prepubescence.

CARPENTER, KATHRYN M., AND J. MARION STEWART.

1962 "Parents take heart at City of Hope." American Journal of Nursing 62 (October):82–85.

Description of facilities and services at the City of Hope Medical Center in a unit for terminally ill children.

CHADWICK, MARY.

1929 "Notes upon the fear of death." International Journal of Psychoanalysis 10 (January):321–334.

Anxiety that occurs without adequate cause may result from fear of death. Such fear may be related to early concerns when mother is absent.

CHANDLER, KENNETH A.

1965   "Three processes of dying and their behavioral effects." Journal of Consulting Psychology 29 (August):296–301.

From the study of groups who were dying differently, 3 major processes are delineated, each with its own behavioral effect.

CHODOFF, PAUL A., STANFORD FRIEDMAN, AND DAVID HAMBURG.

1964   "Stress, defenses and coping behavior: observations in parents of children with malignant disease." American Journal of Psychiatry 120 (February):743–749.

This article is presented to demonstrate examples of persons who handle life's problems and stresses well, describing adaptational techniques and coping strategies employed by a group of parents of fatally ill children.

CHORON, JACQUES.

1963   Death and Western Thought. New York: Collier.

A history of death and dying in Western thought from before Socrates through the Existentialists.

1964   Modern Man and Mortality. New York: Macmillan.

Choron has written a thorough statement on death and dying, including historical, psychological, psychiatric, and philosophic aspects.

CHRIST, ADOLPH E.

1961   "Attitudes toward death among a group of acute geriatric psychiatric patients." Journal of Gerontology 16 (January):56–59.

Analysis of attitudes toward death of 62 acutely psychotic geriatric subjects.

COHEN, SIDNEY.

1965   "LSD and the anguish of dying." Harpers Magazine 231 (September):69–78.

This article presents a discussion of the history of LSD and its possibilities for future use in instances of terminally ill patients who experience great pain and anxiety prior to death.

COREY, LAWRENCE G.

1961   "An analogue of resistance to death awareness." Journal of Gerontology 16 (January):59–60.

Older and younger subjects cope in differing ways with death awareness.

A Briefly Annotated Bibliography [337

COX, PETER R., AND JOHN R. FORD.

1964 "The mortality of widows shortly after widowhood." Lancet 1(January):163–164.

Statistical analysis of expected deaths following widowhood versus actual deaths following widowhood for five years after the death of the spouse suggest that the second year of widowhood may exhibit a somewhat higher mortality rate.

CROWN, BARRY, DENIS O'DONOVAN, AND GALE T. THOMPSON.

1967 "Attitudes toward attitudes toward death." Psychological Reports 20:1181–1182.

Social desirability of attitudes toward death was studied. Attitudes differed on 2 dimensions: healthy-unhealthy and hysterical-obsessive. Healthy sensitivity was found to be most socially desirable.

D

DESICH, ANN S.

1964 "The nurse's most difficult function: terminal care." R.N. 27:45–48.

Analysis of the nurse's approach to terminal care, starting with the fundamental and necessary step of coming to terms with one's individual aversion to death.

DEUTSCH, FELIX.

1936 "Euthanasia: a clinical study." Psychoanalytic Quarterly 5(July): 347–368.

For death to be anything else but a torment, there must be a settlement of differences, a reconciliation among forces of aggression, anxiety, the sense of guilt, and the agencies from which they proceed.

DE VOS, GEORGE, AND HIROSHI WAGATSUMA.

1959 "Psycho-cultural significance of concern over death and illness among rural Japanese." International Journal of Social Psychiatry 5(Summer):5–19.

Illness often seems to be a punishment of self for unacceptable behavior or of unacceptable hostility toward others which cannot be expressed.

DICKSTEIN, LOUIS S., AND SIDNEY J. BLATT.

1966 "Death concern, futurity, and anticipation." Journal of Consulting Psychology 30(February):11–17.

Research results indicate a relationship between heightened death concern and a foreshortened time perspective.

DIGGORY, JAMES C., AND DOREEN Z. ROTHMAN.

1961 "Values destroyed by death." Journal of Abnormal and Social Psychology 63 (July):205–209.

Generally, the consequences of his own death which a person fears most depend upon the role he has or expects to have, and therefore on the goals to which he is committed.

DOVENMUEHLE, ROBERT H.

1965 "Affective response to life-threatening cardiovascular disease." Symposium of the Group for the Advancement of Psychiatry 5 (October):607–613.

The affective changes which accompany cardiac illness include primarily depression. Understanding of depression and other changes can serve as aids to the physician and patient in treating the problem.

E

EASSON, WILLIAM M.

1968 "Care of the young patient who is dying." Journal of the American Medical Association 205 (July):203–207.

Article discusses age-appropriate reactions to imminent death in the very young child, the prepubescent child, and the adolescent.

EATON, JOSEPH W.

1964 "The art of aging and dying." The Gerontologist 4 (June):94–100.

The way of life of the Hutterite religious sect enables them to deal with the 6 universal problems of aging: economic insecurity, the inactivity of retirement, prestige loss, social isolation, loss of health, and death.

EISSLER, KURT R.

1955 The Psychiatrist and the Dying Patient. New York: International Universities Press.

A discussion of psychological aspects, ideas, and theories about death, including case history materials and treatment of patients who are dying.

EKBLOM, BENGT.

1963 "Significance of socio-psychological factors with regard to risk of death among elderly persons." Acta Psychiatrica Scandinavica 39:627–633.

An attempt to calculate how great a risk elderly people who have just lost their spouses run of dying shortly within the following period.

EKMAN, PAUL, LESTER COHEN, RUDOLF MOOS, WALTER RAINE, MARY SCHLESINGER, AND GEORGE STONE.

1963 "Divergent reactions to the threat of war." Science 139 (January): 88–94.

Two types of responses to the possibility of death from atomic attack are examined: the movement toward fallout shelters and the movement toward action for peace. Members of each group are interviewed and tested.

ELIOT, THOMAS D.

1943 "—of the shadow of death." Annals of the American Academy of Political and Social Science 229 (September): 87–99.

This article investigates those respects in which attitudes toward death are different in World War II than in the preceding "peace" and in World War I.

ELLARD, JOHN.

1963 "Emotional reactions associated with death." Medical Journal of Australia 1:979–983.

The physician should be aware of affective changes occurring in the dying patient, and particularly within himself in the course of a terminal illness and its treatment.

EWING, L. S.

1967 "Fighting and death from stress in a cockroach." Science 155 (February):1035–1036.

Illustrates the sequence of events involved in the fighting behavior between pairs of male cockroaches, in which deaths occur independent of external damage.

EXTON-SMITH, A. N.

1961 "Terminal illness in the aged." Lancet 2 (August):305–308.

Pain and distress experienced by a group of elderly patients during terminal illness were measured.

F

FAIRBANKS, ROLLIN J.

1948 "Ministering to the dying." Journal of Pastoral Care 2 (Fall):6–14.

Oriented to ministers, especially those just beginning, the author describes some of the behavior to be expected from dying persons. He classifies them as (1) resigned, (2) impatient, or (3) fearful.

FAUNCE, WILLIAM A., AND ROBERT L. FULTON.

1958 "The sociology of death: a neglected area of research." Social Forces 36(March):205–209.

The sociology of death has been a neglected area of study and this paper points up some of the research possibilities in the area.

FEDER, SAMUEL L.

1965 "Attitudes of patients with advanced malignancy." Symposium of the Group for the Advancement of Psychiatry 5(October): 614–622.

It has been the author's experience that most fatally ill patients "know" they are dying and that the question whether or not to reveal diagnosis is best left to the patient's desire to ask relevant questions and receive honest answers.

FEDERN, PAUL.

1932 "The reality of the death instinct, especially in melancholia." Psychoanalytic Review 19(April):129–151.

The problem of the perfection principle, the problem of religion as an illusion, and the problem of the death instinct are discussed.

FEIFEL, HERMAN.

1954 "Psychiatric patients look at old age: level of adjustment and attitudes toward aging." American Journal of Psychiatry 111(December):459–465.

The results of a study into attitudes of the mentally ill (both open and closed ward patients) toward aging are reported and compared with similar studies involving normal subjects.

1955 "Attitudes of mentally ill patients toward death." Journal of Nervous and Mental Diseases 122(October):375–380.

An exploratory study to augment the limited available data regarding the conscious attitudes toward death of mentally disturbed patients.

1956 "Older persons look at death." Geriatrics 11(March):127–130.

Presentation of some data regarding the conscious attitudes of older persons toward death.

1959 "Attitudes toward death in some normal and mentally ill populations." Pp. 114–130 in Herman Feifel (ed.), The Meaning of Death. New York: McGraw-Hill.

Some general findings on attitudes toward death indicate that women tend to think more frequently about death than men; also, patients want to talk about feelings and thoughts about death but feel that the living close off the avenues for their accomplishing this.

1959 The Meaning of Death. New York: McGraw-Hill.
A collection of articles by prominent scholars in the field of death, ranging from philosophy to the arts to psychology to physiology. The articles themselves are annotated elsewhere in this bibliography.

1962 "Scientific research in taboo areas—death." American Behavioral Scientist 5(March):28–30.
In the course of a study of adaptive and maladaptive reactions to stress and how different individuals cope with severe threat, the author found that "the caretakers of the deathly ill are sometimes 'sicker' than the sick themselves."

1963 "The taboo on death." American Behavioral Scientist 6(May): 66–67.
Psychology and Western culture generally have tended to run, hide, and seek refuge in euphemistic language, in the development of an industry that has a major interest in the creation of greater lifelike qualities in the dead, and in actuarial statistics in the presence of death.

1963 "Death." Pp. 427–450 in Albert Deutsch (ed.), The Encyclopedia of Mental Health, Vol. II. New York: Franklin Watts.
An extensive overview of death in contemporary America, with emphasis upon mental health aspects.

1965 "The function of attitudes toward death." Symposium of the Group for the Advancement of Psychiatry 5(October):633–641.
Discusses (1) physician's fear of death, (2) patients' reactions to their own terminal illnesses, (3) disposition of physicians to talk to their patients about terminal diagnoses, and (4) ways in which individuals attempt to transcend death.

FEIFEL, HERMAN, SUSAN HANSON, ROBERT JONES, AND LAURI EDWARDS.

1967 "Physicians consider death." Proceedings of the 75th Annual Convention of the American Psychological Association 2:201–202.
Study to consider hypothesis that a major reason for some doctors entering medicine is to compensate for inordinate fear of death. In this study, medical students were found to be more fearful of death than either healthy or ill control subjects.

FELDMAN, MARVIN J., AND MICHEL HERSEN.

1967 "Attitudes toward death in nightmare subjects." Journal of Abnormal Psychology 72(October):421–425.
Subjects manifested greater conscious concerns about death in direct proportion to their frequency of nightmares.

FENICHEL, OTTO.

1953 "A critique of the death instinct." Pp. 363–372 in The Collected Papers of Otto Fenichel: First Series. New York: Norton.

Discusses the concepts of instincts and tension reduction generally as well as various other persons' comments and interpretations of the death instinct.

FITTS, WILLIAM T., JR., AND I. S. RAVDIN.

1953 "What Philadelphia physicians tell patients with cancer." Journal of the American Medical Association 153 (November):901–904.

Results of a questionnaire sent to Philadelphia doctors indicate that most do not tell patients they have cancer.

FOLCK, MARILYN M., AND PHYLLIS J. NIE.

1959 "Nursing students learn to face death." Nursing Outlook 7 (September):510–513.

This article makes a case for incorporating sociologic, psychiatric, and religious aspects of death into the nursing curriculum to prepare students to function easier while working with dying patients and their families.

FOLTA, JEANNETTE R.

1965 "The perception of death." Nursing Research 14 (Summer):232–235.

Reports the results of a questionnaire administered to 426 nurses. Scales included semantic differential items related to death, an anxiety scale, and a sacred-secular scale.

FOX, JEAN E.

1966 "Reflections on cancer nursing." American Journal of Nursing 66 (June):1317–1319.

The nurse caring for the patient in the terminal stages of this disease (cancer) has one primary and all-encompassing goal: to guide the patient, with love and understanding, to a peaceful death.

FREUD, SIGMUND.

1949 "The theme of the three caskets." Pp. 244–256 in Collected Papers (5th printing). London: Hogarth Press [original printing: 1913]

Freud translates two scenes from Shakespeare and other stories and fairy tales such as Cinderella as themes in which the symbol of death is represented by one of the choices, always, the pale or silent or dumb one.

1925 "Thoughts for the times on war and death." Pp. 288–317 in Collected Papers, Vol. IV. London: Hogarth Press. [Also pp. 289–300 in Complete Psychological Works of Sigmund Freud, Vol. XIV. London: Hogarth Press, 1957.]

Our unconscious attitude toward death is analogous to that of primeval man in that the unconscious does not recognize its own death but regards itself as immortal. The death of other persons, however, is acknowledged and often desired in the unconscious.

FRIEDMAN, STANFORD B., PAUL CHODOFF, JOHN MASON, AND DAVID HAMBURG.

1963 "Behavioral observations of parents anticipating the death of a child." Pediatrics 32(October):610–625.

The emotional and behavioral aspects of children suffering from neoplastic disease are discussed. Suggestions for medical management are made.

FULTON, ROBERT L.

1965 "The sacred and the secular: attitudes of the American public toward death, funerals, and funeral directors." Pp. 89–105 in Robert L. Fulton (ed.), Death and Identity. New York: Wiley.

Questionnaires and interviews related to death, dying, bereavement, and funerals were administered to about 2,000 persons. Religious affiliation was a pivotal factor in attitudes toward funerals and funeral directors.

1965 Death and Identity. New York: Wiley.

A collection of readings on death and bereavement with extensive editorial commentary by the author, a sociologist.

FULTON, ROBERT L., AND GILBERT GEIS.

1962 "Death and social values." Indian Journal of Social Research 3:7–14. [Also reprinted in Robert L. Fulton (ed.), Death and Identity. New York: Wiley.]

Attitudes toward death reflect the values prevailing within a particular society. However, because of religious overtones, presumably beyond secular inquiry, and the implicit general morbid nature of the subject, avoidance of death research has occurred.

1968 "Social change and social conflict: the rabbi and the funeral director." Sociological Symposium 1(Fall):1–9.

A study aimed at differential attitudes of Protestant, Catholic, and Jewish clergymen toward the purpose and function of the funeral, the duties of the clergyman, the duties of the funeral director, and the conflicts between the two.

G

GAVEY, C. J.

1952 The Management of the Hopeless Case. London: H. K. Lewis.

This book deals with the problem of treatment, both physical and psychological, for the patient with a terminal prognosis.

GLASER, BARNEY G.

1966 "Disclosure of terminal illness." Journal of Health and Human Behavior 7(Summer):83–91.

The descriptive process for understanding disclosure of terminal illness combines both (1) typical stages in the response stimulated by the disclosure and (2) typical forms of patient-hospital staff interaction at each stage.

GLASER, BARNEY G., AND ANSELM L. STRAUSS.

1964 "The social loss of dying patients." American Journal of Nursing 64(June):119–121.

A social value is placed on the patient, and that value has much to do with the impact on the nurse of his dying and, frequently, on the care he receives.

1964 "Awareness contexts and social interaction." American Sociological Review 29(October):669–679.

This paper presents a definition and typology of "awareness contexts" and offers a paradigm for their study.

1965 "Dying on time." Trans-action 2(May–June):27–31.

This article discusses the interplay of forces (both patient's and staff's) which occur when a terminal patient dies.

1965 "Temporal aspects of dying as a non-scheduled status passage." American Journal of Sociology 71(July):48–59.

Dying is the transition between two statuses: living and dead. The transition is marked off by the authors into four areas and passage into these areas is marked by cues.

1965 Awareness of Dying. Chicago: Aldine.

A study of dying in hospitals using a theory of "awareness" and examination of the dying patient and those about him in social interaction.

1968 Time for Dying. Chicago: Aldine.

The authors discuss the dying "trajectory" (the movement of the patient through time eventuating in death). The relationship of the trajectory to the hospital structure is examined.

GOLDFARB, ALVIN I.

1965 "Death and dying: attitudes of patient and doctor." Symposium of the Group for the Advancement of Psychiatry 5(October), 76 pp.
This publication covers 4 topics of discussion at the April, 1963, symposium of GAP: (1) affective response to life-threatening cardiovascular disease, (2) attitudes of patients with advanced malignancy, (3) studies on attitudes toward death, and (4) the fumction of attitudes toward death.

GOLDING, STEPHEN L., GEORGE E. ATWOOD, AND RICHARD A. GOODMAN.

1966 "Anxiety and two cognitive forms of resistance to the idea of death." Psychological Reports 18:359–364.
Study hypothesizes a relationship between affective orientation to death and cognitive resistance to the idea of death. Correlations were found only between measures of perceptual defense and connotative rigidity.

GORDON, NORMAN B.

1965 "Long term and fatal illness and the family." Journal of Health and Human Behavior 6:190–196.
The effects of fatal and long-term illnesses of children on family-life stability are discussed.

GORER, GEOFFREY.

1956 "The pornography of death." Pp. 56–62 in W. Phillips and P. Rahv (eds.), Modern Writing. New York: Berkeley.
In the twentieth century, death rather than sex becomes the pornography. "Ugly" facts of death are hidden and euphemisms are used.

1965 Death, Grief and Mourning in Contemporary Britain. London: Cresset.
The inevitability of death, as well as that of the related responses, grief and mourning, is contrasted with the total inadequacy of guidance available to meet these crises. Survey results are presented.

GREEN, MORRIS, AND ALBERT J. SOLNIT.

1964 "Reactions to the threatened loss of a child: a vulnerable child syndrome." Pediatrics 34(July):58–66.
Children who are expected by their parents to die prematurely are hypothesized to react with a disturbance in psycho-social development.

GREENBERG, IRWIN M.

1964 "Attitudes toward death in schizophrenia." Journal of the Hillside Hospital 13(April):104–113.

Tests and interviews provide data on subjects' ways of coping with their own death as an inevitable event and their methods of coping with inevitable events in general to compare with ego strength and self-esteem.

GREENBERGER, ELLEN.

1965 "Fantasies of women confronting death." Journal of Consulting Psychology 29(June):252–260.

The author advances the hypothesis that death is, itself, a sexual concept and that changes in sexualization may occur, either increasing or decreasing the preoccupation and anxiety toward death.

1966 "'Flirting' with death: fantasies of a critically ill woman." Journal of Projective Techniques 30(April):197–204.

TAT stories are analyzed with particular attention to material suggesting that the fantasy of death as a lover, dating back to antiquity, continues to live in the unconscious.

GREENE, WILLIAM A.

1958 "Role of a vicarious object in the adaptation to object loss." Psychosomatic Medicine 20(September–October):344–350.

A group of 150 patients with leukemia and lymphoma are studied to observe their mechanisms for adapting to object loss.

GREENE, WILLIAM A., AND GERALD MILLER.

1958 "Psychological factors and reticuloendothelial disease: IV: observations on a group of children and adolescents with leukemia: an interpretation of disease development in terms of the mother-child unit." Psychosomatic Medicine 20(March–April):124–144.

The authors consider that "separation from a significant object with ensuing depression may be one of the conditions determining manifest development of leukemia in children."

GROLLMAN, EARL A.

1967 Explaining Death to Children. Boston: Beacon Press.

An anthology, drawing from religion, psychology, sociology, anthropology, biology, and children's literature; the purpose of the book is to help adults and children attain a more mature understanding of death.

GROTJAHN, MARTIN.

1960 "Ego identity and the fear of death and dying." Journal of the Hillside Hospital 9(July):147–155.

Discusses Freud's death instinct and Melanie Klein's system of psychoanalytic thought.

H

HACKETT, THOMAS P.

1966 "How to help the dying patient." Medical Economics 43 (June): 2–6.

The author advances the reasons for telling the terminally ill patient his prognosis and discusses in which situations this is appropriate. The author also emphasizes the importance of "presence" (having relatives and other people around the dying person).

HACKETT, THOMAS P., AND AVERY WEISMAN.

1962 "The treatment of the dying." Pp. 121–126 in Jules Masserman (ed.), Current Psychiatric Therapies. New York: Grune and Stratton.

It is a mistake to assume that everyone feels the same fear of death, and it is almost impossible to withhold the knowledge of death from a dying person; to attempt to do so blindly imposes an unintended exile on someone facing ultimate loneliness.

HAIDER, IJAZ.

1967 "Attitudes toward death of psychiatric patients." International Journal of Neuropsychiatry 3 (February): 10–14.

Fifty psychiatric patients over 50 years of age were examined for their attitude toward death by means of a direct questionnaire.

HALL, G. STANLEY.

1897 "A study of fears." American Journal of Psychology 8 (January): 147–249.

Frequency of feared stimuli by verbal report. Most frequently reported was thunder and lightning; death was ranked fourth.

1915 "Thanatophobia and immortality." American Journal of Psychology 26 (October): 550–613.

A discussion of death anxiety based upon 299 questionnaire responses.

HAMOVITCH, MAURICE B.

1963 "Research interviewing in terminal illness." Social Work 8 (April): 4–9.

Interviews were conducted with parents and hospital staff members in an effort to ascertain the parents' attitude toward the illness and death of their children.

1964 The Parent and the Fatally Ill Child. Los Angeles, Calif.: Delmar.

A brief book describing a parent participation project at the City of Hope. Parents spent considerable time with their fatally ill children, and took care of many of their needs. Interview results are reported.

HARNIK, J.

1930 "One component of the fear of death in early infancy." International Journal of Psychoanalysis 11 (October):485–491.

The author disagrees with Freud that the fear of death derives from fear of the super ego, but says that instead the fear of dying is rooted in the most primitive of all levels and is in some way related to ultimate narcissism.

HARRIS, EDWARD G.

1951 "The physician, the clergyman, and the patient in terminal illness." Pennsylvania Medical Journal 54 (June):541–545.

This article represents a plea for application of the resources of the church to illnesses, as a supplement to medical treatment, and as an aid in providing the patient with a sense of peace, confidence, security, and well-being.

HARTMANN, HEINZ.

1956 "Notes on the reality principle." Psychoanalytic Study of the Child 11:31–53.

"Reality" and the "reality principle" are not simple and unitary, but have many aspects related to ego functions and their interactions.

HEUSCHER, JULIUS E.

1966 "Existential crisis, death, and changing 'world-designs' in myths and fairy tales." Journal of Existentialism 7 (Fall):45–62.

The human being becomes inauthentic because of the dread of death. If he becomes capable of facing courageously the absolute certainty of his death, he grows more authentic and imbues his life with new meaning.

1967 "Death in the fairy tale." Diseases of the Nervous System 28 (July):462–468.

Required growth, the encountering of new patterns of life and their substitution for the familiar old ones, is seen as initiating an existential crisis in the individual. Death can be viewed as a new, if completely unknown, pattern of life.

HICKS, WILLIAM, AND ROBERT S. DANIELS.

1968 "The dying patient, his physician and the psychiatric consultant." Psychosomatics 9:47–52.

This article deals with the role of the psychiatric consultant called in when fatally ill patients develop psychological complications as a result of their impending death.

HINTON, JOHN M.

1963 "The physical and mental distress of the dying." Quarterly Journal of Medicine 32(January):1–21.

After measuring mental and physical distress experienced in terminal illness, the author associated the distress with features of the patient's personal life or illness.

1964 "Problems in the care of the dying." Journal of Chronic Diseases 17(March):201–205.

The author feels that physicians should let good research provide them with some guidance.

1966 "Facing death." Journal of Psychosomatic Research 10(July): 22–28.

This paper discusses (1) the opinions expressed by people about their wish to be told if they have a potentially fatal disease and (2) the reported reactions of patients upon being told that they probably have a fatal illness and the proportion of fatally ill people who become aware that they may be dying.

1966 "Distress in dying." Pp. 180–187 in John N. Agate (ed.), Medicine in Old Age. London: Pitman Medical Publishing.

Awareness of dying, depression, anxiety, physical distress and discomfort, and time (intensity and duration) of physical distress were all compared with 102 dying patients and 102 control patients.

1967 Dying. Baltimore: Penguin Books.

An overview of medical, socio-medical, psychiatric, and psychological aspects of death and dying. This book takes a patient-centered (rather than family-centered, physician-centered, or hospital-centered) point of view.

HOCKING, WILLIAM ERNEST.

1957 The Meaning of Immortality in Human Experience. New York: Harper.

The contents of this book represent lectures by the author on 3 occasions when he was called upon to summarize his view on human destiny.

HOFFMAN, FRANCIS H., AND MORRIS W. BRODY.

1957 "The symptom fear of death." Psychoanalytic Review 44(October):433–438.

The case of a white, married, 39-year-old woman is presented in a discussion of the significance of the symptom, fear of death.

HOFFMAN, FREDERICK J.

1959   "Mortality and modern literature." Pp. 133–156 in Herman Feifel (ed.), The Meaning of Death. New York: McGraw-Hill.

Because of the phenomenon of total war and changes in the balance of expectation in human physical and spiritual organization, the disposition toward death in twentieth-century literature is different from that in any other.

HORDER, T. J.

1948   "Signs and symptoms of impending death." Practitioner 161 (August):73–75.

Medical article dealing with the reliability of symptoms of impending death.

HOWARD, ALAN, AND ROBERT A. SCOTT.

1965   "Cultural values and attitudes toward death." Journal of Existentialism 6(Winter):161–174.

The authors analyze some of the cultural values that appear to affect American attitudes toward death, and explore their social consequences.

HOWARD, JOSEPH D.

1961   "Fear of death." The Journal of the Indiana State Medical Association 54(December):1773–1779.

The psychiatrist and physician must together meet the challenge of fear of death and evolve a service of thanatopsychotherapy.

HOWELL, DORIS A.

1966   "A child dies." Journal of Pediatric Surgery 1(February):2–7.

Two professional goals which reflect the physician's empathy and compassion are: to make death bearable when it is inevitable and to salvage the family after the death.

HUNTER, R. C.

1967   "On the experience of nearly dying." American Journal of Psychiatry 124(July):122–126.

A patient with a hysterical personality unexpectedly encountered a sudden, relatively painless threat to life.

HUTSCHNECKER, ARNOLD A.

1959   "Personality factors in dying patients." Pp. 237–250 in Herman Feifel (ed.), The Meaning of Death. New York: McGraw-Hill.

A relationship appears to exist between the patient's terminal disease picture and his personality characteristics. If this is true, it could be that the basic personality influenced the course of the disease or that the illness affected the personality structure.

I

INGLES, THELMA.

1964 "Death on a ward." Nursing Outlook 12(January):28.

Story of the death of a hospital patient, and the ways in which many persons on his ward were able to share its meaning.

J

JACKSON, EDGAR N.

1963 For the Living. New York: Channel Press.

Answers to questions that are frequently asked regarding death, bereavement, and funerals. Written by a minister for a lay audience.

JAQUES, ELLIOTT.

1965 "Death and the mid-life crisis." International Journal of Psychoanalysis 46(October):502–514.

Association of change in the levels of creativity with the "mid-life crisis" defined as the mid-life encounter with the reality of one's own eventual death.

JEFFERS, FRANCES C., CLAUDE R. NICHOLS, AND CARL EISDORFER.

1961 "Attitudes of older persons toward death: a preliminary study." Journal of Gerontology 16(January):53–56.

Two hundred and sixty community volunteers, 60 years of age and over, were asked as part of a two-day series of examinations, during the course of a two-hour social history interview, "Are you afraid to die?" and "Do you believe in a life after death?"

JELLIFFE, SMITH ELY.

1933 "The death instinct in somatic and psychopathology." Psychoanalytic Review 20(April):121–132.

A discussion of the death instinct and treatment of certain mental illnesses, focusing upon recovery from severe mental illness due to acute somatic illness.

JOSEPH, FLORENCE.

1962 "Transference and countertransference in the case of a dying patient." Psychoanalysis and Psychoanalytic Review 49(Winter): 21–34.

An account of the death of a young woman from cancer who was in the process of terminating her psychoanalysis at the time the illness was diagnosed. The article discusses the involvement of the analyst in helping his patient cope with her fate.

JUNG, CARL G.

1959 "The soul and death." Pp. 3–15 in Herman Feifel (ed.), The Meaning of Death. New York: McGraw-Hill.

Life is an energy process and as such is directed toward a goal—rest or death. Psychological life refuses to conform to the law of biological life, giving rise to fear of death. Religion has complicated the system of preparation for death and has no significance except as such.

K

KALISH, RICHARD A.

1963 "Some variables in death attitudes." Journal of Social Psychology 59(February):137–145.

This study explores attitudes of 210 adult college students toward approaches to the destruction of life (birth control, euthanasia, abortion, wartime killing, capital punishment, fear of death, God and afterlife).

1963 "An approach to the study of death attitudes." American Behavioral Scientist 6(May):68–70.

A factor analysis was performed on some 600 questionnaires consisting of attitude items concerning death, dying, bereavement, funerals, methods of depriving others of life, religious values, and other variables.

1965 "The aged and the dying process: the inevitable decisions." Journal of Social Issues 21(October):87–96.

The dying process requires that numerous decisions be made, either by the dying person himself or by others with whom he has contact, usually family members or health care professionals.

1966 "A continuum of subjectively perceived death." The Gerontologist 6(June):73–76.

The author discusses "social death" (perception of the individual and treatment of him as if he were deceased), "psychological death" (loss of self-awareness and awareness of environment), and "social immortality" (maintenance of life of deceased individual through thoughts of the living).

1966 "Social distance and the dying." Community Mental Health Journal 2(Summer):152–155.

Two hundred and three college students completed a social distance scale indicating their preferred social distance from 14 groups, including nationality groups, social deviate groups, physical disability groups, and so forth.

1968 "Death and the elderly: a modern-day phantasy." Geriatrics 23 (February):60–69.

A number of common assumptions about death and dying have been shown to be wrong when investigated through objective research methods.

1968 "Life and death: dividing the indivisible." Social Science and Medicine 2:249–259.

The definitions of life and of death are often more complex than appear at first inspection. A person can die physically, psychologically, socially, or sociologically.

1969 "The practicing physician and death research." Medical Times 97(January):211–220.

The author encourages practicing physicians to attend more carefully to the variables involved with terminal illness and death, so that they might contribute to the behavioral scientific research on these topics.

KASTENBAUM, ROBERT.

1959 "Time and death in adolescence." Pp. 99–113 in Herman Feifel (ed.), The Meaning of Death. New York: McGraw-Hill.

The adolescent has one frame of reference in terms of which he regards most things but death is separated from his dominant view.

1963 "The reluctant therapist." Geriatrics 18(April):296–301.

Psychotherapists' reluctance to work with elderly persons is based largely upon attitudes and values that have been uncritically absorbed from views prevalent in our society.

1963 "Cognitive and personal futurity in later life." Journal of Individual Psychology 19(November):216–222.

Personal futurity for older subjects is curtailed significantly less than that projected by younger subjects whereas there is no difference between age groups in cognitive futurity.

1965 "The realm of death: an emerging area in psychological research." Journal of Human Relations 13:538–552.

Reliabilities of longevity estimates by physicians are fairly high when evaluating patients in a hospital for the aged.

1966 "Death as a research problem in social gerontology: an overview." The Gerontologist 6(June):67–69.

What is fear of death? How is it detected and verified? The author suggests a closer alliance between clinician and experimenter in an effort to tighten up the meaning of these questions, as well as the method of answering them.

1966 "As the clock runs out." Mental Hygiene 50(July):332–336.

The author presents some tentative conclusions regarding experiences of time, aging, and death derived from a series of investigations and clinical activities conducted by psychologists at an all-geriatric institution.

1966 "On the meaning of time in later life." Journal of Genetic Psychology 109:9–25.

The research literature on time perspective in later life is reviewed and the following topics are selected for particular consideration: two meanings of futurity; living in the past; time and death in later life, etc.

1967 "Multiple perspectives on a geriatric 'death valley.'" Community Mental Health Journal 3(Spring):21–29.

Focuses upon perceptions of an intensive treatment unit in a geriatric hospital. Interviews were conducted with patients and with the unit attendants, with concern directed to the manner in which death was mentioned, with accompanying explanation.

1967 "The mental life of dying geriatric patients." The Gerontologist 7(June):97–100.

Analysis of psychological autopsy findings for 61 geriatric patients failed to support the assumption that most aged persons are in poor mental contact as they are dying.

KATZ, ALFRED H.

1967 "Dilemma of the biological age: who shall survive?" Medical Opinion and Review 3:52–61.

Article examines the extent of social philosophy considerations where new medical aid (e.g., the new artificial kidney center) is expensive, in short supply, and necessary to life.

KAUFMANN, WALTER.

1959 "Existentialism and death." Pp. 39–63 in Herman Feifel (ed.), The Meaning of Death. New York: McGraw-Hill.

An existentialist deals with the most important distinction that makes all the difference in facing death—that one attains his satisfaction with himself. One who has made something of his life can face death without anxiety.

KAY, D. W. K., VERA NORRIS, AND FELIX POST.

1956 "Prognosis in psychiatric disorders of the elderly: an attempt to define indicators or early death and early recovery." Journal of Mental Science 102 (January):129–140.

After an observation period (not exceeding 10 days) it was possible to correctly predict death or discharge from mental care during the subsequent year in about three-quarters of the patients over 60 admitted to a mental observation unit.

KELLETT, THOMAS R.

1965 "The dying patient and the hospital: an attitude sampling." Hospital Administration 10 (Fall):26–37.

One hundred questionnaires were sent to hospital administrators and 100 to college professors, soliciting attitudes on hospital approach to terminal patients.

KELLY, WILLIAM D., AND STANLEY R. FRIESEN.

1950 "Do cancer patients want to be told?" Surgery 27 (June):822–826.

In an opinion survey of 2 groups of patients (100 persons with a diagnosis of cancer and 100 without known cancer), the great majority of each group (80% and 73% respectively) indicated a preference for being told.

KEPHART, WILLIAM M.

1950 "Status after death." American Sociological Review 15 (October):635–643.

Findings indicating that observable differences in class behavior exist "after death"; that is, with reference to funeral and burial customs and in practices associated with bereavement.

KLINGBERG, GOTE.

1957 "The distinction between living and not living among 7–10 year old children, with some remarks concerning the so called animism controversy." Journal of Genetic Psychology 90 (June):227–238.

The author deals with 2 questions: Do children attribute life to non-living objects and, if so, Is it to be assumed that the cause is an animistic tendency based on a primitive mental structure?

KNAPP, ROBERT H.

1960 "A study of the metaphor." Journal of Projective Techniques 24 (December):389–395.

The construction of 6 metaphor scales dealing with time, love, death, success, conscience, and self-image is reported. These scales were administered to 136 women and 87 men and the means and standard deviations for each sex are reported for all items.

KNUDSON, ALFRED G., AND JOSEPH M. NATTERSON.

1960 "Participation of parents in the hospital care of fatally ill children." Pediatrics 26(September):482–490.
Observed benefits of a parent participation program with terminal children differed according to the age of the child.

KOESTENBAUM, PETER.

1964 "The vitality of death." Journal of Existentialism 5(Fall):139–166.
The author states that mortality is an essential characteristic of life and examines how the anticipation of inevitable personal death affects the quality of human existence.

KRAUS, ARTHUR S., AND ABRAHAM M. LILIENFIELD.

1959 "Some epidemiological aspects of the high mortality rate in the young widowed group." Journal of Chronic Diseases 10(August):207–217.
The relationship between marital status and mortality appearing in statistical data on deaths and death rates by marital status, age, color, and sex was reviewed.

L

LANGER, MARION.

1957 Learning to Live as a Widow. New York: Julian Messner.
This handbook of advice for widows provides an empathetic picture of widowhood portrayed within the framework of the prior marriage.

LANGSLEY, DONALD G.

1961 "Psychology of a doomed family." American Journal of Psychotherapy 15(October):531–538.
This paper discusses the psychologic defenses with which one family as a unit (consisting of 10 siblings) and its individual members deal with the threat of premature death from an inherited renal disorder.

LE SHAN, LAWRENCE L., AND MARTHE L. GASSMAN.

1958 "Some observations on psychotherapy with patients suffering from neoplastic disease." American Journal of Psychotherapy 12(October):723–734.
Ten patients with various malignant diseases with self-known prognosis were involved in in-depth psychotherapy, with the recognition of several problems resulting from the special nature of their cases.

LE SHAN, LAWRENCE L., AND EDA J. LE SHAN.

1961 "Psychotherapy and the patient with a limited life span." Psychiatry 24 (November):318–323.

In the course of a research project into the relationships between personality and neoplastic disease, these patients and others were given the opportunity of intensive psychotherapy after their cancers had been diagnosed.

LESTER, DAVID.

1966 "Antecedents of the fear of the dead." Psychological Reports 19:741–742.

The level of fear of the dead is correlated with level of fear of others and with other variables in 75 societies.

1966 "Checking on the Harlequin." Psychological Reports 19:984.

Death-related metaphors were administered to 80 college students and sex differences were reported. The author is critical of the testing instrument.

1967 "The fear of death of suicidal persons." Psychological Reports 20:1077–1078.

Suicidal students feared death less than less suicidal students and were more aware of and concerned with the manipulative aspects of death.

1967 "Inconsistency in the fear of death of individuals." Psychological Reports 20:1084.

Subjects whose response to a death questionnaire were least consistent also indicated significantly more death fear than subjects with the most consistent responses.

1967 "Experimental and correlational studies of the fear of death." Psychological Bulletin 67 (January):27–36.

Focus of the article is survey of experimental and correlational studies on "fear of death."

LEVETON, ALAN.

1965 "Time, death, and the ego-chill." Journal of Existentialism 6 (Fall):69–80.

The ego-chill (". . . a shudder which comes from the sudden awareness that our non-existence . . . is entirely possible") is described in the case history of a woman who sought to avoid thoughts of her own death by frantic action, drugs, sex, and alcohol.

LEVIN, A. J.

1951 "The fiction of the death instinct." Psychiatric Quarterly 25 (April):257–281.

The author attacks Freud's theory of the "death instinct."

LIEBERMAN, MORTON A.

1961 "Relationship of mortality rates to entrance to a home for the aged." Geriatrics 16(October):515–519.

First-year mortality rates in a home for the aged apparently are related to the impact of institutionalization on the aged, but are not related to average age on admission or to the number of chronically ill persons admitted.

1966 "Observations on death and dying." The Gerontologist 6(June): 70–72.

The author views death as an ongoing process in time accompanied by psychological indicators including lowered ego functions. Death is an end point in a complex network of psycho-biological changes.

LIFTON, ROBERT JAY.

1965 "Psychological effects of the atomic bomb in Hiroshima: the theme of death." Pp. 8–42 in Robert L. Fulton (ed.), Death and Identity. New York: Wiley.

Interviews were conducted with survivors of the Hiroshima tragedy, with attention focused on the physical and psychological effects, each from both the long and short term, and the long-term sociological impact.

LINDEMANN, ERICH.

1944 "Symptomatology and management of acute grief." American Journal of Psychiatry 101(September):141–148.

Observations gleaned from 101 patients recently bereaved are presented. The hypothesis that acute grief is a definite syndrome with psychological and somatic symptomatology is offered.

1960 "Psychosocial factors as stressor agents." Pp. 13–16 in J. M. Tanner (ed.), Stress and Psychiatric Disorder. Oxford: Blackwell Scientific Publications.

Bereavement is a stressful situation brought about by the cessation of interaction with an emotionally relevant other person. It leads to patterns of response with physiological, psychological, and social facets.

LIPMAN, AARON, AND PHILIP W. MARDEN.

1966 "Preparation for death in old age." Journal of Gerontology 21 (July):426–431.

One hundred and nineteen residents of Miami, Florida, public housing for senior citizens were asked about concrete provisions for death, and variables were examined.

LOESER, LEWIS, AND THEA BRY.

1960 "The role of death fears in the etiology of phobic anxiety as revealed in group psychotherapy." International Journal of Group Psychotherapy 10(July):287–297.

The authors feel that the fear of death and the significance of death fears in psycho-dynamic processes are severely underestimated in theory and much neglected in practice.

M

MCCLELLAND, DAVID C.

1964 "The Harlequin complex." Pp. 94–119 in Robert W. White (ed.), The Study of Lives. New York: Atherton Press.

A historical study of the mythical Harlequin and an experimental study of the fantasies of women approaching death.

MCCULLY, ROBERT S.

1963 "Fantasy productions of children with a progressively crippling and fatal illness." Journal of Genetic Psychology 102(June): 203–216.

The fantasy productions of a group of children with a progressively crippling and fatal illness were compared with those of children who were crippled but did not face early death, and those of normal children.

MCDONALD, MARJORIE.

1963 "Helping children to understand death: an experience with death in a nursery school." Journal of Nursery School Education 19 (November):19–25.

Children must be helped to understand the facts about death and to experience the feelings it causes though it is difficult to explain and painful to bear.

MCVAY, LINDA.

1966 "An interaction study involving a patient with a guarded prognosis." American Journal of Nursing 66(May):1071–1073.

From analyzing the verbatim data in a series of "purposeful" conversations, this author learned a great deal about the patient's feelings about her illness and also improved her own perceptions.

MACDONALD, ARTHUR.

1921 "Death psychology of historical personages." American Journal of Psychology 32:552–556.

Various distinguished persons were categorized according to age of the individual at death, manner of death, and mood of last communication (i.e., resigned, sardonic, sarcastic, contented) and the average number of words of the last communication.

MACLAURIN, HARRIET.

1959 "In the hour of their going forth." Social Casework 40(February):136–141.

The caseworker with a dying patient must work through feelings about his own death as well as recognize the reactions (i.e., guilt) likely to be touched off by the actual encounter with the death of another.

MADDISON, DAVID.

1968 "The relevance of conjugal bereavement for preventive psychiatry." British Journal of Medical Psychology 41:223–233.

This article discusses research on widows that identifies certain aspects of their life situations which may affect bereavement.

MAGAZU, PETER, JOSEPH GOLNER, AND JOHN ARSENIAN.

1964 "Reactions of a group of chronic psychotic patients to the departure of the group therapist." Psychiatric Quarterly 38(April): 292–303.

A parting therapist creates some of the same responses as does the death of a therapist.

MARCUSE, HERBERT.

1959 "The ideology of death." Pp. 64–76 in Herman Feifel (ed.), The Meaning of Death. New York: McGraw-Hill.

Death is usually viewed as either a natural end process of life or else as the dissolution of bodily life and the beginning of a new life.

MARTIN, DAVID, AND LAWRENCE S. WRIGHTSMAN.

1964 "Religion and fears about death: a critical review of research." Religious Education 59(March–April):174–176.

Authors review past research and suggest ways in which they find it lacking.

1965 "The relationship between religious behavior and concern about death." Journal of Social Psychology 65(April):317–323.

Study of 58 adult members of three Protestant congregations utilizing several measures of religious attitude, religious participation, and concern about death. Those subjects who reported greater religious participation indicated less fear of death on several measures ranging from a Likert-type attitude scale to a sentence-completion technique.

A Briefly Annotated Bibliography [361

MASSERMAN, JULES H.

1954 "Emotional reactions to death and suicide." American Practitioner and Digest of Treatment 5 (November):41–46.

Theoretical discussion characterizing death and suicide as release from pain, tension, stress, and conflict, as opposed to Freud's "death instinct" theory of self-destruction.

MAURER, ADAH.

1961 "The child's knowledge of non-existence." Journal of Existential Psychiatry 2:193–212.

The commonly held belief that children know nothing of death is incorrect. Both a historical and an ontogenetic approach to the development of death awareness and conceptualizing are presented.

1964 "Did little Hans really want to marry his mother?" Journal of Humanistic Psychology 4 (Fall): 139–148.

Article stresses the role of death, rather than sex, in the etiology of phobias.

1964 "Adolescent attitudes toward death." Journal of Genetic Psychology 105 (September):75–90.

An evaluation of 172 high school senior compositions on death; subjects were all female.

1966 "Maturation of concepts of death." British Journal of Medical Psychology 39:35–41.

Children preconceptually "know" of death; this paper traces the evolution of preconceptual awareness about death to the idealism of adolescence.

1967 "The game of peek-a-boo." Diseases of the Nervous System 28 (February):118–121.

Peek-a-boo, one of the earliest of human interpersonal relationships, is seen as allaying primordial anxiety in its concern with life, death, and survival.

MEISL, ARTHUR M., AND MORTON H. HAND.

1965 "Reactions to approaching death." Diseases of the Nervous System 26 (January):15–24.

Twenty-five subjects were asked what they would think or do in 5 imagined and given circumstances involving death or immediate physical danger.

MEISSNER, W. W.

1958 "Affective response to psychoanalytic death symbols." Journal of Abnormal and Social Psychology 56 (May):295–299.

The presentation of stimulus words (found by psychoanalytic methods to be symbolic of the death concept) elicits unconscious emotional responses, indicated by a greater GSR amplitude to such words than to neutral terms.

MIDDLETON, WARREN C.

1936 "Some reactions toward death among college students." Journal of Abnormal and Social Psychology 31(July–September):165–173.

An "analysis of certain thoughts, attitudes and behavior reactions toward death" found among 825 college students of both sexes from two Midwestern universities.

MILLER, PAUL W.

1965 "Provenience of the death symbolism in Van Gogh's cornscapes." Psychoanalytic Review 52(Winter):60–66.

Van Gogh's attempt at an artistic resolution of the problem of death.

MITCHELL, MARJORIE E.

1967 The Child's Attitude to Death. New York: Schocken Books.

An outline of some of the religious, scientific, and sociological influences surrounding the British child today, including the role of myth in determining attitudes to death.

MOELLENHOFF, FRITZ.

1939 "Ideas of children about death." Bulletin of the Menninger Clinic 3(September):148–156.

Some techniques for investigating the death thoughts of children are described.

MONSOUR, KAREM J.

1960 "Asthma and the fear of death." Psychoanalytic Quarterly 29 (January):56–71.

It is postulated that asthma is a somatic expression of anxiety which later appears in psychological form as a phobic fear of death.

MORENO, J. L.

1947 "The social atom and death." Sociometry 10(February):80–84.

Discussion of how the consistency of social atoms changes as we get old, especially the ability to replace loss of membership.

MORRISSEY, JAMES R.

1963 "A note on interviews with children facing imminent death." Social Casework 44(June):343–345.

A report of a pilot study in which a small number of children with a catastrophic illness were interviewed.

1963 "Children's adaptation to fatal illness." Social Work 8 (October): 81–88.

Anxiety was the focal point from which the child's adaptation to his illness and hospitalization was evaluated and was viewed as a key variable in the overall adjustment of the child.

1964 "Death anxiety in children with a fatal illness." American Journal of Psychotherapy 18 (October):606–615.

This study was made to determine death anxiety in children hospitalized with leukemia.

MURPHY, GARDNER.

1959 "Discussion." Pp. 317–340 in Herman Feifel (ed.), The Meaning of Death. New York: McGraw-Hill.

A concluding discussion to *The Meaning of Death* by Feifel. Seven different systems of attitudes toward death are given.

MYERS, FREDERIC W. H.

1919 Human Personality and Its Survival of Bodily Death. London: Longmans, Green.

An attempt to probe the question of man's immortality through the evidence of spiritualists and related people.

N

NAGLER, J. HERBERT.

1956 "Care of the terminal cancer patient." Journal of the American Geriatrics Society 4 (July):699–707.

After stages of diagnosis and choice of treatment, therapy should be applied, not to cure the patient (since this is, by definition, impossible) but to provide comfort and perhaps to prolong life significantly.

NAGY, MARIA.

1948 "The child's theories concerning death." Journal of Genetic Psychology 73:3–27. Reprinted, pp. 79–98 in Herman Feifel (ed.), The Meaning of Death. New York: McGraw-Hill.

Written compositions, drawings, and interviews were employed in a effort to find out how children from 3 to 10 years old think about death.

NATANSON, MAURICE.

1959 "Death and situation." American Imago 16:447–457.

An essay seeking to answer the question "If 'my' death is . . . outside my possible experience, in what sense is my death a possible object for my phenomenological study?" using an analysis of Sartre's philosophy of death.

NATTERSON, JOSEPH M., AND ALFRED G. KNUDSON.

1960 "Observations concerning fear of death in fatally ill children and their mothers." Psychosomatic Medicine 22(November–December):456–465.

Observations concerning the behavior of 33 children fatally ill with leukemia or related disorders and of their mothers are presented.

NEEDLEMAN, JACOB.

1966 "Imagining absence, non-existence, and death: a sketch." Review of Existential Psychology and Psychiatry 6(Fall):230–236.

An analysis of Freud's stated impossibility: "our own death is indeed unimaginable." The question posed is whether the unimaginable is death itself, or ourselves dying.

NEURINGER, CHARLES.

1968 "Divergencies between attitudes towards life and death among suicidal, psychosomatic, and normal hospitalized patients." Journal of Consulting Psychology 32:59–63.

Attitudes toward life and death were gathered from suicidal, psychosomatic, and normal hospitalized adult male patients via semantic differential ratings of the concepts.

NORTON, JANICE.

1963 "Treatment of a dying patient." Pp. 541–560 in The Psychoanalytic Study of the Child. New York: International Universities Press.

A case study of a cancer patient. The treatment can be summarized as a process in which the author helped the patient defend herself against object loss by the development of a regressive relationship to the author.

O

O'CONNELL, WALTER E.

1968 "Humor and death." Psychological Reports 22:391–402.

A study relating the scores of 96 college students on preferences for kinds of humor to 20 death factors on a factor analyzed questionnaire.

O'CONNELL, WALTER E., AND CHARLES COVERT.

1967 "Death attitudes and humor appreciation among medical students." Existential Psychiatry 6(Winter):433–442.

When tested on scales of humor appreciation and of death attitudes, medical students differ from nonmedical students and from each other based on future specialty on the latter, but not on the former.

OKEN, DONALD.

1961 "What to tell cancer patients." Journal of the American Medical Association 175(April):1120–1128.

Most doctors prefer not to inform their patients. Emotional rather than rational reasons are usually responsible for the physicians' policy.

ORBACH, CHARLES E., ARTHUR M. SUTHERLAND, AND MARY F. BOZEMAN.

1955 "Psychological impact of cancer and its treatment: III. The adaptation of mothers to the threatened loss of their children through leukemia: Part II." Cancer 8(January–February):20–33.

Discusses the relationship of the mother and maternal grandmother in a psychoanalytic manner à la Anna Freud, Melanie Klein, and Felix Deutsch.

OSLER, WILLIAM.

1904 Science and Immortality. London: Constable.

Attitudes toward immortality are studied from three perspectives: acceptance of a belief in immortality, rejection of any supernatural part of human existence, and belief in an immortal life.

OSTOW, MORTIMER.

1958 "The death instinct—a contribution to the study of instincts." International Journal of Psychoanalysis 39:5–16.

The author suggests that primitive interspecific tendencies constitute death instinct in man.

P

PARIS, JOYCE, AND LEONARD D. GOODSTEIN.

1966 "Responses to death and sex stimulus materials as a function of repression-sensitization." Psychological Reports 19:1283–1291.

Sensitizers and repressers do not differ in expression of anxiety to death or sex-related materials.

PARSONS, TALCOTT.

1963 "Death in American society—a brief working paper." American Behavioral Scientist 6(May):61–65.

Numerous kinds of attitudes toward death are discussed along with the way they fit into the social structure.

PARSONS, TALCOTT, AND VICTOR LIDZ.

1967   "Death in American society." Pp. 133–170 in Edwin S. Shneidman (ed.), Essays in Self-Destruction. New York: Science House.

Discussion of death and various kinds of death (i.e., symbolic, biological, sociological, etc.) and how it is handled both secularly and religiously in the United States.

PATRY, FREDERICK L.

1965   "A psychiatric evaluation of communicating with the dying." Diseases of the Nervous System 26(November):715–718.

A general listing of facts and factors involved in communicating with dying patients, including a study of the role of the patient-physician relationship.

PATTISON, E. MANSELL.

1967   "The experience of dying." American Journal of Psychotherapy 21(January):32–43.

Focuses on the process of dying and the human experience that culminates in death. One's culture helps to condition the process depending upon whether death is defied, denied, or accepted.

PAZ, OCTAVIO.

1961   "The day of the dead." Pp. 47–64 in Lysander Kemp (trans.), The Labyrinth of Solitude: Life and Thought in Mexico. New York: Grove Press.

Two attitudes toward death are given: (1) pointing forward, conceiving of it as creation and (2) pointing backward, expressing itself as a fascination with nothingness or as a nostalgia for limbo.

PEARSON, LEONARD.

1969   Death and Dying. Cleveland: Case Western Reserve Press.

A collection of 5 articles based upon talks given for a lecture series on death and dying.

PENISTON, D. HUGH.

1962   "The importance of 'death education' in family life." Family Life Coordinator 11(January):15–18.

The author, a pastor, feels that good preparation before the experience of death occurs could mean the possibility of dealing with this event with better understanding and insight preventing the usual difficulties.

Q

QUINT, JEANNE C.

1963 "The impact of mastectomy." American Journal of Nursing 63 (November):88–97.
The focus of this article is on the viewpoint of the woman who experiences mastectomy and the changes that may occur in her psychological outlook and attitudes as a result.

1967 Nurse and the Dying Patient. New York: Macmillan.
Authored by a nurse with extensive experience in doing research and service with terminal patients, this book is addressed primarily to nurses, especially those responsible for the education of other nurses.

1967 "The dying patient: a difficult nursing problem." Nursing Clinics of North America 2(December):763–773.
The author delineates the problems confronting nurses participating in terminal care.

QUINT, JEANNE C., AND ANSELM L. STRAUSS.

1964 "Nursing students' assignments and dying patients." Nursing Outlook 12(January):24–27.
Attention is focused on certain assignment characteristics which affect the kinds of encounters students have with death and dying.

R

RHUDICK, PAUL J., AND ANDREW S. DIBNER.

1961 "Age, personality, and health correlates of death concerns in normal aged individuals." Journal of Gerontology 16(January): 44–49.
Study of certain anticipated correlates of death concerns among a sample of 58 normal aging individuals.

RICHMOND, JULIUS B., AND HARRY A. WAISMAN.

1955 "Psychologic aspects of management of children with malignant diseases." American Journal of Diseases of Children 89(January): 42–47.
The author suggests that parents be allowed to assist in the physical care of their fatally ill child.

RICHTER, CURT P.

1959 "The phenomenon of unexplained sudden death in animals and man." Pp. 302–313 in Herman Feifel (ed.), The Meaning of Death. New York: McGraw-Hill.

Phenomenon of unexplained sudden death in animals can be studied in the laboratory using the Norway rat. Apparently, death results from "excessive stimulation of vagal system rather than sympathetic overactivity."

RIEGEL, KLAUS F., RUTH M. RIEGEL, AND GUNTHER MEYER.

1967 "A study of the dropout rates in longitudinal research on aging and the prediction of death." Journal of Personality and Social Psychology 5 (March) :342–348.

Loss of subjects through death in longitudinal work is not randomly distributed, but occurs to those with certain characteristics more often than chance.

RIES, HANNAH.

1945 "An unwelcome child and her death instinct." International Journal of Psychoanalysis 26:153–161.

A young girl was born to a mother who never wanted children. The author concludes that unwanted children are bound to develop suicidal and destructive wishes.

RILEY, JOHN W. JR.

1968 "Death: death and bereavement." Pp. 19–26 in International Encyclopedia of the Social Sciences. New York: Macmillan and Free Press.

A philosophical, anthropological, and sociological discussion of death and bereavement plus an overview of methodology and research in this area.

RIOCH, DAVID, CHARLES C. HERBERT, NANCY E. MEAD, MAURICE GOLDSTEIN, AND EDWIN A. WEINSTEIN.

1961 "The psychophysiology of death." Pp. 177–225 in Alexander Simon (ed.) The Physiology of Emotions. Springfield, Ill.: Charles C Thomas.

A variety of behavioral phenomena: autonomic, endocrine, symbolic, and social as they relate to one or another aspect of death are discussed.

RIVERS, WILLIAM H. R.

1926 "The primitive conception of death." Pp. 36–50 in Psychology and Ethnology. London: Kegan Paul, Trench, Trubner.

Primitive peoples (Melanesians in this case) do not regard the dichotomy between living and dead as do civilized societies.

ROSE, GILBERT J.

1960 "Analytic first aid for a three year old." American Journal of Orthopsychiatry 30 (January) :200–201.

Manifestations of separation and anxiety and other fears (including fear of dying) in a 3-year-old disappear after the opportunity is presented for verbalization of her fears of death.

ROSENTHAL, HATTIE R.
1957 "Psychotherapy for the dying." American Journal of Psychotherapy 11(July):626–633.
Therapy for a dying patient, whether or not he is totally aware of the seriousness of his situation, can be of great help in preparing the patient to face death and in alleviating various anxieties and guilt feelings before death.

1963 "The fear of death as an indispensable factor in psychotherapy." American Journal of Psychotherapy 17(October):619–630.
This article stresses the need for the psychotherapist to be aware of the universality of the fear and anxiety regarding death.

ROSENTHAL, PAULINE.
1947 "The death of the leader in group psychotherapy." American Journal of Orthopsychiatry 17(April):266–277.
A discussion of the reactions of group therapy patients to the death of Dr. Paul Schilder, himself active in research on reactions to death.

ROSS, ELISABETH KÜBLER.
1969 On Death and Dying. New York: The Macmillan Company.
See Chapter 8.

ROTHENBERG, ALBERT.
1961 "Psychological problems in terminal cancer management." Cancer 14(September–October):1063–1073.
Five prominent interpersonal issues operating in terminal cancer management are defined: loss of control and mastery, denial, grief, sense of failure, and isolation.

RUSSELL, BERTRAND.
1929 "Your child and the fear of death." The Forum 81(March):174–178.
Knowledge of painful hazards of life, including death, should be neither avoided nor obtruded as regards children. They should come when circumstances make it unavoidable.

S

SAFIER, GWEN.
1964 "A study in relationships between the life and death concepts in children." Journal of Genetic Psychology 105(December):283–294.

Study aimed at determining whether or not a person's "animism" score and his "death" score decrease as he ages.

SANDERS, DAVID, AND JESSE DUKEMINIER JR.

1968 "Medical advance and legal lag: hemodialysis and kidney transplantation." UCLA Law Review 15 (February):357–413.

With the advent of advanced techniques for curing biological failures and prolonging otherwise fatal conditions, there are profound legal and ethical considerations and responsibilities.

SARNOFF, IRVING, AND SETH M. CORWIN.

1959 "Castration anxiety and the fear of death." Journal of Personality 27 (September):374–385.

Persons with high castration anxiety show a greater fear of death after the arousal of their sexual feelings than would persons who have a low degree of castration anxiety.

SAUL, LEON J.

1959 "Reactions of a man to natural death." Psychoanalytic Quarterly 28 (July):383–386.

Study of a physician who was faced with fatal cancer, a diagnosis with which he agreed, and his use of denial in the face of such inevitable reality.

SAUNDERS, CICELY.

1965 "The last stages of life." American Journal of Nursing 65 (March):70–75.

The author argues for accepting and preparing, rather than avoiding and negating, death; for focusing on death as life's fulfillment rather than defeat.

SCHILDER, PAUL.

1936 "The attitude of murderers towards death." Journal of Abnormal and Social Psychology 31 (October–December):348–363.

Thirty-one murderers incarcerated at Bellevue Hospital for treatment were administered a standardized questionnaire dealing with various attitudes toward death, dying, killing, etc.

1942 Pp. 61–110 in Goals and Desires of Man: A Psychological Survey of Life. New York: Columbia University Press.

These 4 chapters dealing with death are part of a book based on a large psychiatric experience in both private and public practice.

SCHILDER, PAUL, AND DAVID WECHSLER.

1934 "The attitudes of children toward death." Journal of Genetic Psychology 45 (September):406–451.

A study of the attitudes toward death of 76 children ages 5 to 15, through interviews and responses to pictures.

SCHNECK, JEROME M.

1951 "The unconscious relationship between hypnosis and death." Psychoanalytic Review 38(July):271–275.
From psychotherapeutic case histories, persons equating hypnosis with death are illustrated.

SCHWARTZ, BERNARD J.

1955 "The measurement of castration anxiety and anxiety over loss of love." Journal of Personality 24(December):204–219.
A statistically significant increase in castration anxiety was elicited for subjects who had just viewed a film on subincision rites; a film that was expected to produce a similar change in loss of love anxiety was not successful.

SCOTT, COLIN A.

1896 "Old age and death." American Journal of Psychology 8(October):67–122.
Based upon 226 questionnaire responses, the author concluded that death is an important element in the consciousness of human beings.

SEARLES, HAROLD F.

1961 "Schizophrenia and the inevitability of death." Psychiatric Quarterly 35(October):631–665.
Schizophrenia can be seen as an intense effort to ward off or deny death. The author is convinced of the importance of the concept of death as a source of anxiety in all our lives.

SEGAL, HANNA.

1958 "Fear of death: notes on the analysis of an old man." International Journal of Psychoanalysis 39:178–181.
The author cites a case as evidence for his theory that fear of death underlies many old-age breakdowns.

SHEPS, JACK.

1957 "Management of fear of death in chronic disease." Journal of the American Geriatrics Society 5(September):793–797.
The author stresses the importance of recognizing and managing the fear of death in chronically diseased and dying patients.

SHNEIDMAN, EDWIN S.

1964 "Orientations toward death: a vital aspect of the study of lives." Pp. 201–227 in Robert W. White (ed.), The Study of Lives. New York: Atherton Press.

This is an attempt to create a psychologically oriented classification of death phenomena and to take into account the role of the individual in his own demise.

1964 "Suicide, sleep and death: some possible interrelations among cessation, interruption and continuation phenomena." Journal of Consulting Psychology 28 (April) : 95–106.
Article searches for similarities between sleep phenomena (called interruption) and death phenomena (called cessation).

1967 Essays in Self-Destruction. New York: Science House.
A grouping of essays in the following categories: literary and philosophic, sociological, psychological and psychiatric, and taxonomic and forensic—all dealing with death and, in particular, suicide.

SHONTZ, FRANKLIN C., AND STEPHEN L. FINK.

1959 "'A psychobiological analysis of discomfort, pain and death." Journal of General Psychology 60 (April) : 275–287.
Discussed positive, negative, oscillating, and integrating orientations to comfort, pain, and death.

SHOOR, MERVYN, AND MARY H. SPEED.

1965 "Death, delinquency, and the mourning process." Pp. 201–206 in Robert L. Fulton (ed.), Death and Identity. New York: Wiley. [Also: Psychiatric Quarterly, 1963, 37, 540–558].
Abnormal reactions tending to delinquency are presented as case histories of several young persons, each suffering the loss of a close family member.

SHRUT, SAMUEL D.

1958 "Attitudes toward old age and death." Mental Hygiene 42 (April) : 259–266.
Old people living under conditions approximating previous mode of independent residence in the community reflect a less apprehensive attitude toward death, and are generally better adjusted to the life about them.

SIMMEL, ERNST.

1944 "Self-preservation and the death instinct." Psychoanalytic Quarterly 13 (April) : 160–185.
Simmel considers the destructive energies to be manifestations of an instinct of self-preservation rather than of a death instinct.

SIMMONS, LEO W.

1945 Role of the Aged in Primitive Society. New Haven: Yale University Press. [Pp. 217–244.]

A Briefly Annotated Bibliography

Delineation of some of the attitudes of primitive societies toward death and dying.

SLATER, ELIOT.

1958 "The biologist and the fear of death." The Plain View 12(May): 29–42.

The physician's role is to preserve health but not to prolong life artificially.

SLATER, PHILIP E.

1964 "Prolegomena to a psychoanalytic theory of aging and death." Chap. 2 in Robert Kastenbaum (ed.), New Thoughts on Old Age. New York: Springer.

The combination of experiences that each individual undergoes is unique. This uniqueness creates barriers to the diffusion of libidinal attachments, a tendency which is continually exacerbated by the accelerating frequency with which he experiences losses of love objects.

SOLNIT, ALBERT J., AND MORRIS GREEN.

1959 "Psychologic considerations in the management of deaths on pediatric hospital services, I: the doctor and the child's family." Pediatrics 24(July):106–112.

The doctor's aid to the family extends from before the child's death, through informing the parents of the death, to helping the family after the death and dealing with his own reaction to the death.

1963 "The pediatric management of the dying child: Part II: the child's reaction to the fear of dying." Pp. 217–228 in Albert J. Solnit and Sally A. Provence (eds.), Modern Perspectives in Child Development. New York: International Universities Press.

Three major considerations in the child's psychological reactions to his own dying: Am I safe? Will there be a trusted person to keep me from feeling helpless, alone, and to overcome pain? Will you make me feel all right?

SPILKA, BERNARD, ROBERT J. PELLEGRINI, AND KATHRYN DAILEY.

1968 "Religion, American values and death perspectives." Sociological Symposium 1(Fall):57–66.

Study which attempts to correlate death attitudes with three measures of motivation and life orientation.

SPITZER, STEPHEN P., AND JEANETTE R. FOLTA.

1964 "Death in the hospital—a problem for study." Nursing Forum 3 (March):85–92.

Authors advance the hypothesis that unexpected deaths tend to disrupt hospital routine which lowers the efficiency of the hospital.

STACEY, CHALMERS L., AND KARL MARKIN.

1952 "The attitudes of college students and penitentiary inmates toward death and a future life." Psychiatric Quarterly 26:27–32.

Compared attitudes toward death of engineering, forestry, and law students with prisoners.

STACEY, CHALMERS L., AND MARIE L. REICHEN.

1954 "Attitudes toward death and future life among normal and subnormal adolescent girls." Exceptional Children 20(March):259–262.

Subnormal adolescent girls appear to be more emotional and fearful in their attitudes toward death than a control group of normals.

STEINZOR, BERNARD.

1960 "Death and the construction of reality." Pp. 358–375 in John G. Peatman and Eugene L. Hartley (eds.), Festschrift for Gardner Murphy. New York: Harper.

Attempt at correlating child's development of ideas about death and his adaptation to reality by first, a review of depth psychology, second, presentation of material from the viewpoint of child psychologists and, finally, some suggested proposals for research.

STERBA, RICHARD.

1948 "On Hallowe'en." American Imago 5(April):213–224.

The author contends that since we do not honor the dead on Halloween in this country, we are symbolically sacrificing our children to them on Halloween night by letting them be dead, i.e., the spirits of the dead for that night, and also that we appease them by the goodies we give them at our doors.

STRAUSS, ANSELM L., BARNEY GLASER, AND JEANNE QUINT.

1964 "The nonaccountability of terminal care." Hospitals 38(January): 73–87.

Health services personnel responsible for terminal patients are often seen to have less accountability for their actions than those handling other patients. (See Chapter 7.)

SUDNOW, DAVID.

1967 Passing on: The Social Organization of Dying. Englewood Cliffs, N.J.: Prentice Hall.

Close personal observations of the hospital setting in which people die, how these deaths occur, and how they affect the personalities and social structure of the hospitals. (See Chapter 10.)

SWENSON, WENDELL M.

1959 "Attitudes toward death among the aged." Minnesota Medicine 42(April):399–402.
Responses to a death attitudes checklist divided elderly subjects into 3 groups: those looking forward to death, those avoiding any thought of death, and those fearing death.

1961 "Attitudes toward death in an aged population." Journal of Gerontology 16(January):49–52.
Attitudes toward death can be measured by a structured psychometric device, not only projective techniques.

T

TABACHNICK, NORMAN, AND DAVID KLUGMAN.

1967 "Suicide research and the death instinct." Yale Scientific Magazine (March).
There are many reasons behind suicide other than the wish to die but the ultimate question as to the existence of the death instinct is unanswered by research to date.

TEICHER, JOSEPH D.

1953 "Combat fatigue or death anxiety neurosis." Journal of Nervous and Mental Disease 117(January–June):234–243.
The use of the diagnostic term "combat fatigue" is examined and shown to be inadequate; the term "death anxiety neurosis" is more appropriate for this syndrome.

THURMOND, CHARLES J.

1943 "Last thoughts before drowning." Journal of Abnormal and Social Psychology 38(April):165–184.
A 19-year-old boy who survived an unusual accident only because he was a good swimmer was afterward in a delirious state for hours. His every word, while in delirium, was transcribed and later the transcript was discussed with him.

TILLICH, PAUL.

1959 "The eternal now." Pp. 30–38 in Herman Feifel (ed.), The Meaning of Death. New York: McGraw-Hill.
Time runs from beginning to end but our awareness goes in the opposite direction—that is, it starts with anxious anticipation of end.

TOCH, RUDOLF.

1964 "Management of the child with a fatal disease." Clinical Pediatrics 3(July):418–427.

A physician discusses his personal views of dealing with the question of how to handle information in cases of fatal childhood diseases.

TOLOR, ALEXANDER, AND MARVIN REZNIKOFF.

1967 "Relation between insight, repression-sensitization, internal-external control and death anxiety." Journal of Abnormal Psychology 72:426–430.

Among college males, death anxiety is found related to repression and sensitization, insight, and other variables.

U

ULANOV, BARRY.

1959 Death—A Book of Preparation and Consolation. New York: Sheed and Ward.

Much of the weight and wisdom of a society may be discerned from its attitudes toward death. The news media, advertisements, the popular arts, etc. all offer an indication of the death attitudes of twentieth-century America, but they fail to reveal the thought processes of Americans about death.

V

VERNICK, JOEL, AND MYRON KARON.

1965 "Who's afraid of death on a leukemia ward?" American Journal of Diseases of the Child 109(May):393–397.

The most meaningful way adults can help meet the emotional needs of the fatally ill child is to create an environment in which the child is free to express his fears and receive an honest answer to any question.

VERNON, GLENN M.

1968 "Some questions about the 'inevitable-death orientation.'" Sociological Symposium 1(Fall):74–84.

The author looks at death as a personal, biological, and social phenomenon and questions the perspective which regards death strictly as an inevitable event.

VERWOERDT, ADRIAAN.

1966 Communication with the Fatally Ill. Springfield, Ill.: Charles C Thomas.

A Briefly Annotated Bibliography [377

The circumstances surrounding communication with the fatally ill produce a variety of complications, intense feelings, uncertainties, and distress.

VITANZA, ANGELO A.

1960 "Toward a theory of crying." Psychoanalysis and Psychoanalytic Review 47(Winter):65–77.
Implications for a relationship between crying and death or dying.

VON HUG-HELLMUTH, HERMINE.

1965 "The child's concept of death." Psychoanalytic Quarterly 34 (October):499–516.
"Being dead" to a child means lying quietly for a time, sleeping, being away; but always man has the power to change it.

VON LERCHENTHAL, ERICH.

1948 "Death from psychic causes." Bulletin of the Menninger Clinic 12(January):31–36.
Psychic deaths occur from both hysteria and suggestion. One case is discussed in which a woman predicted her death but it did not occur; other cases are discussed briefly.

W

WAGNER, BERNICE M.

1964 "Teaching students to work with the dying." American Journal of Nursing 64(November):128–131.
A survey of efforts at University of Kansas shows that, there, students are exposed to a variety of material on death and dying, and are then helped to analyze their own attitudes.

WAHL, CHARLES W.

1962 "The physician's management of the dying patient." Pp. 127–136 in Jules Masserman (ed.), Current Psychiatric Therapies. New York: Grune and Stratton.
The physician's primary goal is seen as assuaging the terror of death and dying in the patient, to prevent adverse affect on the disease, to give hope, and to offer death as a dignified process.

1965 "The fear of death." Pp. 56–66 in Robert L. Fulton (ed.), Death and Identity. New York: Wiley. [Also: Bulletin of the Menninger Clinic, 1958, 22:214–223; and pp. 16–29 in Herman Feifel (ed.), The Meaning of Death (New York: McGraw-Hill).]

The use of magic and irrationality as a defensive solution to the inevitability of death is explored with child study forwarded as the most promising research avenue into the subconscious mind.

WALTERS, MARY JANE.

1944 "Psychic death: report of a possible case." Archives of Neurology and Psychiatry 52(July):84–85.

The case of the death of a 42-year-old woman who strongly identified with her mother to the point of dying at almost exactly the same age is discussed.

WARNER, LLOYD.

1959 The Living and the Dead. New Haven: Yale University Press. [Pp. 280–320.]

Description and explanation of the cemetery as an important part of life in "Yankee City," a typical American city.

WEISMAN, AVERY D., AND THOMAS P. HACKETT.

1961 "Predilection to death: death and dying as a psychiatric problem." Psychosomatic Medicine 23(May–June):232–256.

A series of 5 unusual surgical patients is reported in which "predilection" to death at the time of admission to the hospital was a prominent part of the clinical picture.

WEISMAN, AVERY D., AND ROBERT KASTENBAUM.

1969 "The psychological autopsy." Community Mental Health Journal, monograph series.

A study of the dying process through the thorough analysis of the social and psychological events during the period of time preceeding death.

WILKES, ERIC.

1965 "Terminal cancer at home." Lancet 1(April):799–801.

Primarily the article is aimed at the logistics of the dying patient at home, having to do with amount and quality of nursing required, etc.

WILLIAMS, GLANVILLE L.

1957 The Sanctity of Life and the Criminal Law. New York: Knopf.

A full discussion of birth control, abortion, infanticide, euthanasia, and sterilization comparing laws of the United States and England and discussing adequacy of such laws.

WILLIAMS, MARY.

1966 "Changing attitudes to death: a survey of contributions in *Psychological Abstracts* over a thirty year period." Human Relations 19:405–423.

Analyzes contributions listed in the service from subject, field of work, and time points of view.

WILLIAMS, ROBERT L., AND SPURGEON COLE.

1968   "Religiosity, generalized anxiety, and apprehension concerning death." Journal of Social Psychology 75:111–117.

The hypothesis tested was that there would be a strong negative correlation between measures of religiosity and security. The high religiosity group showed the least anxiety on all dimensions (generalized anxiety, apprehension toward death, conscious anxiety, and physiological arousal) and the low religiosity group showed the most generalized insecurity.

WOHLFORD, PAUL.

1966   "Extension of personal time, affective states and expectation of personal death." Journal of Personality and Social Psychology 3 (May):559–566.

An individual's affective state may causally influence his extension of personal time into the future.

WOLFF, KURT.

1967   "Helping elderly patients face the fear of death." Hospital and Community Psychiatry 18(May):142–144.

The nature, frequency, and significance of death fears among the elderly are explored, including the relationships of such fears to the individual's total attitude-personality complex.

WORCESTER, ALFRED.

1940   The Care of the Aged, the Dying, and the Dead. Springfield, Illinois: Charles C Thomas [2nd printing: 1950].

Directed to the general practitioner, this book gives attention to trying to show the value and reasons for working with aged patients. Devotion for the patient and his needs, rather than theoretical knowledge of the disease, is stressed.

Y

YOUNG, WILLIAM H.

1960   "Death of a patient during psychotherapy." Psychiatry 23(February):103–108.

A psychiatrist recounts a case-history of a patient pronounced terminally ill soon after her first visit.

Z

ZELIGS, ROSE.

1967 "Death casts its shadow on a child." Mental Hygiene 51 (January):9–20.

Traces effect of parental shielding of 6-year-old child from the facts of the sudden death of his 1-year-old brother.

1967 "Children's attitudes toward death." Mental Hygiene 51 (January):393–396.

When a parent is overwhelmed by the death of his spouse or child, his living child may absorb his anxiety. If the parent is afraid to talk about the death, his child may repress his own fears, guilt, and confusion, and become seriously disturbed.

ZILBOORG, GREGORY.

1943 "Fear of death." Psychoanalytic Quarterly 12 (October):465–475.

Discussion of various psychological devices used in problem of how one reacts to the fear of death as the fundamental psychological issue involved in the problem of morale during war.

ZINKER, JOSEPH C., AND STEPHEN L. FINK.

1966 "The possibility for psychological growth in a dying person." Journal of General Psychology 74 (April): 185–199.

Authors used an open-end approach to examine in detail one dying subject over a period of 5 months. On a long-term basis, the subject's motivational life did not change as she was dying.

Name Index

After Experience (Snodgrass), 83
Aldrich, C. K., 99
American College of Physicians, 232
American College of Surgeons, 231
American Hospital Association, 232
American Medical Association, 47, 118, 230, 231, 232, 240, 273
American Public Health Association, 243
Anderson, Odin W., 8, 19
Aring, Charles D., 180
Aronson, Gerald J., 60
Arrow, Kenneth J., 279, 280

Bailey, Richard M., 275–302
Baker, J. W., 69
Banting, Frederick, 127
Barnard, Christiaan, 102, 106, 108, 112, 115, 116, 117, 121
Becker, Howard S., 54, 129, 173, 175
Beecher, H. K., 110, 239
Beigler, J. S., 312
Berkson, J., 74
Best, Charles, 127
Billings, Frank, 231
Blaiberg, Philip, 106
Blau, P. M., 309
Blauner, Robert, 32
Blood, R. O., 317
Blue Cross, 119, 278, 300
Blue Shield, 249
Blum, Henrik L., 286
Bohrod, Milton G., 174
Boulogne, Charles, 107
Bowers, M., 314*n*.
Brim, Orville G., Jr., xiii–xxvi
Bruner, D. K., 54
Burgess, A. M., Jr., 246

Cabot, Richard, 185

Cape Town Conference, 110, 117
Cappon, D., 311, 316, 318, 319
Carlin, J. E., 309
Caudhill, W., 309
Chandler, K. A., 316
Charter, Royal College of Physicians (London), 226
Chase, Samuel B., Jr., 276
Chicago Board of Health, 18
Coggeshall, Lowell T., 175
Coleman, J., 309
College of Surgeons, 231
Conn, H. O., 70
Cooley, Denton, 110, 113*n*., 117
Crane, Diana, 303–325
Curran, William, 242, 243

Davidson, Charles S., 186
Death and Dying (Ross), 156
Death Be Not Proud (Gunther), 171
Death of Ivan Ilyich, The (Tolstoy), 179
DeBakey, M. E., 244
Deeley, T. J., 93
Doctor's Dilemma, The (Shaw), 89, 227
Donne, John, xiii
Dorn, Harold F., 9
Downs, Anthony, 279
Dublin, Louis I., 7
Dubos, René, xxi
Duff, Raymond S., 185, 217, 306, 310, 315, 317
Durkheim, E., 318

Edwards, J. M. Rice, 93
Emanuel, R., 95
Emerson, Joan P., 60, 61
Engel, A. G. W., 228

NAME INDEX

Epstein, Jason, 217
Equitable Life Assurance Society of U.S., 33
Estimating the Cost of Illness (Rice), 298, 299
Evening Standard, 88

Farberow, N. L., 312n.
Feifel, Herman, 30, 32, 43, 46, 56, 60, 172, 314
Feinstein, A. R., 68, 70, 71, 72, 73
Flexner Report, 231, 245
Folsom Committee, 244
Foner, Anne, 39n.
Foundation of Thanatology, 156
Fox, Renee C., 133, 174, 307
Freeman, Howard E., xiii–xxvi
Freud, Sigmund, xv, 171
Freyman, Geoffrey, 230, 231
Friedman, Milton, 227, 277
Friedman, Stanley B., 180
Fullarton, J. E., 21
Fulton, Robert L., 31, 311

Garceau, A. J., 70
Glaser, Barney G., 32, 47, 60, 61, 129–155, 174, 182, 306, 307, 309, 310, 311, 313, 314, 315, 317, 318
Glaser, Robert J., 102–128, 191
Gofman, J. W., 87
Gorer, G., 313, 320
Group for the Advancement of Psychiatry, 171

Hackett, Thomas P., 172, 179, 312, 317
Harvard Medical School, 110
Harvard School of Public Health, 242
Haviland, James W., 283
Hazard, J. Beach, 186
Heart Disease, Cancer and Stroke Amendments, 21
Henning, N., 69
Henry VIII, King, 226
Hillery, George A., Jr., 15, 16
Hinton, J., 79, 183, 311, 320
Hollingshead, August B., 185, 217, 306, 310, 315, 317
Hospital Inpatient Inquiry, 184
Howard, Alan, 43
Hubbard, W. N., Jr., 175
Huizinga, J., 171

Jackson, F. C., 70
Jakobovits, Immanuel, 57, 59
Joint Commission on Hospital Accreditation, 231, 233
Jordan, E. P., 236
Jung, Carl G., 55

Kalish, Richard A., 32, 44, 47, 314n., 318
Kaplan, H. S., 94
Kasper, August M., 172, 173
Kasperak, Mike, 119
Kastenbaum, Robert, 47, 316, 319
Kavinovsky, Bernice, 146
King, L. S., 226
Kitagawa, Evelyn M., 17
Klein, Melanie, 61
Knutson, Andie L., 42–64
Kuznets, S., 227

Landau, Lev Davidovitch, 88, 89
Lasagna, Louis, 67–101
Lees, D. S., 278, 286
Lerner, Monroe, 5–29, 172
LeShan, Lawrence, 314n.
Lester, David, 43, 45, 54, 55, 314
Levine, Sol, 211–224
Lidz, Victor, 31, 308, 311
Lieberman, M., 319
Lillihei, Walton, 117
Lindemann, Erich, 61, 320
Lindenmuth, W. W., 70
Lipworth, L., 177, 184
Lister, Joseph, 184
Lutkins, S. G., 80, 320, 321

Magic Mountain (Mann), 183
Manhattan State Hospital, 157
Manning, Bayless, 253–274
Marmor, Theodore, 245
Marshall, J., 87
Maryland State Department of Health, 22, 183
Mayo, Charles, 177
Mayo Clinic, 74
McEvoy, T. L., 312n.
McGuffey's Fifth Eclectic Reader, 171
McLuhan, Marshall, 121
McMath, W. F. T., 88
Medawar, Peter, 105
Medical Research Council, 238
Medicare, 225, 244, 297

NAME INDEX

Ministry of Health (Gt. Britain), 229
Minot, George R., 127
Mirage of Health, The (Dubos), xxi
Mondale, Walter, 111
Moore, Wilbert E., 33
Morgenstern, Oskar, 280
Moses, L. E., 75, 178
Mosteller, Frederick, 75, 178
Murray, Joseph E., 105
Musser, John H., 231

Nader, Ralph, 242
National Health Service, 229, 237
National Heart Institute, 119
National Institutes of Health, 46, 118, 119, 180
National Opinion Research Center (University of Chicago), 33
Neasden Hospital (London), 87
New York Times, 177
Nighswonger, Carl A., 160, 162
Nightingale, Florence, 183, 184

Office of Program Analysis (HEW), 298
Oken, D., 99, 315

Page, Irvine H., 122
Paget, J., 226
Parke, C. M., 320
Parsons, Talcott, 31, 308, 311
Pearson, R. J. C., 234
Peter Bent Brigham Hospital (Boston), 105
Peterson, Osler L., 118, 225–252
Phillips, D., 312
Platt, Robert, 238
Pond, M. Allen, 19
Public Health Service, 238, 244

Quint, Jeanne C., 129, 130n., 145, 147, 314, 317
Qui Numerare Incipit Errere Incipit (Morgenstern), 280

Rabin, David L., 171–190
Rabin, Laurel H., 171–190
Rackenmann, F. M., 127
Rees, W. D., 80, 320, 321
Ribicoff, Abraham, 112
Rice, Dorothy P., 298, 299
Richter, K., 318

Riley, John W., Jr., 30–41, 314
Riley, Matilda White, 39n.
Robinson, Joan, 280
Rosen, George, 19
Ross, Elisabeth Kübler, 145, 156–170, 315

St. Bartholomew's Hospital, 226
Saphir, O., 57
Savage, L. J., 277
Schelling, T. C., 277
Schimmel, Elihu, 184
Scotch, Norman A., 211–224
Scott, C. A., 45
Scott, Robert A., 43
Secretary of Health, 229
Seidel, Henry, 176
Semmelweis, Ignaz, 184
Shapiro, Sam, 176
Shils, E., 307
Shneidman, Edwin S., 45, 311
Shumway, Norman, 117, 118, 119, 121
Simmons, R. G., 307
Simmons, R. L., 307
Sinclair, William J., 184
Snodgrass, W. P., 83
Social Security Act (1965), Amendments to, 288
Spiegel, John P., 211
Spiegelman, Mortimer, 10
Starzl, Thomas E., 107
Stevens, S., 226, 229
Stewart, I., 312
Stewart, William H., 244
Stone, J. E., 243
Strauss, Anselm L., 19, 32, 47, 60, 61, 129–155, 174, 182, 306, 307, 309, 310, 311, 313, 314, 315, 317, 318
Sudnow, David, 32, 44, 51, 180, 191–208, 221, 308, 309
Swazey, J. P., 307

Tarver, James D., 10

Uniform Anatomical Gift Act, 112, 267
Uniform Simultaneous Death Act, 269
United Nations, 9
University of Chicago, 158

Veterans Administration, 76, 83
Volkart, E. H., 61

Wangensteen, Owen, 117, 118
Washkansky, Louis, 116
Weber, Max, 6
Weisbrod, Burton, 283
Weisman, Avery D., 172, 179, 312, 317, 319
Welch, William H., 231
Wennberg, John, 182
Wertenbaker, Lael, 150
Williams, Greer, xiii–xxvi, 121
Williams, Mary, 45, 54
Wolfe, D. M., 317
Wrongful Death Statute, 259–260

Yordy, K. D., 21
Yudkin, S., 100

Subject Index

Abortion, xxiii, 237, 242–243, 273
Afterlife, xxiii, 43, 62, 211, 313
Alcoholism, 205–206
American medicine, mythology of, xxi
Artificial kidney, 76, 95, 105, 213, 221, 306
  selection for, xxi, 90, 162, 239, 283
Autopsy, 56, 81
  cost of, 186
  in different hospitals, 185, 194
  findings of, 152, 180, 184–185
  in medical education, 173, 185
  permits, 185, 193, 194
  religious beliefs and, 57–59
  value of, 186

Bereavement
  adjustment to, 304, 319–321
  mortality following, 80–81
  problems of, 41, 215–216

Cadaver, in medical education, 173
Cancer, 74, 98, 181, 305
  biological predeterminism in, 72
  prognostication of, 68, 70–71
  suicide in terminal, patients', 311–312
  treatment of, 93–94
  as an unappealing disease, 91–92
Cancer radiotherapy, popularity of, 244
Cancer surgery, radical and conservative, 73
Cardiac Disease. *See* Heart disease
Cardiac transplantation. *See* Heart transplantation
Causes of death, 7, 13, 70, 75n.
  in and outside of institutions, 25–26

Causes of death (*cont.*)
  See also Diseases as causes of death
Children
  conception of death of, 32
  death of, 173–174, 176, 180
  economic value of, 282
  experience of, with death, 47, 48, 50, 171
Chronic diseases. *See* Degenerative diseases
Clergy
  dying patient and, 33, 145, 160, 161, 162, 179
  effectiveness of, in helping the dying patient, 147, 316
Clinical research institutes, 238
Communicable diseases, xxii, 7, 12–15, 212
Cost-benefit analysis
  of disease conditions, 300
  of health services system, 213, 289
  limitations of, 295–297
Critical list, 79, 195

Dead body. *See* Autopsy
Dead on arrival, 199
Dead person, ministering to, 196–197
Death
  allocation of, 255, 256, 257–258, 273
  in the arts and mass media, 40, 42, 48, 62
  attitudes toward, xiv, 32, 33–35, 38, 40, 44, 54, 55–56, 168, 175, 307, 314
  avoidance of, xv, xvi, xviii, 30, 33, 48, 171, 211
  bureaucratization of, 215–217
  causes of. *See* Causes of death; Diseases as causes of death
  of children, 173–174, 176, 180

385

386] SUBJECT INDEX

Death (cont.)
  concept of, 266, 268–269
  control of, 31, 42
  cost of, 291–295
  defining. See Defining death
  different medical specialties associated with, xxii, 178
  direct and indirect costs of, 292–295
  discovery of, 197
  disruptions caused by, 212, 215, 303
  dying and, distinctions between, xix, 144, 212, 218, 303–304
  euphemisms for, 61
  experience of, xv, xvi–xvii, 49
  as failure, 174, 188, 204, 211
  family and. See Family
  fear of. See Fear of death
  funeral parlor and, 215, 216
  in hospitals, xix, 80, 184, 215, 321
  images of, 33, 35–36, 37, 38–39, 40, 43, 152
  individual, xiii, 192
  interpretations of, 42, 43–44
  management of, by society, 215, 218
  nurses and, 49, 196–197, 198
  physician and. See Physician, death and
  plans about, 33, 37–38, 39–40
  research on, 40, 45, 46, 47, 54–56
  social consequences of, xxiii, 30, 32, 217, 283
  symbols of, 173
Death and Dying, seminar on, 158–159
Death coma, 194, 196
Death taboo, xvi, 30, 34, 37, 40, 45, 49, 62, 171
Death talk, 144, 147
Death watch, as form of social death, 194
Decisions concerning patient care. See Hospitals, organization of, related to physician decisions; Physician, determinants of, behavior
Defining death, xv, xx, 30, 33, 40, 43, 108, 265–266
  as anthropological death, 44
  as biological death, 44, 191
  as brain death, 44, 109, 110, 125, 191, 239
  as clinical death, 44
  as heart death, 109, 125
  as process, 109, 266

Defining death (cont.)
  as psychological death, 44
  as social death, 44, 191–193, 194, 196, 199–200, 318
Degenerative diseases, xxii, 7, 15–16
Diseases as causes of death, 27, 68, 75–76, 285
  as in cancer. See Cancer
  communicable, decline in, xxii, 12–15, 212
  degenerative, increase in, xxii, 15–16
  in other countries, 16
  in and outside of institutions, 24–26
  pneumonia, 86, 123, 240, 306
  shift from communicable diseases (acute infections) to degenerative (chronic), 46, 179, 217, 303
  as in stroke, 86
Donor, problems concerning, 262, 265–266, 304, 306, 307
  heart, problems concerning, 99, 108–113, 110, 117
  See also Organ transplantation
Drug therapy, 8, 69–70, 76, 96–97, 116, 154, 181, 238–239
  as cause of death, 70, 75, 96
Dying
  changes in character and duration of, 179, 212–213, 217–218
  definition of, 207, 208
  family and. See Family
  at home, xviii, 22, 32, 80, 142, 311
  in institutions. See Institutions
  medical technology and, 213, 217–218, 222, 255, 303
  physician and. See Physician
  quality of, xxiii, 319
  quick dying, 133–135
  as self-fulfilling prophecy, 198, 203
  slow, 137–138
  as a social problem, xx, xxiv, 45, 212–214, 217, 223, 304, 307, 321–322
  time factor in, 131, 217–218
Dying patient
  adjustment of, 46, 79, 145, 167–170, 317–319
  aged as, 83–88, 90, 174, 318
  attitudes toward, 54, 308, 313–314, 316
  awareness of, 140–141, 143, 144, 160–161, 167, 315, 319
  child as, 99, 100

Dying patient (cont.)
  clergy and. See Clergy
  communication with, xviii, 32, 46, 61, 100, 138, 147, 156, 158, 161–170, 218, 304, 313–317, 320
  employers of, 220
  hospital staff and. See Hospital staff, dying patient and
  in institutions. See Institutions, dying in
  isolation of, 32, 147, 148, 157, 159, 180
  loses control, 47, 218, 311, 321
  nurse and, 61, 132–139, 143–144, 145, 158, 159, 160, 182, 198, 314
  physician and, 46, 132–139, 143, 145, 158, 179, 195–196, 220
  prolonging life of. See Prolonging life
  radical procedures used on, 204–205
  religious beliefs and, 159, 164–165, 168–169
  self-medication of, 91
  telling the, 60–61, 78, 99–100, 145, 212, 315
  younger person as, 318
Dying trajectory
  critical junctions in, 131–132, 143, 206
  definition of, 131
  kinds of, 133–139
  planning for, 153–154

Economic system, impact of, on health services, 275
Economic value
  of children, 282
  of elderly, 282–283, 296
Epidemiologist, xxi, 298
Euthanasia
  definition of, 198
  need for, xxiii, xxiv, 97–99, 125, 207–208, 311
  opposition to, 127, 257, 273

Family, 100, 141–142
  after patient's death, 41, 151, 180, 215–216, 321. See also Bereavement; Grief reaction
  difficulties of, 218–219
  grief of, 140–142
  hospital staff and, 141–142

Family (cont.)
  leave-takings, 134, 143
  nurse and, 134–135, 140–142, 182, 195
  physician and, 61, 78–80, 90, 139–140, 150, 158, 180, 195, 199, 201, 220, 309, 320
  role of, 48–49, 167
Fear of death, xix, 40–41, 45, 54–55, 100, 172, 314
  religious beliefs and, 32, 55
Future, 211, 293, 313

Grief reaction, 320
Grief-workers, 141–142
Group for the Advancement of Psychiatry, 171

Habits, need for changes in, xxi, 122
Health insurance, 229, 249
  national, 278
Health services system
  changes in, 223–224, 300–301
  economic analysis of, 247–248, 283–301
  organization of, 28, 284–286, 288–289
Heart disease, 92, 122, 300, 305
Heart disease, cancer, and stroke, xv, 15–16, 246
Heart transplantation, 102, 106–107, 208, 306
  cost-benefit analysis of, 90, 112–113, 119–120, 213, 248, 300
  definition of death in, 191
  heart-lung machine in, 106, 114
  problems of, 77, 99, 108, 111–112, 113, 117–118, 122, 239, 247
  public opinion concerning, 120–121
  substitutes for human heart in, 113–115
  See also Donor
Hippocratic oath, 108, 225, 260, 262
Home, dying at, xviii, 22, 32, 80, 142, 311
Hospitals
  death in, xix, 80, 184, 215, 321
  expensive equipment in, 244, 285
  organization of, related to physician decisions, 149, 174, 208, 220–221, 304, 309–310
  self-regulation of, 232–236, 243
  standards for, 231

Hospitals (*cont.*)
 types of, 79, 174, 181–182, 184, 200–202, 206–207, 220–221, 235, 310
Hospital staff
 dying patient and, 46, 132–139, 143–145, 153, 157–158, 182–183, 219–220, 313–316
 standards of, under different staff organizations, 228, 229
House staff training, 202
Humanitarianism, xxiii, 297, 299, 308–309

Immortality, xiv, 104
Infectious diseases. *See* Communicable diseases
Institutions
 death in, by cause, 24–26
 death in, by color and geography, 23–24
 dying in, xvii, xxiii, 7, 21–22, 32, 47, 79, 129, 183, 217, 255
 suppression of death in, 183
Interesting patient, 79, 135, 202–203
Invisible acts, 306

Kidney transplantation, 105, 106, 248. *See also* Organ transplantation
Killing, man's instinct for, 253–254

Last days, 135, 138–139, 148, 151
Life-chances, differences in, 6
Life expectancy, 5–6, 7, 8, 9–10, 269, 316
 definition of, 5, 10
 increase in, xxi, 5, 8, 9, 37, 87, 172
 of U.S. compared with other countries, 9, 26–27
 See also Mortality rates
Life insurance, 38, 215, 219, 277
Life, quality of, xiv, 128, 218, 242, 294–297
Life-style, 6, 7, 17–20
Life, value of individual, xiii. *See also* Physician, determinants of, behavior
 economic, 276–277, 279–283, 293–294, 299, 300
 high, 120, 135, 211
 related to risk-taking, 241–242, 277, 293
 related to social differentiation, 50–

Life, value of individual (*cont.*)
 54, 83–89, 90–91, 199, 206, 283, 299, 306, 308, 309, 311
 to society, 241–242, 279, 293. *See also* Vietnam War
Liver transplantation, 102–103

Medical care
 as comfort care, 135, 139, 140, 142, 306
 demands for, 227, 285–286
 direct and indirect costs of, 299–300
 governmental interest in, 228, 232, 278
 moral issues in, xix, 207–208
 as palliative care, 198–199
 quality of, xviii, xxi, 89, 187, 230, 244, 316
 related to place of death, 21, 182–183
 as a right, 288–289, 298–299
 role of, xxi, 278
 termination of, 254–259, 260–261, 262, 264, 270, 272
Medical education
 autopsy in, 173, 185
 cadaver in, 173
 emphasis on diagnostic work and complex diseases in, 285
 need for training concerning death and dying in, xviii, xxiii, 78, 99, 129, 153, 172, 175, 315
 orientation of, 120, 187, 286
 reform of, 231–232
Medical ethics, 123, 242, 309–310
Medical research, 95–96, 122, 246, 248, 271, 273, 297, 308–309
Medical resources, allocation of, 249–250, 286–287, 291, 292, 295–298, 299
 choice in, between young and aged, 240, 242, 246, 271
 innovational procedures, 122, 247, 300, 306
 need for more widespread, 120, 222, 273
 prolonging life and, 213–214, 275, 306, 312–313
 social differentiation in, 279, 308
Medical technology
 dying and, 213, 217–218, 222, 255, 303

SUBJECT INDEX [389

Medical technology (cont.)
    problems caused by advances in, 268, 270, 274
Mercy killing. See Euthanasia
Mondale proposal, 111, 112, 118
Mortality rates
    decline in, xvi, 10–12, 31, 171–172, 312
    by disease, 7, 18–20
    in infancy and childhood, xv, xvi, 11–12, 172, 246
    institutional, 75, 178, 184–185
    by medical specialties, 175–178
    in old age, 12
    for the poverty populations, 7, 18–19, 120
    by sex, 12, 20
    by socioeconomic status, 7, 17–20

National Health planning, 246–247
Necropsy. See Autopsy
Nurses
    death and, 49, 196–197, 198
    decision to terminate life and, 150
    dying patient and, 61, 132–139, 143–144, 145, 158, 159, 160, 182, 198, 314
    family and, 134–135, 140–142, 182, 195
Nurses' aides, 147, 158, 196, 197–198

Organ transplantation
    cost of, 118–120
    donor in. See Donor
    drama of, xx, 104, 212, 285
    immortality and, 104
    need for guidelines in, 240, 267–268
    position of American Medical Association concerning, 47, 118
    problems of, xx, xxi, 115–116, 207–208, 221–222, 270–271
    survival rates for, 106–108

Physician
    death and, 33, 46, 49, 56, 99, 171, 172, 179, 186–187, 196, 314, 316
    determinants of, behavior, 77–78, 83–87, 88–89, 90–95, 149, 174, 199, 204–207, 208, 220–221, 304, 305, 309–310
    diagnostic skill of, 67–68, 174, 180, 203–204
    dying patient and, 46, 132–139,

Physician (cont.)
    143, 145, 158, 179, 195–196, 220
    family and. See Family, physician and
    role of, 79, 92, 174–175, 180, 181–182, 195, 220–221, 222
    self-government of, 230–245
    therapeutic choices of, 77–78, 94–95
    See also Medical education; House staff training
Post-mortem stories, 151–152
Poverty populations, xvii, 18–19, 89, 120, 248, 273, 289, 299
Premature death, 31, 40, 41, 83, 281, 283, 299
Prognosis, 67–68, 70–75, 203–207, 305–306, 312
Prolonging life, xiv, xix, xxiii–xxiv, 62, 212, 213, 306, 269
    allocation of medical resources and, 213–214, 275, 306, 312–313
    contraindications for, 123, 125–127, 150, 154, 174, 262, 303
    in different hospitals, 125, 149, 310
    economic costs of, 123, 261, 272
    means available for, xxi, 123–125, 127, 128, 303
    need for criteria in, 126–127, 222, 240–241, 260, 307
    participants in decision of, 52–53, 149–150
    reasons for, 125, 127, 135, 273, 304–305, 308–309
    suffering in, 154, 214, 307
    See also Hospital, organization of, related to physician decision; Life, value of individual, related to social differentiation; Medical ethics; Medical technology; Physician, determinants of, behavior; Physician, role of
Psychiatrists, 141, 145, 172, 316, 321

Regional medical planning, 21, 243–245, 249
Religious beliefs
    autopsy and, 57–59
    dying patient and, 159, 164–165, 168–169
    fear of death and, 32, 55
Renal dialysis machine. See Artificial kidney
Right to die, 40, 98, 175, 241, 243

Royal colleges, 228

Sanctity of life, 221, 309, 310
Scientific medicine, ideal of, 174, 181
Self-preservation, 256, 277
Senility and senile dementia, 93, 240, 241
Social differentiation, 50–54, 83–89, 90–91, 199, 206, 279–283, 299, 306, 308, 309, 311
Social institutions, 31
Social welfare function, 279–280
Social willing, 146
Social workers, 141, 316
Soul, beliefs about, 58–59
Suffering
    avoidance of, xxiii, 31, 40, 214, 311
    in prolonging life, 154, 214, 307
Suicide, xxiii, 45, 96, 149, 258–259, 273, 318–319
    in terminal cancer patients, 311–312
Surgery, quality of care in, 234–235

Terminal care
    definition of, 198, 217
    psychological and social aspects of, 129–130, 153
Terminal illness. *See* Diseases as causes of death
Terminally ill patient. *See* Dying patient

Terminal period, uncertainty of, 219
Terminating life, 124–125, 241, 243, 281
    need for criteria in, 126–127
    patient participation in, 149, 310
    prohibitions against, 221, 306
Therapy. *See* Drug therapy; Treatment
Time, conception of, 146–147, 217–218, 269, 312
Treatment
    of aged, 88, 90, 174
    of cancer, 73–74, 81
    cost-benefit analysis of, 298–300
    disagreement about, 69–70
    effects of, 256–257
    See also Physician, determinants of, behavior

Veterans Administration hospital, 83
Veterans Administration study group, 76
Vietnam War, xx, 293

Ward
    death on, 195–196
    dying patient on, 130–131, 136, 198
    sentimental order of, 132–133, 134–135
Welfare economics, government intervention in, 287–288